# Head and Neck Disorders (Fourth Series) Test and Syllabus

Peter M. Som, M.D.
*Section Chairman*

Hugh D. Curtin, M.D.
William P. Dillon, M.D.
Anton N. Hasso, M.D.
Mahmood F. Mafee, M.D.

acr  American College of Radiology
Reston, Virginia  1992

**Sets Published**

Chest Disease
Bone Disease
Genitourinary Tract Disease
Gastrointestinal Disease
Head and Neck Disorders
Pediatric Disease
Nuclear Radiology
Radiation Pathology and
    Radiation Biology
Chest Disease II
Bone Disease II
Genitourinary Tract Disease II
Gastrointestinal Disease II
Head and Neck Disorders II
Nuclear Radiology II
Cardiovascular Disease
Emergency Radiology
Bone Disease III
Gastrointestinal Disease III
Chest Disease III
Pediatric Disease II
Nuclear Radiology III
Head and Neck Disorders III

Genitourinary Tract Disease III
Diagnostic Ultrasound
Breast Disease
Bone Disease IV
Pediatric Disease III
Chest Disease IV
Neuroradiology
Gastrointestinal Disease IV
Nuclear Radiology IV
Magnetic Resonance
Radiation Bioeffects and
    Management
Genitourinary Tract Disease IV
Head and Neck Disorders IV

**Sets in Preparation**

Musculoskeletal Disease
Pediatric Disease IV
Diagnostic Ultrasonography II
Breast Disease II
Chest Disease V
Neuroradiology II
Gastrointestinal Disease V
Emergency Radiology II

---

**Note:** While the American College of Radiology and the editors of this publication have attempted to include the most current and accurate information possible, errors may inadvertently appear. Diagnostic and interventional decisions should be based on the individual circumstances of each case.

# SET 34:
## Head and Neck Disorders (Fourth Series) Test and Syllabus

*Editor in Chief*
BARRY A. SIEGEL, M.D., Professor of Radiology and Medicine and Director, Division of Nuclear Medicine, Mallinckrodt Institute of Radiology, Washington University School of Medicine, St. Louis, Missouri

*Associate Editor*
ANTHONY V. PROTO, M.D., Professor of Radiology and Chairman, Department of Radiology, Medical College of Virginia, Virginia Commonwealth University, Richmond, Virginia

*Section Editor*
PETER M. SOM, M.D., Professor of Radiology and Otolaryngology, The Mount Sinai School of Medicine of the City University of New York, and Director of Head and Neck Radiology, The Mount Sinai Hospital, New York, New York

*Co-Authors*
HUGH D. CURTIN, M.D., Professor of Radiology and Otolaryngology, University of Pittsburgh, and Director of Radiology, Eye and Ear Institute, Pittsburgh, Pennsylvania
WILLIAM P. DILLON, M.D., Associate Professor of Radiology, Neurology, and Otolaryngology, University of California at San Francisco, San Francisco, California
ANTON N. HASSO, M.D., Professor of Radiology and Otolaryngology/Head and Neck Surgery, Director, Section of Neuroradiology, and Associate Director for Research, Section of Magnetic Resonance Imaging, Loma Linda University, Loma Linda, California
MAHMOOD F. MAFEE, M.D., Professor of Radiology, Department of Radiology, University of Illinois, and Director, MRI Center, and Director, Radiology Section, Eye and Ear Infirmary, University of Illinois Hospital, Chicago, Illinois

AMERICAN COLLEGE OF RADIOLOGY
PROFESSIONAL SELF-EVALUATION AND CONTINUING EDUCATION PROGRAM

| | |
|---|---|
| *Publishing Coordinators:* | *G. Rebecca Haines Gardner and Thomas M. Rogers* |
| *Administrative Assistant:* | *Marcy Olney* |
| *Production Editor:* | *Sean M. McKenna* |
| *Copy Editors:* | *Yvonne Strong and John N. Bell* |
| *Text Processing:* | *Fusako T. Nowak* |
| *Composition:* | *Karen Finkle* |
| *Index:* | *Editorial Experts, Inc., Alexandria, Va.* |
| *Lithography:* | *Lanman Progressive, Washington, D.C.* |
| *Typesetting:* | *Publication Technology Corp., Fairfax, Va.* |
| *Printing:* | *John D. Lucas Printing, Baltimore, Md.* |

**Library of Congress Cataloging-in-Publication Data**

Head and neck disorders (fourth series) test and syllabus / Peter M. Som, section chairman ; Hugh D. Curtin ... [et al.]

    p. cm. — (Professional self-evaluation and continuing education program ; set 34)

    "Committee on Professional Self-Evaluation and Continuing Education, Commission on Education, American College of Radiology"—Cover.

    Includes bibliographical references and index.

    ISBN 1-55903-034-8 : $175.00. — ISBN 1-55903-000-3 (series)

    1. Head—Radiography—Examinations, questions, etc. 2. Neck—Radiography—Examinations, questions, etc. I. Som, Peter M. II. Curtin, Hugh D. III. American College of Radiology. Commission on Education. Committee on Professional Self-Evaluation and Continuing Education. IV. Series.

    [DNLM: 1. Head—Radiography—Examination questions, etc. 2. Head and Neck Neoplasms—radiography—examination questions. W1 PR606 set 34]

    RC936.H424 1992

    617.5'107572'076—dc20

    DNLM/DLC                                          92-48821

for Library of Congress                                 CIP

# ACR COMMITTEE ON PROFESSIONAL SELF-EVALUATION AND CONTINUING EDUCATION, COMMISSION ON EDUCATION

Anthony V. Proto, M.D., *Chairman and Associate Editor*

Jack Edeiken, M.D.

Harold G. Jacobson, M.D.

Barry A. Siegel, M.D.
*Editor in Chief*

David H. Stephens, M.D.
*Associate Editor*

Elias G. Theros, M.D.
*Editor Emeritus*

Jerome F. Wiot, M.D.

## SECTIONS

**HEAD & NECK DISORDERS IV**
Peter M. Som, M.D.,
  *Chairman*
Hugh D. Curtin, M.D.
William P. Dillon, M.D.
Anton N. Hasso, M.D.
Mahmood F. Mafee, M.D.

**MUSCULOSKELETAL DISEASE**
William A. Murphy, Jr.,
  M.D., *Chairman*
Lawrence W. Bassett, M.D.
Terry M. Hudson, M.D.
Phoebe A. Kaplan, M.D.
Sheila G. Moore, M.D.

**PEDIATRIC DISEASE IV**
Marilyn J. Siegel, M.D.,
  *Chairman*
George S. Bisset, M.D.
Robert H. Cleveland, M.D.
James S. Donaldson, M.D.
Kenneth H. Fellows, M.D.
Heidi B. Patriquin, M.D.

**DIAGNOSTIC ULTRASONOGRAPHY II**
Thomas L. Lawson, M.D.,
  *Chairman*
Richard Bowerman, M.D.
Beverly Coleman, M.D.
Gary Kellman, M.D.
William K. Middleton,
  M.D.

**BREAST DISEASE II**
Edward A. Sickles, M.D.,
  *Chairman*
Judy M. Destouet, M.D.
G. William Eklund, M.D.
Stephen A. Feig, M.D.
Valerie P. Jackson, M.D.

**CHEST DISEASE V**
Robert H. Choplin, M.D.,
  *Chairman*
Heber M. MacMahon,
  M.D.
Theresa C. McLoud, M.D.
Nestor L. Müller, M.D.,
  Ph.D.
James C. Reed, M.D.

**NEURORADIOLOGY II**
Solomon Batnitzky, M.D.,
  *Chairman*
Anthony J. Barkovich,
  M.D.
Allen D. Elster, M.D.
Robert R. Lukin, M.D.
Eric J. Russell, M.D.

**GASTROINTESTINAL DISEASE V**
Dr. Dennis M. Balfe, M.D.,
  *Chairman*
Judith L. Chezmar, M.D.
R. Brooke Jeffrey, M.D.
Robert E. Koehler, M.D.
Marc S. Levine, M.D.

v

# Additional Contributors

MONIKA L. KIEF-GARCIA, M.D., Clinical Assistant in Radiology, Loma Linda University Medical Center, Loma Linda, California

THU-ANH HOANG, M.D., Instructor in Radiology, Loma Linda University Medical Center, Loma Linda, California

PAUL S. KIM, M.D., Clinical Assistant in Radiology, Loma Linda University Medical Center, Loma Linda, California

ALIX VINCENT, M.D., Clinical Assistant Professor in Radiology, Loma Linda University School of Medicine, Loma Linda, California

THOMAS E. WILEY III, M.D., Clinical Assistant in Radiology, Loma Linda University Medical Center, Loma Linda, California

# Section Chairman's Preface

The coming of age of head and neck radiology as a separate radiologic subspecialty is illustrated by the progressive changes in the four self-evaluation series volumes published by the American College of Radiology (ACR). The first head and neck syllabus, published in 1974, contained plain films, multidirectional tomograms, intracranial angiography, myelography, and pneumoencephalography; the discussion topics focused entirely on what is now considered classical neuroradiology. The second volume (1978) presented essentially the same modalities, with the addition of a few early CT scans, and the cases still reflected an emphasis on classical neuroradiology. The third self-evaluation syllabus (1985) contained mainly CT scans, and the case topics included both clinical neuroradiology and head and neck disorders in approximately equal measure. In the current syllabus, the fourth volume of the ACR's Professional Self-Evaluation and Continuing Education series, MR and high-resolution CT scans are used exclusively, and the case material is devoted entirely to head and neck radiology.

These changes parallel the growing recognition that disorders involving the skull base, orbit, facial structures, temporomandibular joints, salivary glands, oral cavity, pharynx, larynx, and remaining soft tissues of the neck are clinically quite distinct from diseases of the brain and spine. The demands placed upon the radiologist are also much different, requiring a detailed understanding of the anatomy, pathophysiology, and current treatment techniques of the head and neck.

The cases presented in *Head and Neck Disorders (Fourth Series) Test and Syllabus* were carefully chosen to reflect some of the most important issues that now challenge the radiologist evaluating head and neck pathology. Although some radiologists may feel that a few of these cases will only be seen in a major academic center, many of the disorders described here were first detected in private practice radiology offices or in small community hospitals. Thus, all radiologists can expect to encounter patients with a wide variety of head and neck disorders. *Head and Neck Disorders IV* was designed to give exposure to the scope of pathology encountered and to review these topics in detail.

I am greatly indebted to the series editors, Drs. Barry A. Siegel and Anthony V. Proto, for their invaluable insight, knowledge, and advice. They both quickly adapted to the realm of head and neck terminology and disease. Not only did they help us to organize the material, but they did so with style, humor, and panache.

Equally important were the efforts and guidance of the ACR staff, especially Ms. Rebecca Haines Gardner, Director of Publications, and Mr.

Thomas M. Rogers, the Associate Director of Publications. Without their assistance, this volume could never have been published. Their patience, specialized talents, and good humor helped the project run smoothly.

Most of all, I want to thank my co-contributors on this syllabus: Drs. Hugh D. Curtin, William P. Dillon, Anton N. Hasso, and Mahmood F. Mafee. All of them gave freely of their time and enthusiastically shared their clinical and teaching expertise and case material. In the final analysis, such expert radiologists are the foundation upon which this syllabus was built.

Peter M. Som, M.D.
*Section Chairman*

# Editor's Preface

On behalf of the editors of the American College of Radiology's Professional Self-Evaluation and Continuing Education Program, I am delighted to introduce the *Head and Neck Disorders (Fourth Series) Test and Syllabus* to program participants. This 34th volume in the series of diagnostic radiology syllabi is also the first exclusively devoted to radiology of the head and neck, as distinct from neuroradiology. This syllabus focuses on important developments in head and neck radiology that have occurred since the previous volume on this topic, which was published in 1985. As noted by Dr. Peter Som in his preface, this volume also reflects the remarkable transformation of head and neck radiology that has occurred in recent years, with nearly all examinations now in the domain of high-resolution computed tomography and magnetic resonance imaging. Radiologic evaluation is now a cornerstone of the workup of patients with many otolaryngologic and ophthalmologic disorders. It is incumbent upon radiologists whose practices include imaging of patients with head and neck diseases to understand these disorders thoroughly so that the wealth of information available from modern imaging methods can be used to the maximum benefit of patients. The editors believe that this syllabus will help, at least in some small measure, to attain this goal.

As our readers work through this self-evaluation program, they will unquestionably acknowledge that great thanks are due to Dr. Peter Som and to his co-authors: Drs. Hugh D. Curtin, William P. Dillon, Anton N. Hasso, and Mahmood F. Mafee. This lively group of talented radiologists worked long and hard to produce this self-evaluation package. The members of the American College of Radiology are indeed fortunate to be able to learn from the voluntary efforts of expert radiologists of this caliber. As Section Chairman, Peter Som clearly demonstrated himself to be a self-evaluation maven, making my job and that of my colleague, Dr. Anthony V. Proto, so much easier during the development and editing of this volume.

As always, the editors deeply appreciate the consummate efforts of the Publications Department staff of the American College of Radiology. Their work is critical to the success of the self-evaluation program. Special thanks are due to Ms. G. Rebecca Haines Gardner and Mr. Thomas Rogers, who are primarily responsible for the overall coordination of the self-evaluation program and for the editing and production of the syllabi, respectively. Their attention to detail and devotion to quality make the self-evaluation program a source of pride for all College members.

Finally, the editors and authors express our continuing thanks to our "customers," namely the many practicing radiologists and residents who have enthusiastically supported the Self-Evaluation Program for the past 21 years. Since the initiation of the series, nearly 182,000 subscriptions have been delivered into the hands of radiologists. As the series editors, we hope that this program will continue to fill an important niche in the education of radiologists and contribute to the intellectual growth of our specialty.

Barry A. Siegel, M.D.
*Editor in Chief*

# Head and Neck Disorders (Fourth Series) Test

For you to derive the maximum benefit from this program, you should complete the following test, and send your answer sheet to the ACR for scoring, before you proceed to the syllabus.

If for any reason you refer to the syllabus material, or any other references, in answering the questions, please be sure to so indicate when answering Question 111, the first demographic question. Your score will then not be used in developing the norm tables.

NOTE: You must return your answer sheet for scoring, whether or not you use reference materials, in order to claim the 20 hours of Category I credit.

Category I credit is valid for this publication from January 1993 through January 1996. Category I credit review will be conducted in January 1996 and every three years thereafter.

## CASE 1: Questions 1 through 3

This 43-year-old man presented with a left parotid mass. You are shown a postcontrast CT scan (A) and a T2-weighted axial MR image (B) (Figure 1-1).

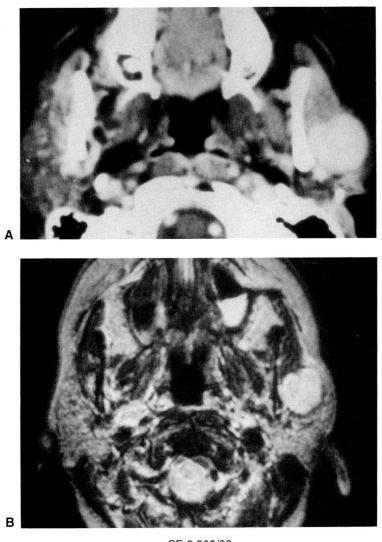

SE 2,500/80

**Figure 1-1**

1. Which *one* of the following is the MOST likely diagnosis?

   (A) Adenocarcinoma
   (B) Pleomorphic adenoma
   (C) Branchial cleft cyst
   (D) Facial nerve schwannoma
   (E) Metastasis

QUESTIONS 2 AND 3: MARK YOUR ANSWER SHEET TRUE (T) OR FALSE (F) FOR EACH OF THE RESPONSE CHOICES.

2. Concerning adenocarcinoma of the head and neck,

   (A) the palate is a common site of origin
   (B) a high-grade lesion in a salivary gland is more likely to represent metastatic colon cancer than a primary tumor
   (C) workers in hardwood industries have an increased incidence of sinonasal tumors
   (D) high-grade lesions usually have high signal intensities on T2-weighted MR images
   (E) it is the most common parotid gland cancer

3. Concerning pleomorphic adenomas,

   (A) they are the most common parotid gland neoplasm
   (B) recurrences are related to violation of the tumor capsule
   (C) the most commonly associated cancer is carcinoma ex pleomorphic adenoma
   (D) facial nerve paralysis is found in about 30% of cases
   (E) dystrophic calcifications are common
   (F) multiple tumors are uncommon in patients who have not had prior surgery
   (G) when small, they have low and high signal intensities on T1- and T2-weighted images, respectively

## CASE 2: Questions 4 through 7

This 71-year-old man has laryngeal carcinoma. You are shown two coronal T1-weighted MR scans (Figure 2-1).

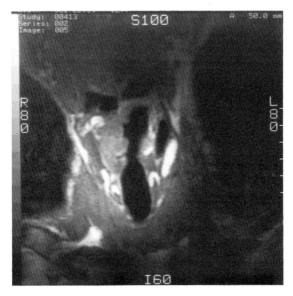

SE 600/20

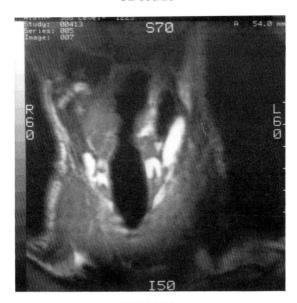

SE 600/20

**Figure 2-1**

QUESTIONS 4 THROUGH 7: MARK YOUR ANSWER SHEET TRUE (T) OR FALSE (F) FOR EACH OF THE RESPONSE CHOICES.

4. The test images demonstrate involvement of the:

   (A) epiglottis
   (B) false cord
   (C) paraglottic space
   (D) cricoid cartilage
   (E) subglottic mucosa

5. Contraindications for a classic supraglottic laryngectomy include:

   (A) involvement of the thyroid cartilage
   (B) involvement of the cervical lymph nodes
   (C) extension to the postcricoid area
   (D) extension across the ventricle
   (E) extension to the vallecula

6. Concerning the lymphatic drainage of the larynx,

   (A) the supraglottic larynx drains to the upper jugular nodes
   (B) the subglottic mucosa drains to the paratracheal nodes
   (C) the true cord has almost no drainage
   (D) all of the laryngeal lymphatics eventually terminate in the jugulodigastric node
   (E) subglottic tumors spread to the Delphian node

## CASE 2 (Cont'd)

7. An axial image through the true cord will identify:

   (A) the superior margin of the arytenoid cartilage
   (B) the superior margin of the cricoid cartilage
   (C) the thyroarytenoid muscle
   (D) the thyroid cartilage
   (E) the ventricular appendix (saccule)

This 46-year-old man presented with right-sided conductive hearing loss and fifth-nerve dysesthesia. You are shown axial T1-weighted (A) and T2-weighted (B) MR scans and a coronal T1-weighted MR scan (C) (Figure 3-1).

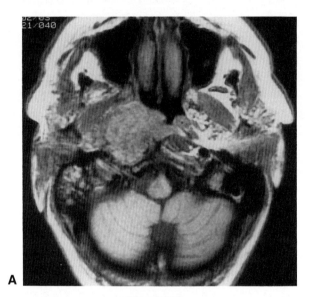

SE 600/20

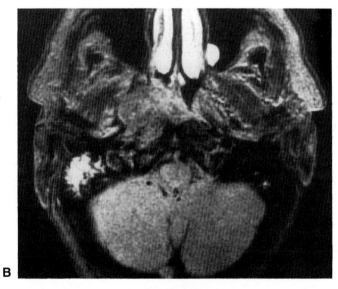

SE 2,800/80

**Figure 3-1**

## CASE 3 (Cont'd)

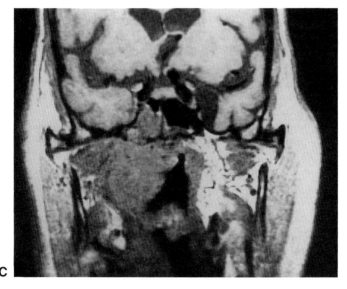

SE 600/20

8. Which *one* of the following is the MOST likely diagnosis?

    (A) Necrotizing otitis externa
    (B) Adenoidal hypertrophy
    (C) Cellulitis of the retropharyngeal space
    (D) Carcinoma of the nasopharynx
    (E) Rhabdomyosarcoma of the nasopharynx

## CASE 3 (Cont'd)

QUESTIONS 9 THROUGH 11: MARK YOUR ANSWER SHEET
TRUE (T) OR FALSE (F) FOR EACH OF THE RESPONSE
CHOICES.

9. Concerning necrotizing otitis externa,

    (A) it is usually caused by *Pseudomonas aeruginosa*
    (B) it generally occurs in diabetic patients
    (C) seventh-nerve palsy is an ominous sign
    (D) cranial neuropathy usually indicates extension into the posterior fossa
    (E) extension into the masticator space usually occurs

10. Concerning the retropharyngeal space,

    (A) it is posterior to the prevertebral space
    (B) it contains no lymph nodes
    (C) it communicates with the mediastinum
    (D) in children, tonsillitis is the most common antecedent illness preceding cellulitis of this space
    (E) juvenile angiofibromas usually involve this space

11. Concerning nasopharyngeal carcinomas,

    (A) more than 80% are squamous cell carcinomas
    (B) they are not related to cigarette smoking
    (C) most begin in the fossa of Rosenmüller
    (D) nodal metastases are infrequent at presentation
    (E) surgery is the primary treatment of choice

# CASE 4: Questions 12 through 16

This 36-year-old man has nasal obstruction and headache. You are shown sagittal (A) and coronal (B) T1-weighted MR images (Figure 4-1).

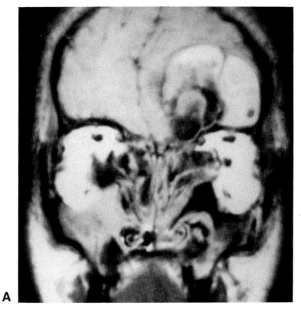

SE 900/30

**Figure 4-1**

12. Which *one* of the following is the MOST likely diagnosis?

   (A) Squamous cell carcinoma
   (B) Polyposis and mucocele
   (C) Melanoma
   (D) Esthesioneuroblastoma
   (E) Extramedullary plasmacytoma

CASE 4 (Cont'd)

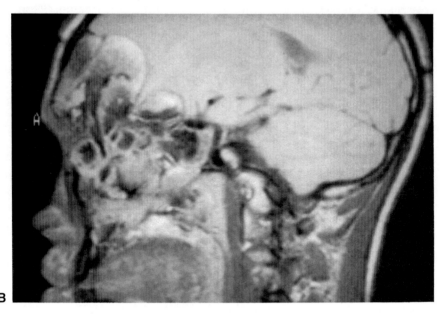

SE 900/30

QUESTIONS 13 THROUGH 16: MARK YOUR ANSWER SHEET TRUE (T) OR FALSE (F) FOR EACH OF THE RESPONSE CHOICES.

13. Concerning nasal polyps,

(A) they are local upheavals of mucosa
(B) the major cause of enlargement is an accumulation of extracellular fluid
(C) most small ones have high signal intensity on T2-weighted MR images
(D) the coexistence of multiple polyps and mucoceles usually occurs in atopic patients
(E) about 25% are antrochoanal lesions

# CASE 4 (Cont'd)

14. Concerning sinonasal melanomas,

    (A) they account for 10% of melanomas
    (B) epistaxis is a common complaint
    (C) about 60% are amelanotic
    (D) about 95% have high signal intensity on T1-weighted MR images
    (E) the 10-year survival rate is about 35%

15. Concerning esthesioneuroblastomas,

    (A) most patients are under 20 years of age
    (B) intracranial extension demonstrable by CT or MRI is present in most patients
    (C) most present as unilateral nasal masses
    (D) bone remodeling around the tumor is common
    (E) tumoral calcification identifiable by CT is present in most cases

16. Concerning extramedullary plasmacytomas,

    (A) about 80% occur in the head and neck
    (B) most occur in patients over 40 years of age
    (C) subsequent development of multiple myeloma is rare
    (D) they are highly vascular tumors
    (E) they usually have high signal intensity on T1-weighted images

For each of the numbered CT scans (Figures 5-1 through 5-4), select the *one* lettered diagnosis (A, B, C, D, or E) that is MOST closely associated with it. Each diagnosis may be used once, more than once, or not at all.

17. Figure 5-1
18. Figure 5-2
19. Figure 5-3
20. Figure 5-4

    (A) Retinoblastoma
    (B) Drusen of the optic nerve head
    (C) Coats's disease
    (D) Colobomatous cyst
    (E) Retinopathy of prematurity

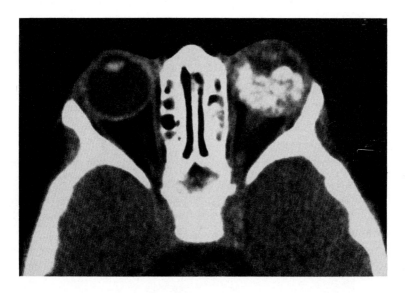

**Figure 5-1**

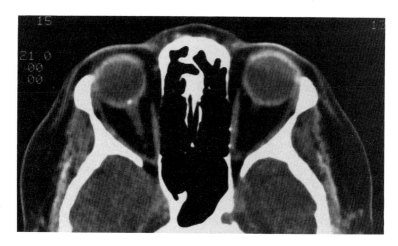

**Figure 5-2**

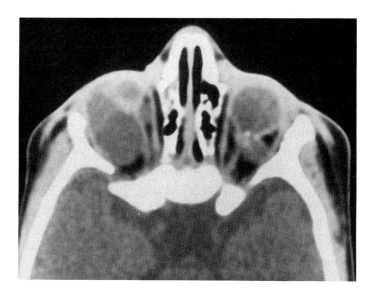

**Figure 5-3**

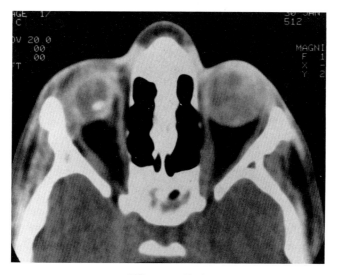

**Figure 5-4**

## CASE 5 (Cont'd)

QUESTIONS 21 THROUGH 27: MARK YOUR ANSWER SHEET TRUE (T) OR FALSE (F) FOR EACH OF THE RESPONSE CHOICES.

21. Concerning retinoblastoma,

    (A) it arises from the pigmented layer of the retina
    (B) it is the most common intraocular malignant tumor in childhood
    (C) it is bilateral in about 70% of cases
    (D) all patients with bilateral retinoblastoma harbor the retinoblastoma gene

22. Concerning imaging of retinoblastoma,

    (A) CT demonstrates calcification in about 90% of cases
    (B) intense contrast enhancement on CT is characteristic
    (C) retinoblastomas are hypointense relative to the vitreous in T1-weighted MR images
    (D) the tumor margin is easily differentiated from retinal detachment by CT
    (E) extraocular extension of retinoblastoma is reliably detected by both CT and MRI
    (F) involvement of Tenon's capsule is characterized as optic nerve enlargement with subarachnoid seeding

23. Concerning persistent hyperplastic primary vitreous,

    (A) it occurs when the embryonic hyaloid vascular system (primary vitreous) fails to regress
    (B) it presents clinically as leukokoria
    (C) calcification is rare
    (D) it often presents as a dense globe on CT

# CASE 5 (Cont'd)

24. Concerning Coats's disease,

   (A) it is more common in boys than in girls
   (B) it is a congenital telangiectasia of the retina
   (C) MRI is superior to CT for the diagnosis
   (D) calcification is a common finding on CT

25. Drusen of the optic nerve head:

   (A) occur in the intraocular portion of the optic nerve
   (B) are usually bilateral
   (C) are rarely detected by CT in early childhood
   (D) simulate papilledema on clinical examination
   (E) appear on CT as a well-defined calcification beneath the surface of the optic disk

26. Concerning optic nerve coloboma and colobomatous cyst,

   (A) optic nerve coloboma arises from failure of closure of the embryonic fissure
   (B) isolated coloboma of the optic nerve is a common congenital disorder
   (C) microphthalmus with colobomatous cyst is an anomaly seen in an eye with a retinochoroidal coloboma
   (D) optic nerve coloboma characteristically appears on CT and MRI as an area of excavation of the disk
   (E) calcification commonly occurs within a colobomatous cyst

27. Concerning retinopathy of prematurity,

    (A) it usually develops as a response to prolonged supplemental oxygen therapy

    (B) pathologically, there is retinal neovascularization

    (C) both retinal detachment and vitreous hemorrhage are common

    (D) calcification is common

## CASE 6: Questions 28 through 31

This 23-year-old woman presented with progressively worsening episodes of decreased acuity in her left eye. You are shown coronal T1-weighted (A), adjacent axial T2-weighted (B and C), and coronal postcontrast T1-weighted (D) MR scans (Figure 6-1).

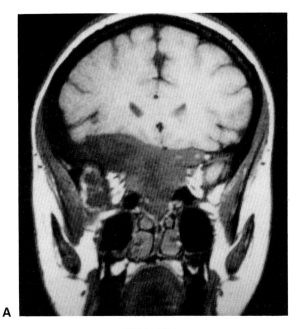

SE 600/20

**Figure 6-1**

28. Which *one* of the following is the MOST likely diagnosis?

   (A) Fibrous dysplasia
   (B) Mucocele of the sphenoid sinus
   (C) Langerhans cell histiocytosis
   (D) Mucormycosis
   (E) Meningioma

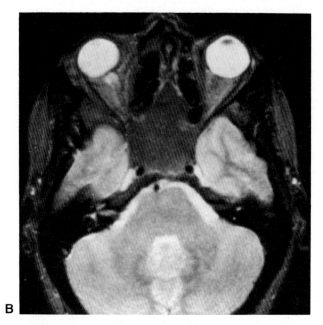

SE 2,200/80

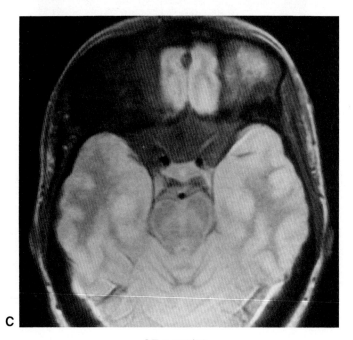

SE 2,200/80

## CASE 6 (Cont'd)

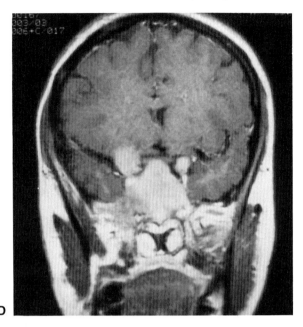

D

SE 600/20

QUESTIONS 29 THROUGH 31: MARK YOUR ANSWER SHEET TRUE (T) OR FALSE (F) FOR EACH OF THE RESPONSE CHOICES.

29. Concerning fibrous dysplasia,

   (A) the calvarium is involved in about 50% of patients with the monostotic form of the disease
   (B) fewer than 20% of patients with the polyostotic form of the disease have involvement of the skull and facial bones
   (C) the temporal bone is the most commonly involved skull bone
   (D) involvement of the base of the skull is usually sclerotic
   (E) enhancement after administration of gadolinium DTPA is a typical MR finding

## CASE 6 (Cont'd)

30. Concerning mucoceles,

    (A) the sphenoid sinus is the most commonly involved sinus
    (B) an air-fluid level is usually present
    (C) expansion of the sinus is characteristic
    (D) they occasionally arise within the middle turbinate
    (E) their signal intensity on T1-weighted images is variable


31. Concerning Langerhans cell histiocytosis,

    (A) the chronic recurring (Hand-Schüller-Christian) variety is characterized by monostotic osseous lesions
    (B) the osseous lesions are characteristically sclerotic
    (C) the temporal bone is involved in about 30% of cases
    (D) enlargement of the pituitary infundibulum is an associated finding
    (E) diabetes insipidus is most commonly associated with the localized (eosinophilic granuloma) form of the disease

# CASE 7: Questions 32 through 37

You are shown a series of direct sagittal CT images from an air-positive contrast arthrogram of a normal left temporomandibular joint (Figure 7-1). For each numbered arrow (Questions 32 through 36), select the *one* lettered part of the anatomy (A, B, C, D, or E) that is MOST closely associated with it.

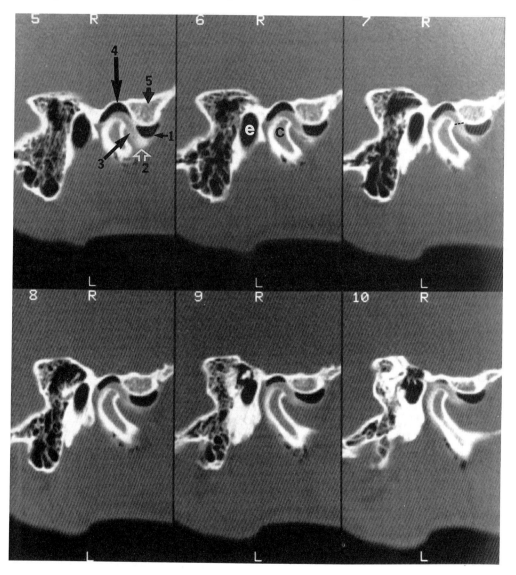

**Figure 7-1**

CASE 7 (Cont'd)

32. Arrow 1
33. Arrow 2
34. Arrow 3
35. Arrow 4
36. Arrow 5

   (A) Meniscus
   (B) Anterior recess of superior joint space
   (C) Articular eminence
   (D) Posterior recess of superior joint space
   (E) Anterior recess of inferior joint space

QUESTION 37: MARK YOUR ANSWER SHEET TRUE (T) OR FALSE (F) FOR EACH OF THE RESPONSE CHOICES.

37. Concerning the temporomandibular joint meniscus,

   (A) it is a fibrous articular disk
   (B) it divides the joint into superior and inferior compartments
   (C) the fibrous joint capsule is attached to its medial and lateral margins
   (D) the tendon of the superior head of the lateral pterygoid muscle inserts into it
   (E) the tendon of the inferior head of the lateral pterygoid muscle inserts into it
   (F) the posterior band is thinner than the anterior band

# CASE 8: Questions 38 through 40

You are shown an axial postcontrast CT scan of a 32-year-old man with multiple palpable cervical lymph nodes and bilateral parotid gland enlargement (Figure 8-1). You are also shown a coronal T2-weighted MR scan of another patient, a 28-year-old man with the same clinical findings (Figure 8-2).

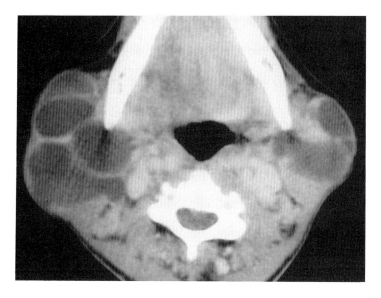

**Figure 8-1**

38. Which *one* of the following is the MOST likely diagnosis in these two patients?

   (A) Sarcoidosis
   (B) Lymphoepithelial parotid cysts
   (C) Warthin's tumors (papillary cystadenoma lymphomatosum)
   (D) Non-Hodgkin's lymphoma
   (E) Abscesses

## CASE 8 (Cont'd)

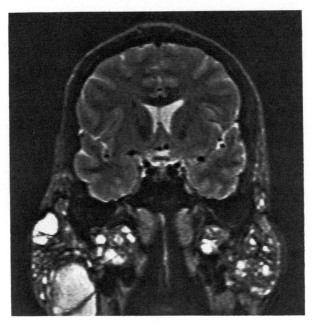

SE 2,000/90

**Figure 8-2**

QUESTIONS 39 AND 40: MARK YOUR ANSWER SHEET TRUE (T) OR FALSE (F) FOR EACH OF THE RESPONSE CHOICES.

39. Concerning lymphoepithelial parotid cysts,

    (A) patients are nearly always infected with human immunodeficiency virus
    (B) enlarged adenoids are an associated finding
    (C) they are often associated with diffuse reactive cervical lymphadenopathy
    (D) they are a direct precursor of Kaposi's sarcoma

40. Concerning parotid tumors,

    (A) they usually have low signal intensity on T1-weighted MR images
    (B) most high-grade malignant ones have high signal intensity on T2-weighted MR images
    (C) most benign ones lie deep to the facial nerve
    (D) the Warthin's variety rarely enhances following intravenous administration of contrast agents

# CASE 9: Questions 41 through 44

You are shown a series of three-dimensional CT images of the calvarium and face of a 6-year-old boy (Figure 9-1).

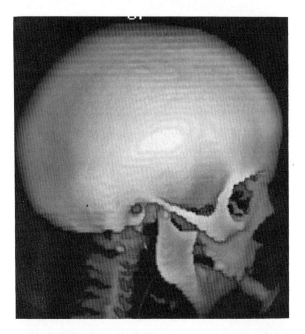

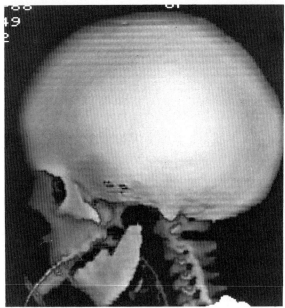

**Figure 9-1**

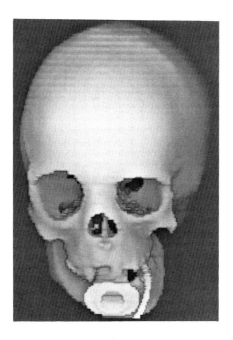

41. Which *one* of the following is the MOST likely diagnosis?

    (A) Crouzon's disease
    (B) Treacher Collins syndrome
    (C) Pierre Robin syndrome
    (D) Hemifacial microsomia
    (E) Apert's syndrome

QUESTIONS 42 THROUGH 44: MARK YOUR ANSWER SHEET TRUE (T) OR FALSE (F) FOR EACH OF THE RESPONSE CHOICES.

42. Features of the Treacher Collins syndrome include:

   (A) antimongoloid slant of the palpebral fissures
   (B) colobomas of the eyelids
   (C) deformed auricles
   (D) stenosis of the external auditory canals
   (E) abnormal course of the facial nerve
   (F) mandibular hypoplasia

43. Concerning hemifacial microsomia,

   (A) the external auditory canal is hypoplastic
   (B) macrostomia is typically present
   (C) the inner ear is usually involved
   (D) the temporomandibular joint is typically involved
   (E) the lateral orbital rim is hypoplastic

44. Concerning craniosynostosis of the skull,

   (A) head dimensions perpendicular to the affected suture are increased
   (B) involvement of the sagittal suture results in brachy-cephaly
   (C) involvement of the coronal sutures results in scapho-cephaly
   (D) it is usually associated with one of the craniofacial syndromes
   (E) most patients have a symmetric cranial deformity

## CASE 10: Questions 45 through 48

This 42-year-old woman has painful proptosis of the right eye. You are shown proton-density (A), T2-weighted (B), fat-suppressed STIR (C), and postcontrast T1-weighted (D) MR scans (Figure 10-1).

SE 2,200/20

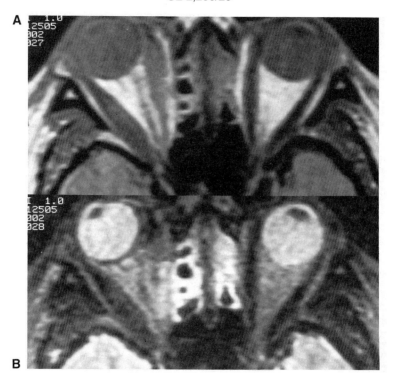

SE 2,200/80

**Figure 10-1**

45. Which *one* of the following is the MOST likely diagnosis?

(A) Dysthyroid orbitopathy
(B) Myositic orbital pseudotumor
(C) Lymphoma
(D) Metastasis
(E) Rhabdomyosarcoma

STIR 2,000/40/160

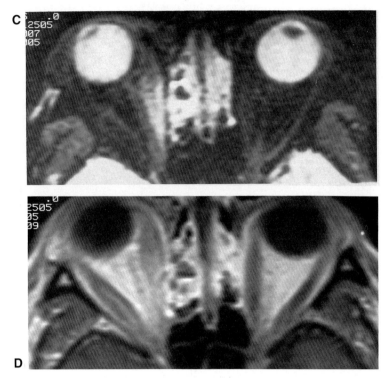

SE 600/20

QUESTIONS 46 THROUGH 48: MARK YOUR ANSWER SHEET TRUE (T) OR FALSE (F) FOR EACH OF THE RESPONSE CHOICES.

46. Concerning dysthyroid orbitopathy,

(A) it is an autoimmune disorder
(B) pain is a common clinical presentation
(C) the lateral rectus muscles are most commonly involved
(D) enlargement of the muscle is usually limited to its belly
(E) bilateral enlargement of the extraocular muscles is less common than in pseudotumor

## CASE 10 (Cont'd)

47. Concerning orbital lymphoma,

    (A) it accounts for 10 to 15% of orbital masses

    (B) it commonly occurs in the anterior portions of the orbit

    (C) when limited to extraocular muscles, it generally cannot be differentiated from myositic pseudotumor by CT or MRI

    (D) it demonstrates intense contrast enhancement on MRI

48. Concerning rhabdomyosarcoma of the orbit,

    (A) it is the most common primary orbital cancer in children

    (B) it arises from the pluripotential mesenchymal elements

    (C) it commonly presents as a rapidly progressive unilateral proptosis

    (D) it is resistant to both radiation therapy and chemotherapy

## CASE 11: Questions 49 through 53

This 26-year-old woman presented with a headache and left-sixth-nerve palsy. You are shown a contrast-enhanced CT scan photographed at soft tissue (A) and bone (B) window settings (Figure 11-1), a coronal T1-weighted MR scan (Figure 11-2), an axial proton density MR scan (Figure 11-3), and two T1-weighted axial contrast-enhanced MR scans (Figure 11-4).

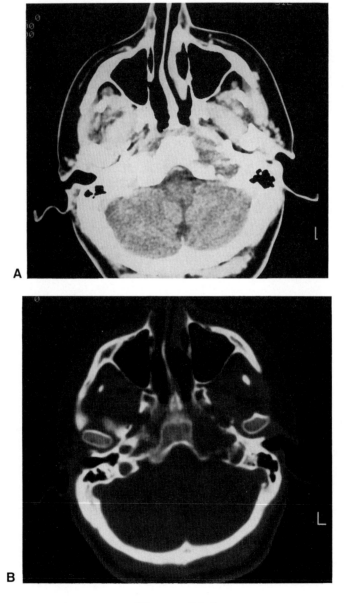

**Figure 11-1**

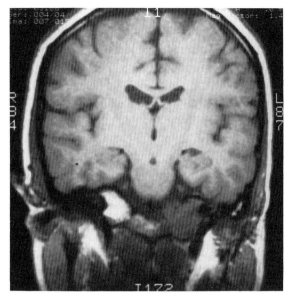

SE 600/20

**Figure 11-2**

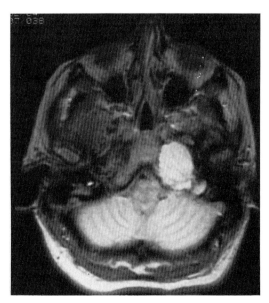

SE 2,000/35

**Figure 11-3**

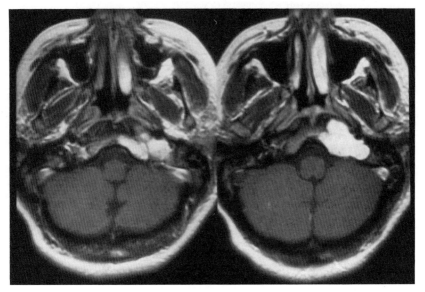

SE 600/20

**Figure 11-4**

49. Which *one* of the following is the MOST likely diagnosis?

   (A) Glomus jugulare tumor
   (B) Cholesterol granuloma
   (C) Intrapetrous carotid aneurysm
   (D) Chondrosarcoma
   (E) Intraosseous epidermoid tumor

## CASE 11 (Cont'd)

QUESTIONS 50 THROUGH 53: MARK YOUR ANSWER SHEET TRUE (T) OR FALSE (F) FOR EACH OF THE RESPONSE CHOICES.

50. Concerning cholesterol granuloma,

   (A) it usually occurs in an obstructed air cell of the petrous apex
   (B) it occasionally occurs in the middle ear
   (C) it contains blood products
   (D) it typically causes third cranial nerve palsy
   (E) CT is as specific as MRI for the diagnosis

51. Concerning intrapetrous carotid artery aneurysm,

   (A) it is usually traumatic in origin
   (B) CT is as specific as MRI for the diagnosis
   (C) mature thrombus within the aneurysm has a decreased signal intensity relative to brain on T2-weighted images
   (D) carotid occlusion is an accepted treatment

52. Concerning chondrosarcoma of the skull base,

   (A) it usually arises in the midline of the clivus
   (B) it is easily distinguished histologically from chordoma
   (C) it is a rapidly progressive lesion
   (D) enhancement on MRI is typical

53. Concerning epidermoid tumor,

   (A) it is a congenital tumor of epithelial tissue
   (B) it usually arises in the mastoid antrum
   (C) it frequently erodes into the middle ear
   (D) it usually has low signal intensity on T2-weighted MR images

## CASE 12:  Questions 54 through 57

This 77-year-old man presented with hoarseness. You are shown a T1-weighted axial MR image (Figure 12-1).

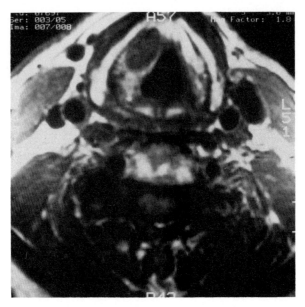

SE 600/25

**Figure 12-1**

54.  Which *one* of the following is the MOST likely diagnosis?

 (A)  Obstructed laryngocele
 (B)  Thyroglossal duct cyst
 (C)  Chondrosarcoma
 (D)  Squamous cell carcinoma
 (E)  Tuberculosis

# CASE 12 (Cont'd)

QUESTIONS 55 THROUGH 57: MARK YOUR ANSWER SHEET TRUE (T) OR FALSE (F) FOR EACH OF THE RESPONSE CHOICES.

55. An obstructed laryngocele:

   (A) leaves the larynx via the thyroid notch
   (B) passes through the thyrohyoid membrane
   (C) frequently involves the true cord
   (D) ascends in the paraglottic space
   (E) arises from the laryngeal ventricular saccule (appendix)

56. Concerning thyroglossal duct cysts,

   (A) a prominent intralaryngeal component is usually present
   (B) when surgically excised, a portion of the hyoid bone is removed
   (C) when infrahyoid, they have an intimate association with the strap muscles
   (D) malignant lesions related to thyroglossal duct remnants are usually carcinomas

57. Concerning laryngeal chondrosarcomas,

   (A) most arise from the epiglottic cartilage
   (B) the involved cartilage is expanded
   (C) metastasis is common
   (D) when they involve the thyroid cartilage, a total laryngectomy is usually required

# CASE 13: Questions 58 through 61

This 46-year-old man has submandibular pain and swelling. You are shown a series of postcontrast axial CT scans (Figure 13-1) and a bone-window axial image of the most superior section in the series (Figure 13-2).

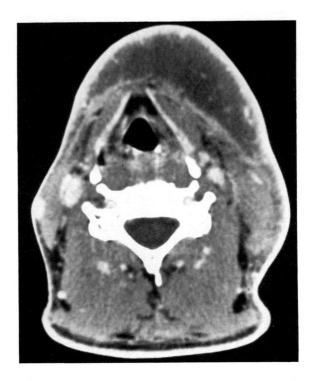

**Figure 13-1**

58. Which *one* of the following is the MOST likely diagnosis?

    (A) Squamous cell carcinoma
    (B) Plunging ranula
    (C) Epidermoid cyst
    (D) Abscess
    (E) Cystic hygroma

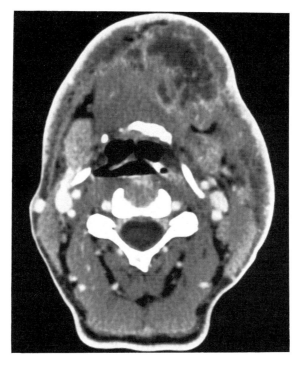

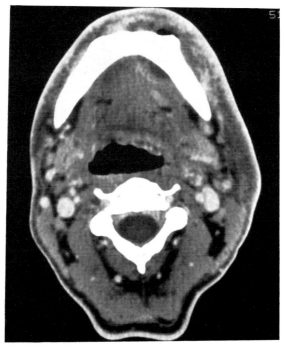

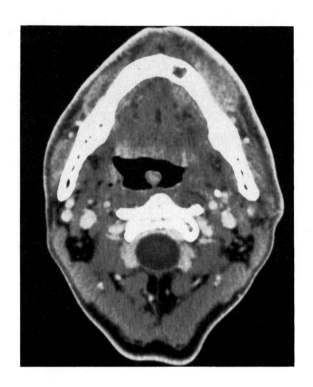

**Figure 13-1 (Continued)**

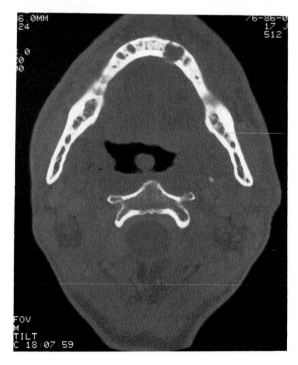

**Figure 13-2**

## CASE 13 (Cont'd)

QUESTIONS 59 AND 60: MARK YOUR ANSWER SHEET TRUE (T) OR FALSE (F) FOR EACH OF THE RESPONSE CHOICES.

59. Concerning ranulas,

   (A) they most commonly originate in the sublingual glands
   (B) the plunging variety usually extend into the masticator space
   (C) a location medial to the mylohyoid muscle is typical
   (D) they are common in trumpet players


60. Concerning epidermoid cysts of the head and neck,

   (A) they represent ectodermal inclusions
   (B) they occur along the lines of embryologic fusion
   (C) they contain skin appendages
   (D) they are attached to the tongue and hyoid bone


61. A midline mass in the floor of the mouth is MOST likely to represent:

   (A) an epidermoid cyst
   (B) a ranula
   (C) a salivary duct stone
   (D) an odontogenic cyst
   (E) an enlarged lymph node

This 19-year-old woman has recurrent episodes of right facial palsy. You are shown two bone-algorithm axial CT scans through the temporal bones (Figures 14-1 and 14-2).

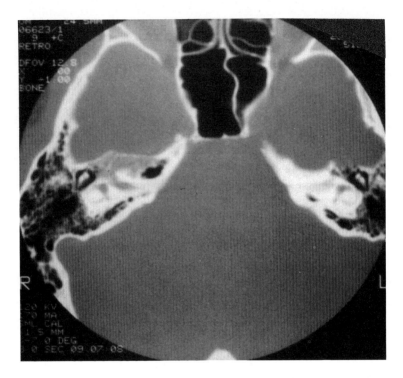

**Figure 14-1**

62. Which *one* of the following is the MOST likely diagnosis?

   (A) Facial nerve schwannoma
   (B) Perineural extension of adenoid cystic carcinoma
   (C) Hemangioma
   (D) Glomus faciale tumor
   (E) Cholesteatoma

## CASE 14 (Cont'd)

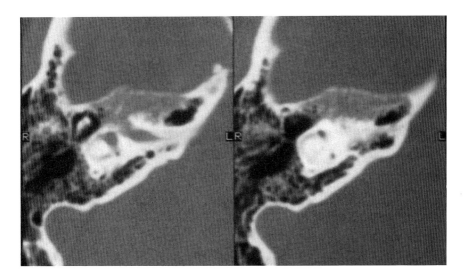

**Figure 14-2**

63. An acute onset of facial nerve paralysis is MOST commonly due to:

   (A) facial nerve schwannoma
   (B) hemangioma of the temporal bone
   (C) meningioma of the facial canal
   (D) acute otitis media
   (E) Bell's palsy

## CASE 14 (Cont'd)

QUESTIONS 64 AND 65: MARK YOUR ANSWER SHEET TRUE
(T) OR FALSE (F) FOR EACH OF THE RESPONSE CHOICES.

64. Concerning the course of the facial nerve canal through the
normal temporal bone,

   (A) the labyrinthine segment passes superior to the cochlea
   (B) the tympanic segment passes superior to the horizontal
   semicircular canal
   (C) the tympanic segment passes inferior to the oval window
   (D) the second or pyramidal turn is more posterior than the
   geniculate turn

65. Concerning cholesteatoma,

   (A) the most common location is in the inferior tympanic
   cavity
   (B) the posterior semicircular canal is the most likely canal
   to be eroded
   (C) an automastoidectomy is the defect left when a chole-
   steatoma evacuates into the external canal
   (D) a normal scutum excludes this diagnosis
   (E) it usually has low signal intensity on T1-weighted MR
   images
   (F) the central portion enhances on MRI with gadolinium
   DTPA

# CASE 15: Question 66

This 53-year-old woman presented with pain referable to her left temporomandibular joint. You are shown a sagittal CT scan (Figure 15-1), a sagittal T1-weighted MR image (Figure 15-2), several coronal T1-weighted MR images (Figure 15-3), and a coronal T2-weighted MR image (Figure 15-4) of the left temporomandibular joint.

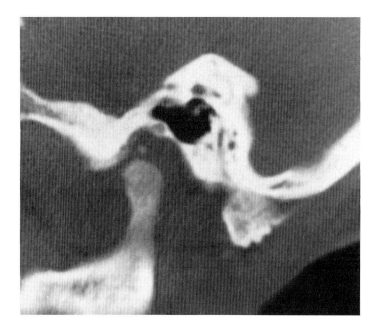

**Figure 15-1**

66. Which *one* of the following is the MOST likely diagnosis?

    (A) Meniscal dislocation
    (B) Synovial chondromatosis
    (C) Septic arthritis
    (D) Post-traumatic joint hemorrhage
    (E) Rheumatoid arthritis

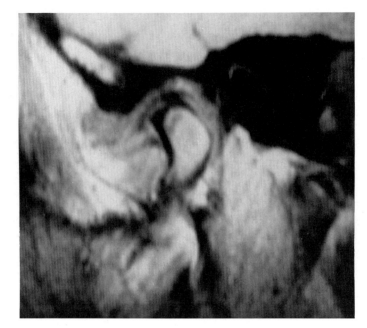

SE 800/20

**Figure 15-2**

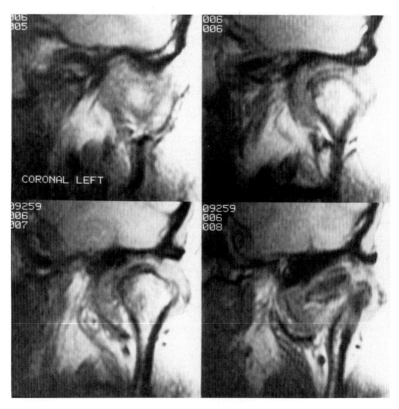

SE 800/20

**Figure 15-3**

# CASE 15 (Cont'd)

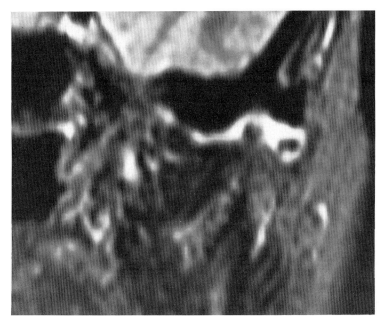

SE 2,000/80

**Figure 15-4**

This 56-year-old man presented with dysphagia. You are shown T1-weighted axial (A) and sagittal (B) MR images (Figure 16-1).

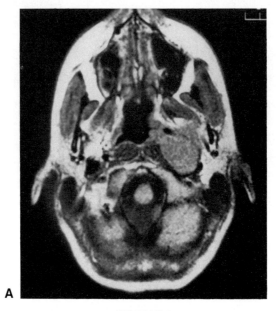

SE 700/25

**Figure 16-1**

67. Which *one* of the following is the MOST likely diagnosis?

   (A) Glomus vagale tumor
   (B) Schwannoma
   (C) Minor salivary gland tumor
   (D) Deep-lobe parotid tumor
   (E) Carotid aneurysm

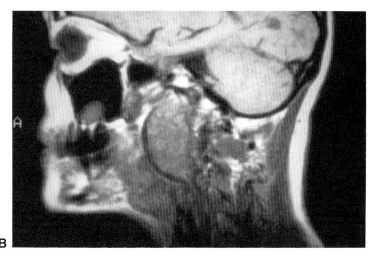

SE 550/20

QUESTIONS 68 THROUGH 71: MARK YOUR ANSWER SHEET TRUE (T) OR FALSE (F) FOR EACH OF THE RESPONSE CHOICES.

68. Concerning schwannomas of the parapharyngeal space,

   (A) they usually arise in the third division of the trigeminal nerve
   (B) they usually displace the internal carotid artery posteriorly
   (C) they are hypovascular lesions
   (D) they usually develop in the prestyloid compartment
   (E) they often contain scattered calcification

# CASE 16 (Cont'd)

69. Concerning extraparotid salivary gland tumors of the para-pharyngeal space,

    (A) they usually arise in salivary rest tissue
    (B) they usually develop in the prestyloid compartment
    (C) they usually are benign mixed tumors
    (D) MRI usually shows a fat plane separating the tumor from the parotid gland

70. Concerning deep-lobe parotid tumors,

    (A) they frequently extend into the prestyloid compartment
    (B) they usually are malignant mixed tumors
    (C) if dumbbell shaped, they extend through the styloman-dibular tunnel
    (D) they often have calcifications along their periphery

71. Concerning the parapharyngeal space,

    (A) it is immediately posteromedial to the masticator space
    (B) its boundaries run from the skull base to the level of the hard palate
    (C) mycotic aneurysm is a potential complication of an abscess within it
    (D) the surgical approach to a mass within it is determined by the intraparotid or extraparotid origin of the mass

This 17-year-old girl has a history of recent mastoiditis. You are shown two axial postcontrast CT scans (Figures 17-1 and 17-2), as well as axial (Figure 17-3) and coronal (Figure 17-4) high-resolution CT scans.

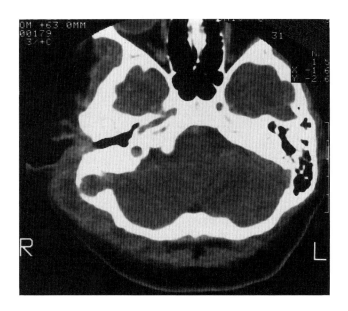

**Figure 17-1**

QUESTIONS 72 THROUGH 74: MARK YOUR ANSWER SHEET TRUE (T) OR FALSE (F) FOR EACH OF THE RESPONSE CHOICES.

72. The images demonstrate:

   (A) serous otitis media
   (B) subperiosteal mastoid abscess
   (C) perisinus abscess
   (D) coalescent mastoiditis
   (E) cerebellar abscess

# CASE 17 (Cont'd)

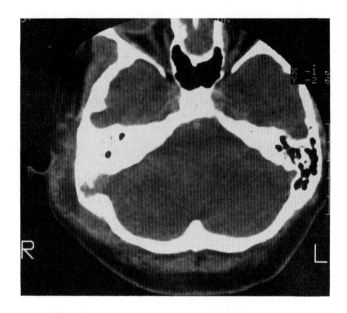

**Figure 17-2**

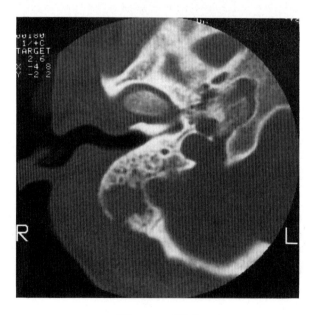

**Figure 17-3**

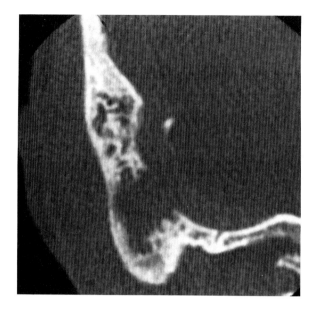

**Figure 17-4**

73. Complications of acute otomastoiditis include:

   (A) thrombosis of lateral and sigmoid sinuses
   (B) thrombosis of petrosal and cavernous sinuses
   (C) facial nerve palsy
   (D) leptomeningitis
   (E) labyrinthitis
   (F) Gradenigo syndrome

74. Features of Gradenigo syndrome include:

   (A) apex petrositis
   (B) abducens nerve paresis
   (C) gasserian ganglionitis
   (D) facial paralysis

This 26-year-old woman has had decreased hearing on the left side for several years and on the right side for the past 7 to 8 months. You are shown a series of MR scans, including T1-weighted images without enhancement (A) and with gadolinium DTPA enhancement (B and C) and T2-weighted images (D through F) (Figure 18-1).

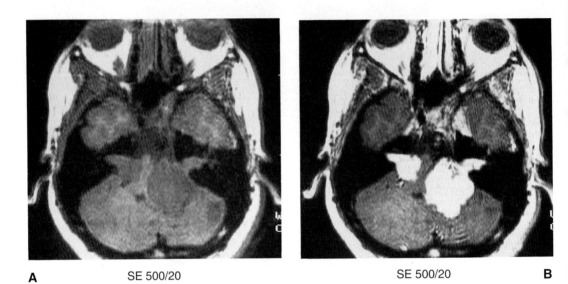

A          SE 500/20          SE 500/20          B

**Figure 18-1**

75. Which *one* of the following is the MOST likely diagnosis?

(A) Neurofibromatosis 2
(B) Multiple leptomeningeal metastases
(C) Ruptured dermoid cyst
(D) Meningiomatosis
(E) Lymphoma

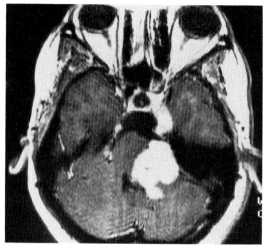

C                    SE 500/20

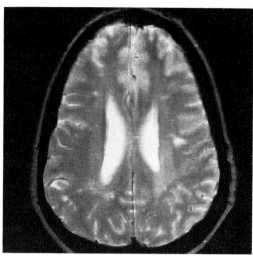

SE 2,500/90                    D

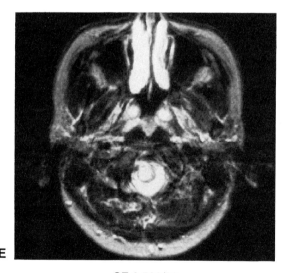

E

SE 2,500/90

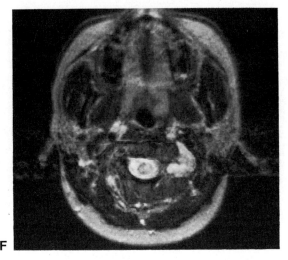

SE 2,500/90

QUESTIONS 76 THROUGH 78: MARK YOUR ANSWER SHEET TRUE (T) OR FALSE (F) FOR EACH OF THE RESPONSE CHOICES.

76. Typical features of neurofibromatosis 2 include:

    (A) a genetic locus on chromosome 22
    (B) plexiform neurofibromas
    (C) white matter lesions
    (D) bilateral acoustic schwannomas
    (E) multiple meningiomas
    (F) optic nerve glioma

## CASE 18 (Cont'd)

77. Concerning multiple leptomeningeal metastases,

   (A) most patients have hydrocephalus
   (B) they typically result from further dissemination of an intraventricular metastasis
   (C) involvement of the cranial nerves is best evaluated by T2-weighted MRI
   (D) in adults they are most commonly seen with adenocarcinoma
   (E) they are usually asymptomatic

78. Concerning meningiomatosis,

   (A) it is usually a manifestation of dissemination from a single neoplasm
   (B) it is usually a familial disease
   (C) it is a specific form of phakomatosis
   (D) it is a common component of neurofibromatosis 1

## CASE 19: Questions 79 and 80

This 50-year-old man has a newly diagnosed carcinoma of the tongue. You are shown T1- and T2-weighted axial MR scans (Figure 19-1A and B) as well as axial and coronal T1-weighted scans obtained after intravenous administration of gadolinium DTPA (Figure 19-1C and D).

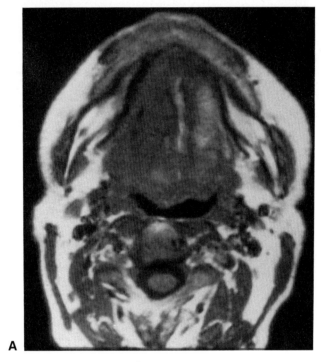

SE 800/20

**Figure 19-1**

QUESTION 79: MARK YOUR ANSWER SHEET TRUE (T) OR FALSE (F) FOR EACH OF THE RESPONSE CHOICES.

79. The tumor involves the:

   (A) free margin of the tongue
   (B) contralateral tongue
   (C) mandible
   (D) floor of the mouth
   (E) pterygoid plate

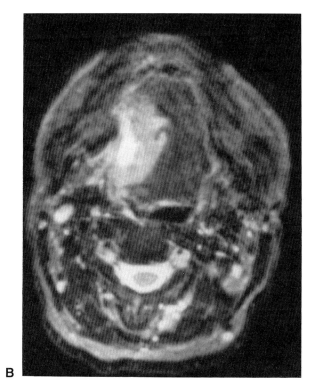

B

SE 2,727/80

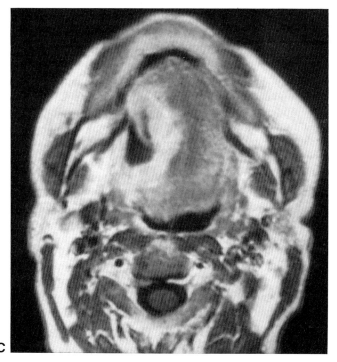

C

SE 800/20

T-59

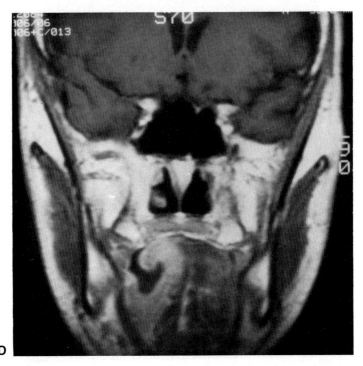

SE 2,727/80

80. Which *one* of the following is LEAST likely in a patient with carcinoma of the tongue base?

    (A) Metastasis to a jugulodigastric node
    (B) Involvement of the supraglottic larynx
    (C) Perineural spread to the pterygopalatine fossa
    (D) Simultaneous carcinoma of the esophagus
    (E) Involvement of the mandible

## CASE 20: Questions 81 through 84

This 55-year-old man presented with chronic nasal stuffiness and pain. You are shown coronal T1-weighted MR images through the nasal vault without (A) and with (B) fat saturation (Figure 20-1), a coronal postcontrast T1-weighted MR image (Figure 20-2), and an axial noncontrast CT scan through the maxillary sinuses and nasal vault (Figure 20-3).

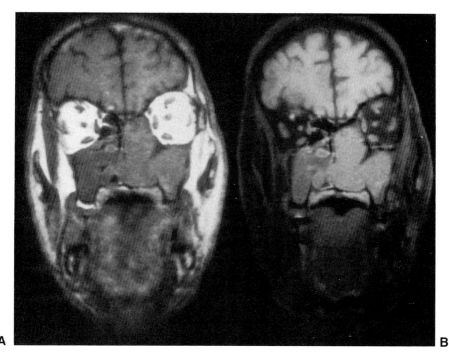

A   B

SE 600/15

**Figure 20-1**

81. Which *one* of the following is the MOST likely diagnosis?

    (A) Concha bullosa
    (B) Inverted papilloma
    (C) Squamous cell carcinoma
    (D) Hemangioma of the nasal turbinate
    (E) Nasopharyngeal angiofibroma

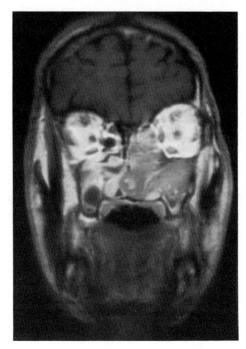

SE 600/15

**Figure 20-2**

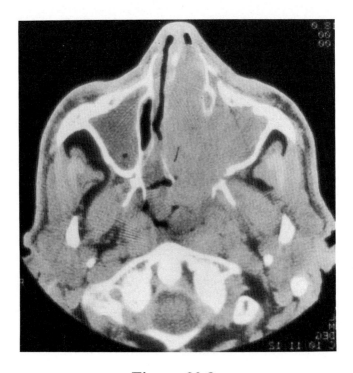

**Figure 20-3**

QUESTIONS 82 THROUGH 84: MARK YOUR ANSWER SHEET TRUE (T) OR FALSE (F) FOR EACH OF THE RESPONSE CHOICES.

82.  Concerning inverted papilloma,

    (A) the most common site is within the ethmoid sinuses

    (B) it is associated with the development of squamous cell carcinoma

    (C) it is often confused clinically with a benign nasal polyp

    (D) bone invasion is common

    (E) it recurs after surgical resection in about 50% of cases

83.  Concerning carcinoma of the nasal cavity and paranasal sinuses,

    (A) adenocarcinoma is the most frequent histologic type

    (B) extension into the tonsillar pillar is typical

    (C) the lesions usually have a higher signal intensity than mucous secretions on T2-weighted MR sequences

    (D) it cannot be reliably differentiated from lymphoma by CT

84.  Concerning fat suppression in MRI,

    (A) it results in high signal intensity of fat on T1-weighted sequences

    (B) it improves contrast between enhancing lesions and fat on gadolinium-enhanced MR images

    (C) it has a lower frequency of susceptibility artifacts than does conventional spin-echo imaging

    (D) it can be used to verify a diagnosis of lipoma

This 38-year-old man has painful swelling of the right side of his face and numbness in the right side of his jaw and chin. You are shown axial (Figure 21-1) and coronal (Figure 21-2) MR images with gadolinium DTPA enhancement and fat saturation.

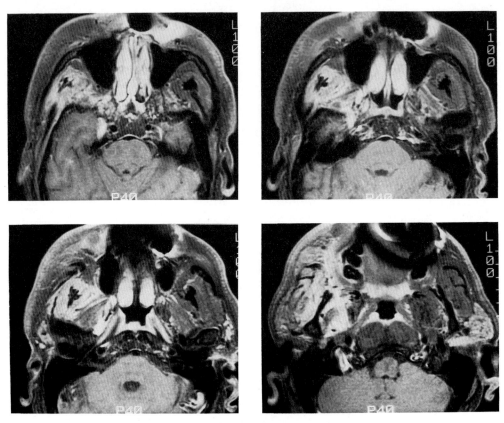

SE 800/20

**Figure 21-1**

85. Which *one* of the following is the MOST likely diagnosis?

   (A) Lipoma
   (B) Denervation atrophy
   (C) Malignant schwannoma
   (D) Lymphangioma
   (E) Abscess

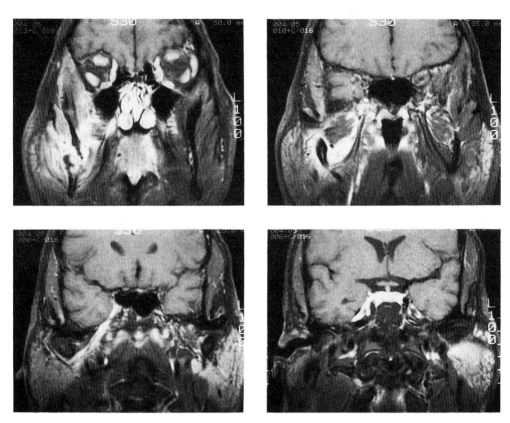

SE 800/20

**Figure 21-2**

QUESTIONS 86 THROUGH 88: MARK YOUR ANSWER SHEET TRUE (T) OR FALSE (F) FOR EACH OF THE RESPONSE CHOICES.

86. Concerning malignant schwannomas of the head and neck,

    (A) they often arise in the trigeminal nerve
    (B) they follow the course of a cranial nerve
    (C) they rarely cause pain
    (D) they are usually sensitive to radiation therapy

87. Concerning hemangiomas and lymphangiomas of the head and neck,

    (A) lymphangiomas typically disseminate along the drainage pathways of the cervical lymphatics
    (B) large ones usually involve multiple spaces
    (C) hemangiomas are typically pulsatile
    (D) lymphangiomas typically destroy adjacent bone
    (E) the presence of phleboliths indicates the cavernous variety of hemangioma

88. Concerning an abscess of the masticator space,

    (A) it is commonly associated with dental infections
    (B) it presents as a mass in the cheek
    (C) trismus is rarely present
    (D) it rarely spreads to the buccal space

This 12-year-old boy presented with pulsatile tinnitus and a mass behind the left tympanic membrane. You are shown an axial CT scan (Figure 22-1).

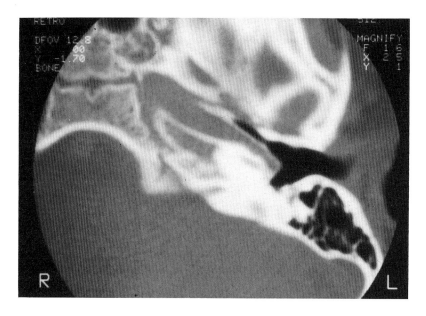

**Figure 22-1**

89. Which *one* of the following is the MOST likely diagnosis?

    (A) Cholesterol granuloma (cholesterol cyst)
    (B) Glomus tympanicum
    (C) Aberrant carotid artery
    (D) Dehiscent jugular fossa
    (E) Facial nerve sheath tumor

90. Which *one* of the following is LEAST likely to cause a conductive hearing loss?

    (A) Aberrant carotid artery
    (B) Otosclerosis
    (C) Acoustic neuroma
    (D) Atresia of the external auditory canal
    (E) Cholesteatoma

QUESTIONS 91 AND 92: MARK YOUR ANSWER SHEET TRUE (T) OR FALSE (F) FOR EACH OF THE RESPONSE CHOICES.

91. Concerning paragangliomas (glomus tumors),

    (A) a glomus jugulare tumor is more likely to present with a conductive hearing loss than with a sensorineural hearing loss
    (B) on CT, a glomus tympanicum tumor is differentiated from a glomus jugulare tumor by the demonstration of the intact bony lateral wall of the jugular bulb with the former
    (C) most glomus jugulare tumors present with symptoms relating to the nerves that pass through the jugular foramen
    (D) a glomus jugulare tumor has the same histology as a carotid body tumor

92. Aberrant carotid artery is frequently associated with absence of the:

    (A) lateral wall of the jugular canal
    (B) lateral wall of the carotid canal
    (C) foramen spinosum
    (D) facial nerve canal
    (E) auditory ossicles

This 38-year-old woman has left facial discomfort. You are shown axial proton-density (A) and T2-weighted (B) MR scans (Figure 23-1).

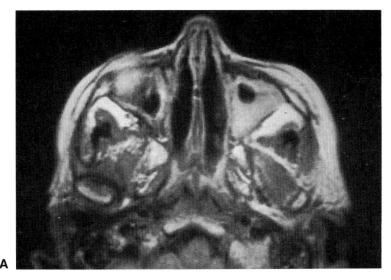

SE 1,800/30

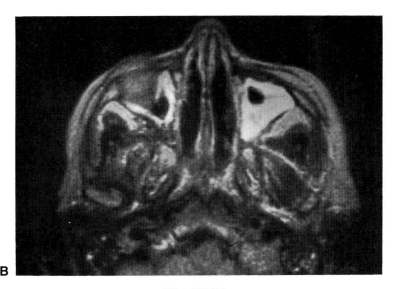

SE 1,800/90

**Figure 23-1**

93. Which *one* of the following is the LEAST likely diagnosis?

    (A) Sinusitis with aeration
    (B) Aspergilloma
    (C) Sinusitis with dried secretions
    (D) Subacute sinus hemorrhage
    (E) Dentigerous cyst

QUESTIONS 94 THROUGH 97: MARK YOUR ANSWER SHEET TRUE (T) OR FALSE (F) FOR EACH OF THE RESPONSE CHOICES.

94. Concerning sinusitis,

    (A) about 20% of cases of acute maxillary bacterial sinusitis are secondary to dental infections
    (B) opacification of a sinus in a child under 2 years of age usually indicates the presence of infection
    (C) acute disease is characterized on MRI by low and high signal intensities on T1- and T2-weighted images, respectively
    (D) allergic disease usually involves just the maxillary sinus
    (E) generalized headache is a common symptom

95. Concerning aspergillosis of the sinuses,

    (A) it occurs in both immunosuppressed and otherwise healthy individuals
    (B) it causes small-vessel thrombosis
    (C) an aspergilloma has high signal intensity on both T1- and T2-weighted MR images
    (D) the mucosal disease is easily distinguished from bacterial sinusitis on MRI
    (E) it is often diagnosed as a result of its failure to respond to routine antibiotic therapy

96. Concerning chronic sinonasal secretions,

    (A) with time there is an increase in the bound-water fraction
    (B) their protein content can be inferred from the signal intensities of T1- and T2-weighted MR scans
    (C) dried secretions often give signal voids on T1- and T2-weighted MR scans
    (D) on MRI, dried secretions can be routinely differentiated from an aspergilloma
    (E) when they have low signal intensity on T1- and T2-weighted MR scans, they have high attenuation on CT

97. Concerning sinus hemorrhage,

    (A) it is a common finding in patients with hemophilia
    (B) it is the cause of pain in barotrauma
    (C) when subacute, it is usually distinguishable on MRI from secretions of acute sinusitis
    (D) when subacute, it has a high attenuation on CT scans

This 38-year-old woman presented with fullness in the right neck. You are shown axial T1-weighted (A) and T2-weighted (B) MR scans (Figure 24-1).

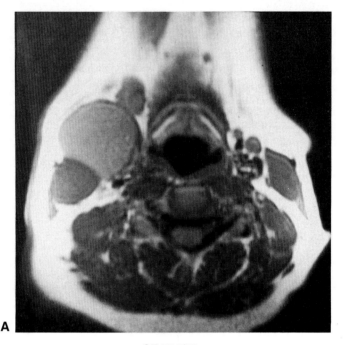

SE 500/30

**Figure 24-1**

98. Which *one* of the following is the MOST likely diagnosis?

    (A) Metastatic carcinoma
    (B) Thyroglossal duct cyst
    (C) Submandibular gland tumor
    (D) Branchial cleft cyst
    (E) Carotid body tumor

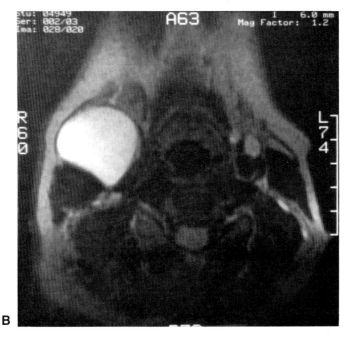

SE 2,500/100

QUESTIONS 99 THROUGH 101: MARK YOUR ANSWER SHEET TRUE (T) OR FALSE (F) FOR EACH OF THE RESPONSE CHOICES.

99. Concerning cervical lymphadenopathy,

    (A) central necrosis is common in a node involved by Hodgkin's lymphoma
    (B) tuberculous adenitis rarely shows central necrosis
    (C) nodes involved by Castelman's disease nearly always enhance
    (D) extracapsular spread of tumor indicates a poor prognosis
    (E) by size criterion only, a 1-cm node in the jugulodigastric area is considered abnormal

100. Concerning tumors of the submandibular gland,

    (A) they are more likely to be malignant than are those of the parotid gland

    (B) the most common tumor is squamous cell carcinoma

    (C) perineural extension of malignant tumors is uncommon

    (D) extraglandular extension involves the mylohyoid muscle more frequently than it does the lateral pterygoid muscle

101. Concerning carotid body tumors,

    (A) the internal carotid artery is frequently displaced anteriorly

    (B) about 30% have symptomatic hypersecretion of catecholamines

    (C) multiple lesions occur in approximately 50% of patients

    (D) they usually have a homogeneous signal intensity on MRI

## CASE 25: Questions 102 through 106

This 65-year-old woman has a long-standing history of progressive loss of vision in her left eye. A fundoscopic examination revealed an elevated pale disk with optociliary shunt vessels. The right eye was normal. You are shown a postcontrast coronal CT scan (Figure 25-1), a T1-weighted coronal MR scan (Figure 25-2A), and a T1-weighted postcontrast axial MR scan (Figure 25-2B).

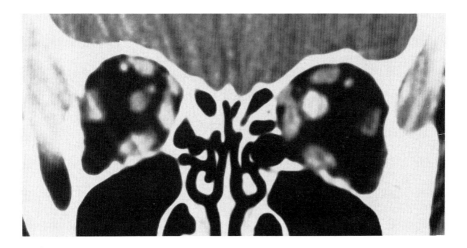

**Figure 25-1**

102. Which *one* of the following is the MOST likely diagnosis?

   (A) Optic nerve sheath meningioma
   (B) Optic nerve glioma
   (C) Optic neuritis
   (D) Optic nerve sarcoidosis
   (E) Orbital pseudotumor

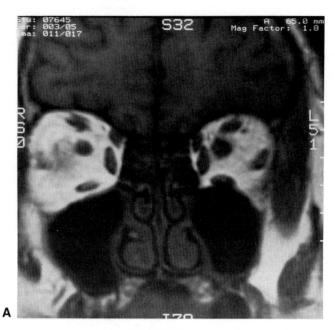

SE 600/20

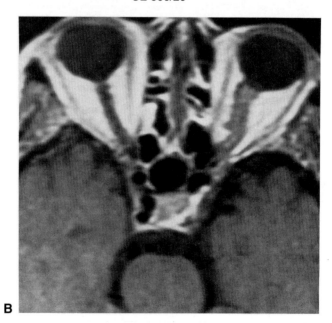

SE 800/20

**Figure 25-2**

QUESTIONS 103 THROUGH 106: MARK YOUR ANSWER SHEET TRUE (T) OR FALSE (F) FOR EACH OF THE RESPONSE CHOICES.

103.  Concerning optic nerve sheath meningiomas,

  (A)  they usually occur in middle-aged women
  (B)  those occurring in children behave aggressively
  (C)  bilateral lesions are diagnostic of neurofibromatosis
  (D)  the presence of tumoral calcification allows their distinction from optic nerve gliomas

104.  Concerning optic nerve gliomas,

  (A)  they occur most frequently in children
  (B)  those occurring in adults are frequently high-grade astrocytomas
  (C)  bilateral lesions are characteristic of neurofibromatosis 1
  (D)  kinking and buckling of the enlarged optic nerve are frequently present

105.  Concerning optic neuritis,

  (A)  it is commonly a manifestation of multiple sclerosis
  (B)  it occurs in patients with malnutrition
  (C)  it occurs in both the acute and chronic forms of sarcoid involvement of the nervous system
  (D)  it commonly causes diffuse enlargement of the optic nerve

106. Concerning optic nerve pseudotumor (perineuritis),

    (A) it presents clinically as a painful eye associated with decreased vision

    (B) it is rarely associated with involvement of the adjacent retrobulbar fat

    (C) CT shows enhancement of the optic nerve

    (D) MRI shows ragged, edematous enlargement of the optic nerve-sheath complex

## CASE 26: Questions 107 through 110

This 8-year-old boy has an enlarging mass in the left side of the mandible. You are shown two transaxial postcontrast CT scans filmed with soft tissue windows (A and B) and transaxial and coronal postcontrast CT scans filmed with bone windows (C and D) (Figure 26-1).

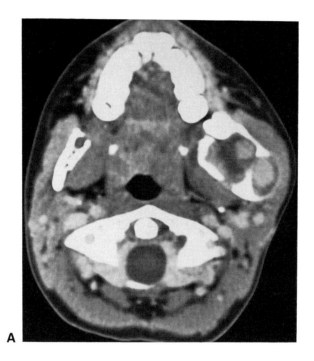

**Figure 26-1**

107. Which *one* of the following is the MOST likely diagnosis?

    (A) Ameloblastoma
    (B) Dentigerous cyst
    (C) Aneurysmal bone cyst
    (D) Actinomycosis
    (E) Metastatic neuroblastoma

## CASE 26 (Cont'd)

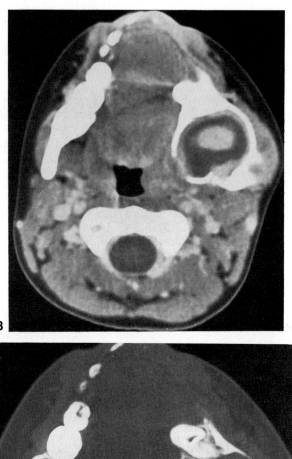

B

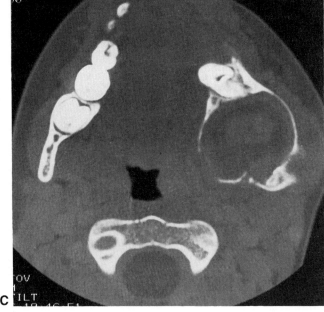

C

CASE 26 (Cont'd)

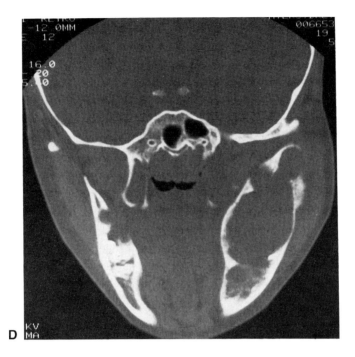

QUESTIONS 108 THROUGH 110: MARK YOUR ANSWER SHEET TRUE (T) OR FALSE (F) FOR EACH OF THE RESPONSE CHOICES.

108. Concerning dentigerous cysts,

    (A) a tooth remnant is identified in the cyst wall
    (B) most are located in the maxilla
    (C) extracystic soft tissue masses are typical
    (D) they are often multilocular

## CASE 26 (Cont'd)

109. Concerning aneurysmal bone cysts,

    (A) in the craniofacial region, they are typically found in the maxilla
    (B) fluid-fluid levels are a common feature
    (C) they commonly arise after trauma
    (D) the most common presenting symptom is painless swelling

110. Common imaging features of mandibular actinomycosis include:

    (A) periosteal reaction
    (B) involvement of adjacent soft tissues
    (C) low signal intensity of the medullary cavity on T1-weighted images
    (D) expansile lesion
    (E) cervical lymphadenopathy

# DEMOGRAPHIC DATA QUESTIONS

*Please answer all of the questions below.* The data you provide will be used to supply information that will allow you to compare your performance on the examination with that of others at similar levels of training and with similar backgrounds, and for purposes of planning continuing education projects. Please answer each question as accurately and as objectively as possible. Please mark the *one* BEST response for each question. Recall, of course, that we do *not* want individual names. Our analyses will reflect only categories and groups; everything will remain completely anonymous and no attempt will be made to identify any specific individual.

111. The ACR will be evaluating the questions in this examination to determine their degree of difficulty and to determine the success of the examination as an instrument of self-evaluation and continuing education. To assist the ACR, please indicate in which of the following ways you took this examination.

   (A) Used reference materials or read the syllabus portion of this book to assist in answering some portion of the examination
   (B) Did not use reference materials and did not read the syllabus portion of this book while taking the examination

112. How much residency and fellowship training in Diagnostic Radiology have you completed as of December 1992?

   (A) None
   (B) Less than 1 year
   (C) 1 year
   (D) 2 years
   (E) 3 years
   (F) 4 or more years

113. When did you finish your residency training in Radiology?

(A) Prior to 1982
(B) 1982–1986
(C) 1987–1991
(D) 1992
(E) Not yet completed
(F) Radiology is not my specialty

114. Have you been certified by the American Board of Radiology in Diagnostic Radiology?

(A) Yes
(B) No

115. Which one of the categories listed below BEST describes the setting of your practice in the immediate past 3 years? (For residents and fellows, in which one did you or will you spend the major portion of your residency or fellowship?)

(A) Community or general hospital—less than 200 beds
(B) Community or general hospital—200 to 499 beds
(C) Community or general hospital—500 or more beds
(D) University-affiliated hospital
(E) Office practice

116. In which one of the following general areas of Radiology do you consider yourself MOST expert?

(A) Chest radiology
(B) Bone radiology
(C) Gastrointestinal radiology
(D) Genitourinary radiology
(E) Head and neck radiology
(F) Neuroradiology
(G) Pediatric radiology
(H) Cardiovascular radiology
(I) Other

117. In which one of the following radiologic modalities do you consider yourself MOST expert?

  (A) General angiography
  (B) Interventional radiology
  (C) Magnetic resonance imaging
  (D) Nuclear radiology
  (E) Ultrasonography
  (F) Computed tomography
  (G) Radiation therapy
  (H) Other

# Head and Neck Disorders
## (Fourth Series)

# Table of Contents

The Table of Contents is placed in this unusual location so that the reader will not be distracted by the answers before completeing the test. A detailed index of the areas considered in this syllabus is provided (beginning on p. 621) for further reference.

# Head and Neck Disorders (Fourth Series) Syllabus

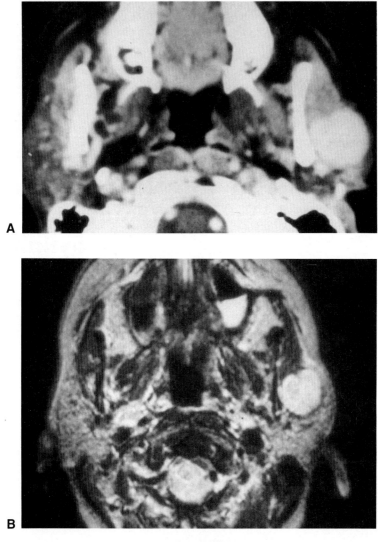

SE 2,500/80

*Figure 1-1.* This 43-year-old man presented with a left parotid mass. You are shown a postcontrast CT scan (A) and a T2-weighted axial MR image (B).

# Case 1:  Pleomorphic Adenoma of the Parotid Gland

## Question 1

Which *one* of the following is the MOST likely diagnosis?

(A) Adenocarcinoma
(B) Pleomorphic adenoma
(C) Branchial cleft cyst
(D) Facial nerve schwannoma
(E) Metastasis

The axial postcontrast CT scan (Figure 1-1A) shows a solitary solid mass in the superficial portion of the left parotid gland (Figure 1-2A, arrow). The lesion has sharp, clear margins separating it from the adjacent parotid tissue. The T2-weighted MR image (Figure 1-1B) shows the mass to have a fairly high signal intensity (Figure 1-2B, wide arrow), and again its borders are clearly identified and separated from the adjacent parotid tissue. Incidentally noted is an unrelated retention cyst in the lower left maxillary sinus (Figure 1-2B, thin arrow).

The sharp margins of this solid, noncystic lesion suggest that it is either a benign mass with a well-defined capsule or a low-grade tumor with a pseudocapsule. It is usually not possible to distinguish between these two categories of lesion on either CT or MRI. Since 75 to 80% of all parotid tumors are benign and 70 to 80% of all salivary gland benign tumors are pleomorphic adenomas (benign mixed tumors), the most likely diagnosis is pleomorphic adenoma **(Option (B) is correct).** These tumors are usually well-differentiated lesions with considerable amounts of serous and mucinous material, which is the major factor in their typical MR appearance of low signal intensity on T1-weighted images and high signal intensity on T2-weighted sequences (Figure 1-3).

Adenocarcinomas of the parotid gland (Option (A)) represent only 3% of all parotid neoplasms. Most of these are high-grade tumors with infiltrative margins (Figure 1-4). In addition, such high-grade tumors are poorly differentiated, highly cellular masses that tend to have low to

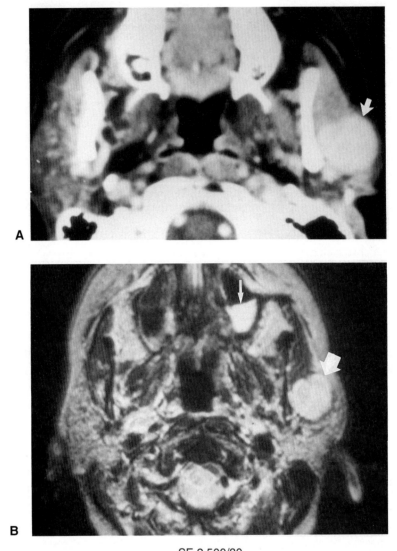

SE 2,500/80

*Figure 1-2* (Same as Figure 1-1). Pleomorphic adenoma. (A) Axial post-contrast CT scan showing a solid left parotid soft tissue mass (arrow) with homogeneous contrast enhancement. The lesion is in the superficial portion of the gland and has sharp margins separating it from the adjacent parotid tissue. (B) Axial T2-weighted MR scan showing the left parotid mass (wide arrow) as an area of high signal intensity. The mass is clearly delineated from the adjacent parotid tissue. An incidental retention cyst (thin arrow) is present in the left maxillary sinus.

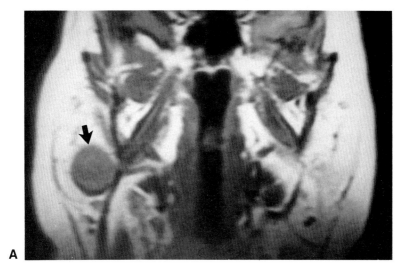

SE 700/30

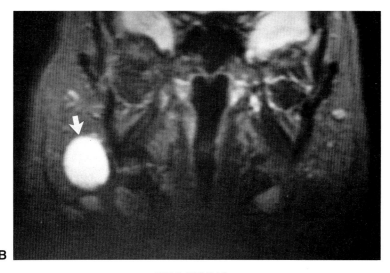

SE 2,000/110

*Figure 1-3.* Pleomorphic adenoma. Coronal T1-weighted (A) and T2-weighted (B) MR scans showing a well-defined right parotid mass (arrow) with low T1-weighted and high T2-weighted signal intensities. This is the typical MR appearance of a small benign salivary gland mass.

intermediate MR signal intensities on T1- and T2-weighted sequences (Figure 1-5).

Most branchial cleft cysts that involve the parotid gland (Option (C)) have been classified as type II cysts. Their hallmark on CT is a central

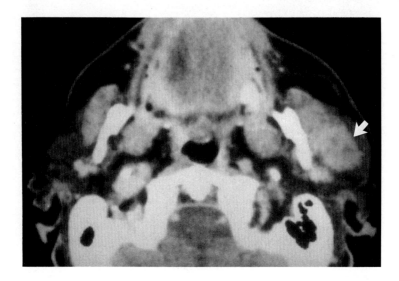

*Figure 1-4.* Adenocarcinoma. Axial postcontrast CT scan showing a left parotid mass (arrow) that has slightly irregular margins with the adjacent parotid tissue. There are also two areas of lower attenuation (necrosis) within the tumor.

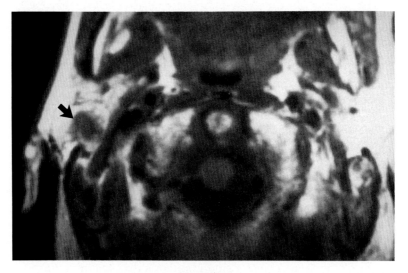

SE 700/20

*Figure 1-5.* Adenocarcinoma. Axial T1-weighted MR scan showing a right parotid retromandibular mass (arrow) with indistinct infiltrative margins and low signal intensity. This mass also had low signal intensity on T2-weighted scans.

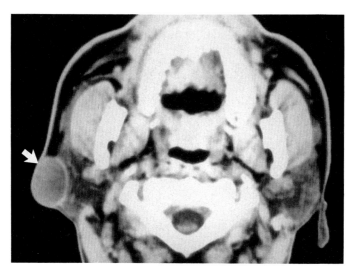

*Figure 1-6.* Noninfected branchial cleft cyst in the parotid gland. Axial CT scan showing a right parotid cystic mass (arrow). The mass has a lower attenuation than muscle and a higher attenuation than fat. There is a thin, well-defined rim.

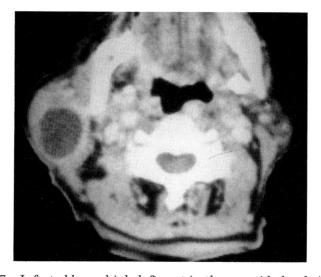

*Figure 1-7.* Infected branchial cleft cyst in the parotid gland. Axial post-contrast CT scan showing a large cystic mass in the right parotid gland. There is a thick, enhancing rim (compare with Figure 1-6).

homogeneous low-attenuation (10 to 20 HU) region surrounded by a uniform, clearly identifiable rim (Figures 1-6 and 1-7). Since the test CT scan (Figure 1-1) shows a solid rather than a cystic mass, this diagnosis

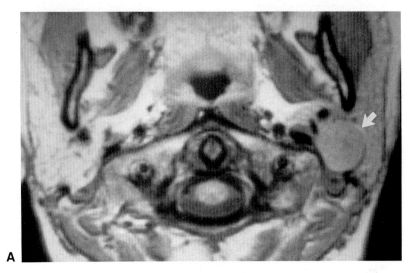

SE 700/30

*Figure 1-8.* Schwannoma of the left facial nerve. Axial T1-weighted (A) and T2-weighted (B) MR scans showing a well-delineated left parotid mass (arrow, panel A) with low T1-weighted and high T2-weighted signal intensities. This has the MR appearance of a benign mass. Note the similarity to Figures 1-1B, 1-2B, and 1-3.

is unlikely. On MRI, these cysts have homogeneous low T1-weighted and high T2-weighted signal intensities due to their high water content.

Facial nerve schwannomas (Option (D)) are rare lesions that often present with a facial nerve paresis or paralysis. In view of their rarity and because the history of the test patient did not include any facial nerve dysfunction, this diagnosis is not likely. However, the basic CT and MR appearances of such a schwannoma (Figure 1-8) are the same as in the test case (Figure 1-1).

Metastasis to the parotid gland (Option (E)) is rare. The metastatic foci can be located either in the parotid gland parenchyma or within one or more intraparotid lymph nodes. It is almost always known that a primary tumor exists. Usually the responsible tumor is highly malignant and the parotid metastasis has irregular or indistinct infiltrative margins and contains areas of tumor necrosis (Figure 1-9). In addition, multiple metastases to the parotid gland are evident in most cases.

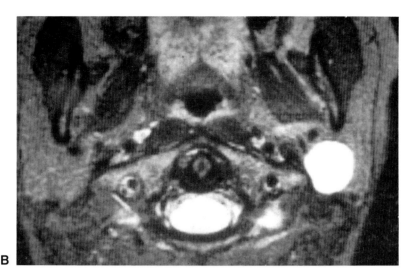

SE 2,500/100

*Figure 1-8 (Continued)*

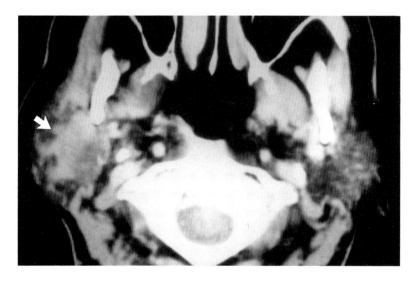

*Figure 1-9.* Metastatic squamous cell carcinoma of the lung. Axial CT scan showing an irregularly marginated right parotid mass (arrow). The lesion also has an area of lower attenuation (necrosis) on its medial margin. This lesion has the CT appearance of a malignant tumor.

## Question 2

Concerning adenocarcinoma of the head and neck,

(A) the palate is a common site of origin

(B) a high-grade lesion in a salivary gland is more likely to represent metastatic colon cancer than a primary tumor

(C) workers in hardwood industries have an increased incidence of sinonasal tumors

(D) high-grade lesions usually have high signal intensities on T2-weighted MR images

(E) it is the most common parotid gland cancer

Adenocarcinomas of the head and neck arise in the major and minor salivary glands. These tumors are more common in the minor salivary glands, and the greatest concentration of minor salivary glands is in the palate **(Option (A) is true)**. Adenocarcinomas represent only about 3% of parotid gland neoplasms.

Adenocarcinomas of the head and neck are almost all high-grade malignancies that have a histologic similarity to adenocarcinomas of the gastrointestinal tract, and when such tumors are discovered in the head or neck, a search for a primary tumor below the clavicles should be made. However, it is estimated that only about 3% of all primary tumors below the clavicles metastasize to the head and neck. Since most of these metastatic sites are to lymph nodes, only a small percentage of tumors metastasize to the salivary glands. Thus, very few adenocarcinomas in the head and neck actually represent metastases from a primary carcinoma in the colon **(Option (B) is false)**.

There is a clearly established increase in the incidence of adenocarcinoma of the paranasal sinuses and nasal fossae in hardwood-furniture makers. Epidemiologic studies have shown that the fine dust from these hardwoods is the causative agent **(Option (C) is true)**. Accordingly, furniture makers now wear masks to filter these particles.

The high-grade tumors are highly malignant lesions with little cellular differentiation, and there is virtually no serous or mucinous material. There is also a high mitotic ratio, which results in little intracellular water. Thus, these tumors usually have low to intermediate signal intensities on both T1- and T2-weighted sequences (Figure 1-10). The high T2-weighted signal intensities associated with the benign neoplasms and low-grade better-differentiated tumors are not seen **(Option (D) is false)**.

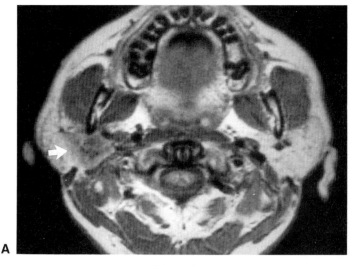

SE 500/20

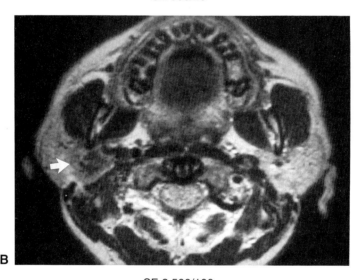

SE 2,500/100

*Figure 1-10.* Adenocarcinoma. Axial T1-weighted (A) and T2-weighted (B) MR scans showing a poorly defined right parotid mass (arrow) in the deep or retromandibular portion of the gland. The mass has low signal intensity on all sequences. This is the MR appearance of a high-grade malignant tumor.

As noted above, adenocarcinomas account for only about 3% of parotid gland neoplasms; they represent 8 to 12% of malignant parotid tumors. The most common parotid gland cancer is the mucoepidermoid carcinoma

**(Option (E) is false).** It represents about one-third of all malignant salivary gland tumors, and nearly 60% of mucoepidermoid carcinomas arise in the parotid glands.

## Question 3

Concerning pleomorphic adenomas,

(A) they are the most common parotid gland neoplasm
(B) recurrences are related to violation of the tumor capsule
(C) the most commonly associated cancer is carcinoma ex pleomorphic adenoma
(D) facial nerve paralysis is found in about 30% of cases
(E) dystrophic calcifications are common
(F) multiple tumors are uncommon in patients who have not had prior surgery
(G) when small, they have low and high signal intensities on T1- and T2-weighted images, respectively

Pleomorphic adenomas represent 70 to 80% of all benign tumors in the major salivary glands, and 84% of them occur in the parotid gland. Since 75 to 80% of parotid gland tumors are benign, pleomorphic adenomas, which are the most common benign tumors, are the most common parotid gland neoplasm **(Option (A) is true).**

The true frequency of multiple primary pleomorphic adenomas occurring in a parotid gland in a patient who has not undergone surgery is low, often estimated to be about 1% of all parotid pleomorphic adenomas. However, the occurrence of multiple pleomorphic adenomas has been ostensibly shown to be secondary to prior surgery during which the capsule of the tumor was violated and tumor cells spilled into the operative field **(Option (F) is true).** Such seeding was fairly common in previous years when enucleation of these tumors was the procedure of choice. These multiple tumors are usually clustered like a bunch of grapes (Figure 1-11). However, once parotidectomy became the procedure of choice, the incidence of such recurrent tumors became almost nonexistent **(Option (B) is true).** Such "seeded" tumors may take 10 or more years after surgery to become clinically evident.

The true malignant mixed tumor is very rare. It contains both epithelial and stromal malignant elements and is therefore a true carcinosarcoma with a grave prognosis. The most common carcinomatous change associated with a pleomorphic adenoma occurs when a portion of the adenoma undergoes carcinomatous degeneration. When this happens the lesion is referred to as carcinoma ex pleomorphic adenoma **(Option (C)**

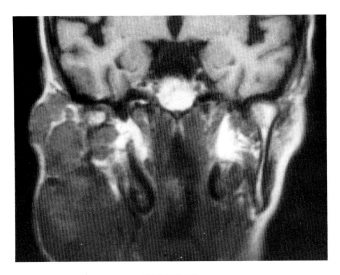

SE 700/30

*Figure 1-11.* Multiple pleomorphic adenomas. Coronal T1-weighted MR scan showing a cluster of well-defined right parotid masses. This patient had a pleomorphic adenoma removed 15 years earlier.

**is true)** (Figure 1-12). The old estimates are that such malignant change occurs in 2 to 5% of all pleomorphic adenomas. However, this has recently been reevaluated, and it is now estimated that as many as 25% of all pleomorphic adenomas will undergo malignant change if left untreated.

Facial nerve paralysis in association with a parotid mass almost always suggests that the tumor is malignant. Only rarely is a benign lesion associated with a facial nerve paralysis. Examples of such cases include a hemorrhagic cystic hygroma involving the parotid gland with compression of the facial nerve, parotid gland sarcoidosis with a granulomatous mass causing facial nerve paralysis as found in Heerfordt's syndrome, and, rarely, a suppurative parotid lymph node associated with an ipsilateral acute otitis media causing a facial nerve paralysis. Facial nerve paralysis is only anecdotally associated with pleomorphic adenoma **(Option (D) is false).**

Calcifications in salivary gland tumors are uncommon. Even though dystrophic calcifications are more commonly associated with pleomorphic adenomas than they are with other neoplasms (Figure 1-13), such calcifications occur in less than 20% of pleomorphic adenomas **(Option (E) is false).** Calcifications can also be seen in some hemangiomas and rarely in some mucoepidermoid carcinomas.

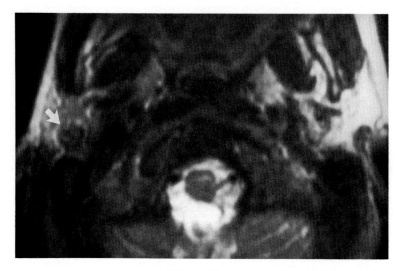

SE 2,500/100

*Figure 1-12.* Pleomorphic adenoma that has been almost entirely replaced by an undifferentiated carcinoma. Axial T2-weighted MR scan showing a well-demarcated right parotid mass (arrow). The lesion has low signal intensity; it also had low signal intensity on T1-weighted scans. This represents a carcinoma ex pleomorphic adenoma.

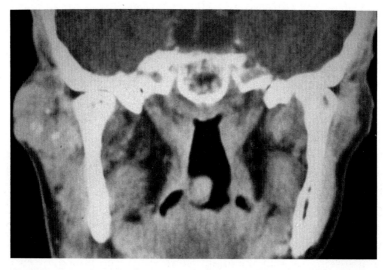

*Figure 1-13.* Pleomorphic adenoma. Coronal CT scan showing a large right parotid mass containing several areas of calcification. This appearance is most suggestive of a pleomorphic adenoma. If it were a large parotid hemangioma, the lesion would have been soft (rather than firm) to palpation and there most probably would have been a bluish discoloration of the overlying skin.

Pleomorphic adenomas are benign, well-differentiated tumors that contain serous and mucinous secretions. When they are small, their MR characteristics reflect this high water content, i.e., low signal intensity on T1-weighted images and high signal intensity on T2-weighted sequences (Figure 1-3) **(Option (G) is true).** When these tumors are large, areas of necrosis and hemorrhage occur, creating heterogeneous MR signal intensities.

*Peter M. Som, M.D.*

## SUGGESTED READINGS

1. Mandelblatt SM, Braun IF, Davis PC, Fry SM, Jacobs LH, Hoffman JC Jr. Parotid masses: MR imaging. Radiology 1987; 163:411–414
2. Mirich DR, McArdle CB, Kulkarni MV. Benign pleomorphic adenomas of the salivary glands: surface coil MR imaging versus CT. J Comput Assist Tomogr 1987; 11:620–623
3. Rabinov K, Weber AL. Radiology of the salivary glands. Boston: GK Halt; 1985:292–367
4. Som PM. Salivary glands. In: Som PM, Bergeron RT (eds), Head and neck imaging, 2nd ed. St. Louis: Mosby-Year Book; 1991:320–348
5. Som PM, Biller HF. High-grade malignancies of the parotid gland: identification with MR imaging. Radiology 1989; 173:823–826
6. Som PM, Shugar JM, Sacher M, Stollman AL, Biller HF. Benign and malignant parotid pleomorphic adenomas: CT and MR studies. J Comput Assist Tomogr 1988; 12:65–69

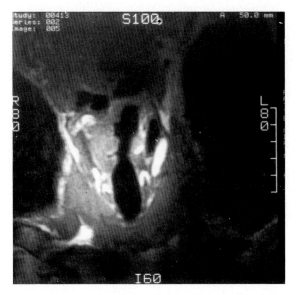

SE 600/20

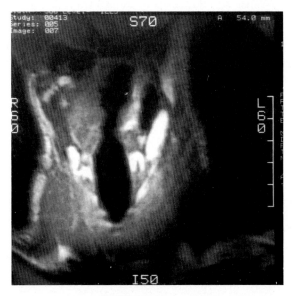

SE 600/20

*Figure 2-1.* This 71-year-old man has laryngeal carcinoma. You are shown two coronal T1-weighted MR scans.

# Case 2: Laryngeal Carcinoma

## Question 4

The test images demonstrate involvement of the:

(A) epiglottis
(B) false cord
(C) paraglottic space
(D) cricoid cartilage
(E) subglottic mucosa

The tumor shown on the test images (Figure 2-1) arises in the supraglottic larynx and extends through the paraglottic space around the ventricle into the lateral part of the true cord (see Figure 2-2).

The larynx is subdivided into three regions that are important both clinically and radiologically: the supraglottic, glottic, and subglottic regions. These terms are used to describe the relationship of a tumor to the true cord, the ventricle, and the false cord (Figures 2-3 and 2-4); the position of the tumor relative to these key structures is important in planning treatment.

The primary mucosal landmarks of the supraglottic larynx are the epiglottis, aryepiglottic folds, and false cords. The epiglottis, right aryepiglottic fold, and right false cord are thickened and nodular in the test images, indicating their involvement by tumor **(Options (A) and (B) are true).**

The term "paraglottic space" refers to the area deep to the mucosa. At the level of the false cord this is made up almost completely of fatty tissue (Figure 2-5). In the test images, the bright MR signal characteristic of fat on T1-weighted images is obliterated by the tumor on the right side, indicating involvement of the paraglottic space **(Option (C) is true).**

The glottic region refers to the true vocal cord. The boundary between the glottic and subglottic regions is considered to be 1 cm caudal to a horizontal plane passing through the most lateral part of the ventricle

---

Figures 2-1 and 2-2 are reprinted with permission from Curtin [1].

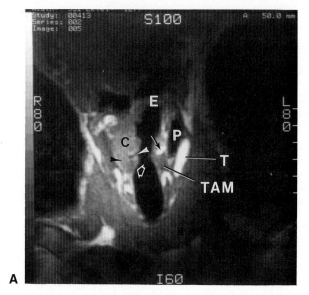

SE 600/20

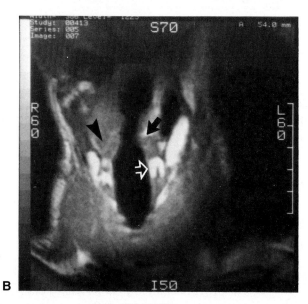

SE 600/20

*Figure 2-2* (Same as Figure 2-1). (A) Coronal T1-weighted MR scan shows a supraglottic cancer (C) extending around the ventricle into the lateral part (black arrowhead) of the true cord. This tumor passes through the paraglottic region. Note the paraglottic fat (solid arrow) on the normal left side and normal thyroarytenoid muscle (TAM), ventricle (white arrowhead), thyroid cartilage (T), pyriform sinus (P), epiglottis (E), and normal subglottic mucosa (open arrow). The thyroid cartilage is ossified and has high signal intensity because of fat in its medullary cavity. (B) Coronal scan slightly posterior to that in panel A. The tumor (arrowhead) extends into the lateral part of the true cord. On this image the ventricle cannot be seen. Its level is indicated on the normal side by the upper edge (solid arrow) of the thyroarytenoid muscle. Note the cricoid cartilage on the normal side (open arrow).

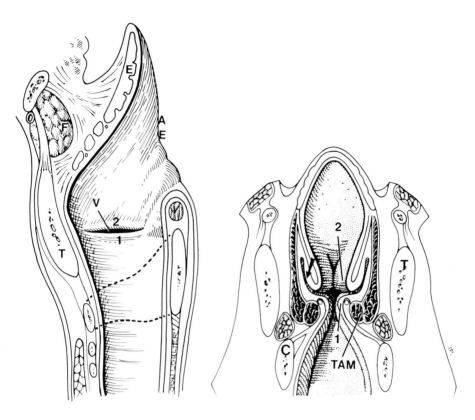

*Figure 2-3*                    *Figure 2-4*

*Figures 2-3 and 2-4.* Figure 2-3 is a diagram of a midline sagittal section of the larynx. The true cord (1) and false cord (2) are indicated. Note the slitlike ventricle (V) between these two parallel structures. The upper edge of the posterior cricoid cartilage is at the level of the true cord. The thyroid cartilage (T), pre-epiglottic fat (F), epiglottis (E), and aryepiglottic fold (AE) are also indicated. Figure 2-4 is a coronal diagram of the larynx. The true cord (1) and false cord (2) are indicated, separated by the ventricle. The thyroarytenoid muscle (TAM), thyroid cartilage (T), and cricoid cartilage (C) are also indicated. The paraglottic space represents the soft tissue (mostly fat) between the mucosa and the thyroid cartilage. The appendix of the ventricle (arrow) is indicated. The supraglottic larynx represents everything above the ventricle. The glottic larynx represents the area of the true cord. The subglottic larynx begins 1 cm below the level of a plane that passes through the midportion of the ventricle and continues to the inferior edge of the cricoid cartilage. (Reprinted with permission from Curtin [2].)

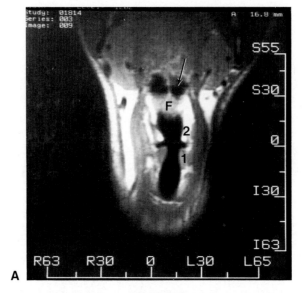

SE 800/20

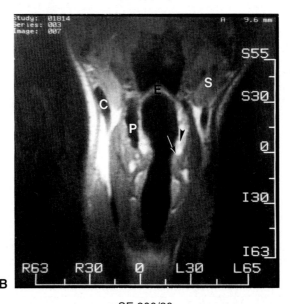

SE 800/20

*Figure 2-5.* Coronal T1-weighted images of the normal larynx. (A) The true cord (1) is predominantly the signal intensity of muscle. The false cord (2) shows the bright signal of fat. The ventricle is easily seen in this anterior section through the larynx. The vallecula (arrow) and pre-epiglottic fat (F) are also indicated. (B) Slightly posterior coronal scan. At this level the ventricle cannot be seen. Its position is at the upper margin of the thyroarytenoid muscle (arrow), which is seen as intermediate signal intensity. Again, the paraglottic fat at the level of the false cord has a bright signal (arrowhead). The epiglottis (E), pyriform sinus (P), carotid artery (C), and submandibular gland (S) are indicated. (Reprinted with permission from Curtin [1].)

(midportion of the ventricle), which in turn separates the supraglottic larynx from the glottic larynx.

Tumors can follow the paraglottic space around the ventricle to reach the level of the true cord or glottic region. This brings the tumor to the lateral margin of the thyroarytenoid muscle, which makes up the bulk of the true cord. In the test images, the tumor is situated beneath the mucosa at the true cord; however, the mucosal surface of the true cord is smooth and thus likely to be normal. The subglottic mucosa is inferior in location to this and is also normal in appearance **(Option (E) is false)**.

The test images show parts of both the thyroid and cricoid cartilages. The tumor is against the thyroid cartilage but is clearly separate from the more caudal cricoid cartilage; the test images do not show involvement of the cricoid cartilage **(Option (D) is false)**.

## *Question 5*

Contraindications for a classic supraglottic laryngectomy include:

(A) involvement of the thyroid cartilage
(B) involvement of the cervical lymph nodes
(C) extension to the postcricoid area
(D) extension across the ventricle
(E) extension to the vallecula

The treatment options for laryngeal cancer include radiation and surgery. Surgical options include total laryngectomy and various voice-sparing partial laryngectomies.

Small lesions of the true cord can be excised by a cord-stripping procedure. Larger lesions require a vertical hemilaryngectomy, which removes the entire involved true cord, as well as a part of the ipsilateral thyroid cartilage. The most relevant contraindications to such a vertical hemilaryngectomy are the inferior extension of the tumor below the upper margin of the cricoid cartilage (Figure 2-6) and involvement of the thyroid cartilage, including anterior extension at the region of the anterior commissure (Figure 2-7). The anterior commissure is the point where the true cords converge anteriorly and attach to the thyroid cartilage.

A supraglottic laryngectomy is considered for treating lesions that arise above the ventricle in the so-called supraglottic larynx. The key incision is made through the laryngeal ventricle (Figure 2-8), and thus

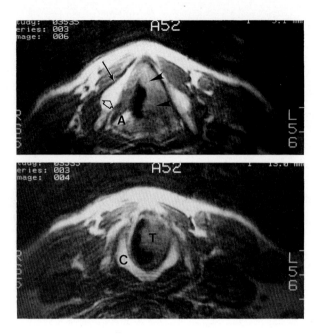

*Figure 2-6.* Glottic carcinoma with subglottic extension. T1-weighted axial MR images. The upper image shows the lesion (arrowheads) of the left true cord. Normal cortex (solid arrow) and fat-filled medullary cavity (open arrow) of the right thyroid cartilage are also indicated, as is the arytenoid (A). In the lower image the tumor (T) is seen within the cricoid ring, and thus the lesion has definitely extended below the upper margin of the cricoid cartilage (C). (Reprinted with permission from Curtin [1].)

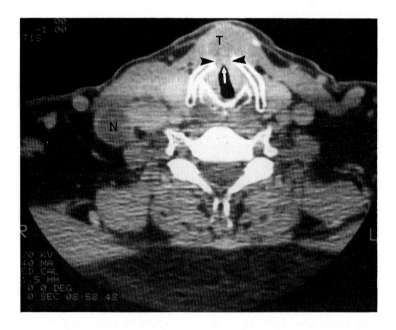

*Figure 2-7.* Carcinoma of the anterior commissure. Axial CT scan shows tumor at the anterior commissure (arrow) and extending through the lower thyroid cartilage (arrowheads) and cricothyroid membrane into the extralaryngeal soft tissues. Extralaryngeal tumor (T) and metastatic lymph node (N) are also indicated. (Reprinted with permission from Curtin [1].)

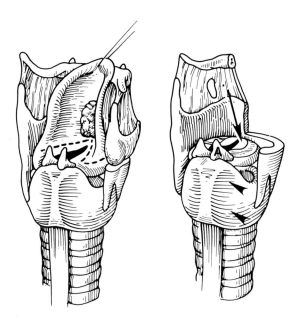

*Figure 2-8.* Diagrams of a supraglottic laryngectomy. On the left diagram the dotted line shows the incision passing through the ventricle and over the posterior aryepiglottic folds. The right diagram shows the residual tissue after the resection. Normally the true cords remain (arrow), as do the arytenoids (A), which are perched on the top of the cricoid cartilage. The postcricoid region is indicated (arrowheads). (Reprinted with permission from Curtin [1].)

the most important requirement for this procedure is that the tumor be limited to the region cranial to the laryngeal ventricle. If the tumor crosses or even reaches the ventricle, the standard supraglottic partial laryngectomy would leave tumor behind at the ventricular margin; therefore, extension across the ventricle is a contraindication for this procedure **(Option (D) is true).**

Some investigators are extending the limits of the various partial laryngectomies, but currently most otolaryngologists consider involvement of the thyroid or the cricoid cartilages to be a contraindication for partial laryngectomy **(Option (A) is true).**

Portions of the thyroid cartilage are removed during either a supraglottic laryngectomy or a vertical hemilaryngectomy. However, the cricoid cartilage, which is the only complete cartilage ring in the respiratory tract, is so important to the structural support of the larynx that removal of this important cartilage compromises the airway. If a tumor involves the cricoid cartilage or is so close to the cartilage that adequate surgical

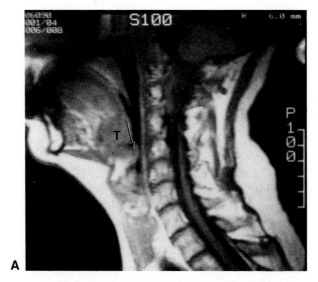

SE 400/20

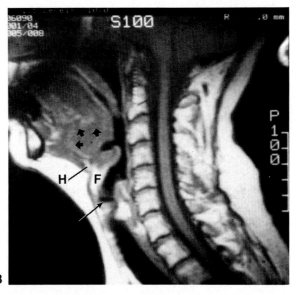

SE 400/20

*Figure 2-9.* Tumor of the base of the tongue and valleculae. Sagittal T1-weighted MR scans. (A) The tumor (T) involves the base of the tongue and spreads into the valleculae to involve the epiglottis (arrow). (B) The tumor does not extend into the pre-epiglottic fat (F), which retains its normal bright signal. The epiglottis is obviously thickened. The hyoid bone (H) and ventricle (long arrow) are indicated. This patient presented with a fairly small lesion visible on the epiglottis. It extended extensively into the tongue base (small arrows). (Reprinted with permission from Curtin [2].)

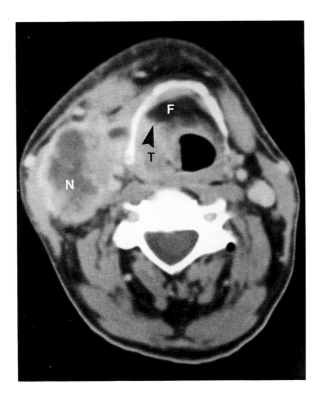

*Figure 2-10.* Carcinoma of the pyriform sinus and aryepiglottic fold. This axial CT scan shows the tumor (T) extending partially (arrowhead) into the pre-epiglottic fat (F). Most of the pre-epiglottic fat is clear. Note the enlarged lymph node (N) involved by metastatic disease in the lateral aspect of the neck. There is low-density central necrosis in this node. (Reprinted with permission from Curtin [2].)

margins would require resection of a part of the cartilage, most surgeons would recommend that a total laryngectomy be performed. Tumors of the supraglottic larynx often involve the pyriform sinus and can spread inferiorly into the postcricoid area (arrowheads, Figure 2-8). Since this brings the tumor into contact with the cricoid cartilage, a supraglottic laryngectomy is contraindicated **(Option (C) is true).**

Enlarging supraglottic tumors may involve the valleculae and the pre-epiglottic fat (space) (Figures 2-9 and 2-10). Involvement of these structures is not a contraindication to a supraglottic laryngectomy because they can easily be resected en bloc with the laryngeal tumor **(Option (E) is false).**

The supraglottic larynx has a rich lymphatic drainage, and lymph node metastasis is common with tumors arising in this region. Lymph node metastasis is related to a worse prognosis and is associated with a lower rate of survival, but it is not a contraindication to performing a supraglottic laryngectomy **(Option (B) is false).** Supraglottic partial laryngectomies are often performed in combination with neck dissections.


## Question 6

Concerning the lymphatic drainage of the larynx,

(A) the supraglottic larynx drains to the upper jugular nodes
(B) the subglottic mucosa drains to the paratracheal nodes
(C) the true cord has almost no drainage
(D) all of the laryngeal lymphatics eventually terminate in the jugulodigastric node
(E) subglottic tumors spread to the Delphian node

The larynx has an elaborate system of lymphatic networks. These lymphatic networks figure prominently in the rationale for the various partial laryngectomies.

The free margin of the true cord has almost no lymphatic drainage **(Option (C) is true),** and so a superficial tumor of the true cord is very unlikely to undergo lymph node metastasis.

The rich lymphatic system of the supraglottic larynx drains through the thyrohyoid membrane to the upper jugular lymph nodes, including the jugulodigastric node (Figures 2-11 and 2-12) **(Option (A) is true).**

Tumors of the subglottic larynx are rare. The mucosa of the subglottic larynx does contain lymphatics, and these channels drain inferolaterally to the paratracheal nodes as well as occasionally to other superior mediastinal nodes **(Option (B) is true).**

Tumors involving the subglottis can spread anteriorly to the Delphian node, which is situated anterior to the cricothyroid membrane. Involvement of the Delphian node and its immediate region can be the result of tumor passage along the lymphatic channels or of direct extension of tumor from the anterior subglottis or the anterior commissure of the larynx. By either route, subglottic lesions can invade the Delphian node region **(Option (E) is true)** (Figure 2-7).

The paratracheal nodes do not drain to the jugulodigastric node **(Option (D) is false).** They drain into the lower jugular chain or into the superior mediastinal nodes.

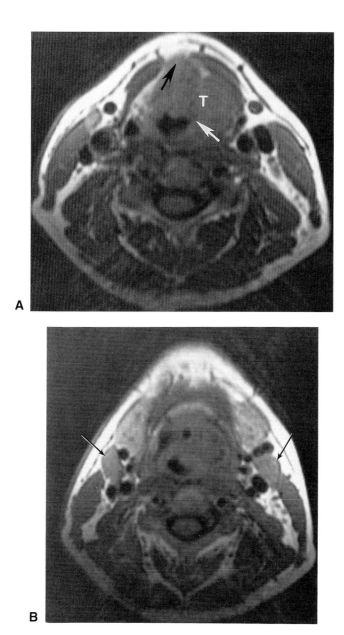

*Figure 2-11.* Supraglottic carcinoma with metastasis to lymph nodes. (A) Large tumor involving the supraglottic larynx (T). The lesion involves the aryepiglottic fold (white arrow). The lesion also extends completely through the pre-epiglottic fat (black arrow). (B) Slightly higher slice shows lymph nodes in the jugular chains (arrows). These nodes are borderline in size but were positive for malignancy upon histologic examination.

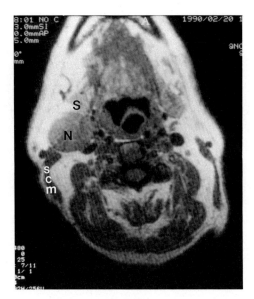

SE 480/25

*Figure 2-12.* Axial MR T1-weighted image. Metastatic disease involving a jugulodigastric node (N) from a tumor of the right pharyngeal wall and pyriform sinus. Note the relationship of the tumor to the submandibular gland (S) and the sternocleidomastoid muscle (scm).

## Question 7

An axial image through the true cord will identify:

    (A) the superior margin of the arytenoid cartilage
    (B) the superior margin of the cricoid cartilage
    (C) the thyroarytenoid muscle
    (D) the thyroid cartilage
    (E) the ventricular appendix (saccule)

Coronal MR images give an excellent demonstration of the important region of the true cord, ventricle, and false cord. CT is limited to the axial plane; however, certain landmarks visible in this plane can help determine the craniocaudal level of the scan.

At the level of the false cord, the paraglottic space is made up almost entirely of fat (Figure 2-13). This fat density is obvious on the CT scan and is the primary indicator that the slice is at the level of the supraglottic larynx.

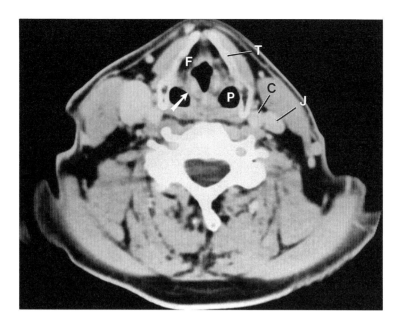

*Figure 2-13.* Axial CT scan through the level of the false cord shows the fat (F) in the upper paraglottic region. The aryepiglottic fold (arrow), pyriform sinus (P), thyroid cartilage (T), carotid artery (C), and internal jugular vein (J) are also indicated. (Reprinted with permission from Curtin [2].)

The bulk of the true cord is made up of the thyroarytenoid muscle, and so the paraglottic region at the level of the true cord is of muscle density (Figure 2-14). On CT this muscle density indicates that the slice is at the level of the true cord **(Option (C) is true)**.

The arytenoid cartilage spans the regions of the true cord, ventricle, and false cord. The vocal ligament extends from the anterior commissure to the vocal process of the arytenoid cartilage. This process is located at the anterior and caudal margin of the arytenoid cartilage, at the level of the cricoarytenoid joint. Thus the lower part of the arytenoid cartilage is at the level of the true cord. However, the superior margin of the arytenoid is above the ventricle at the level of the false cord **(Option (A) is false)** (Figure 2-15).

Most of the cricoid cartilage is caudal to the level of the true cord. The arytenoid cartilage rests on the upper (cranial) edge of the lamina of the cricoid cartilage. This superior margin of the cricoid is at the cricoarytenoid joint level, and thus the upper cricoid lamina is seen on the axial image through the true cord **(Option (B) is true)** (Figure 2-14).

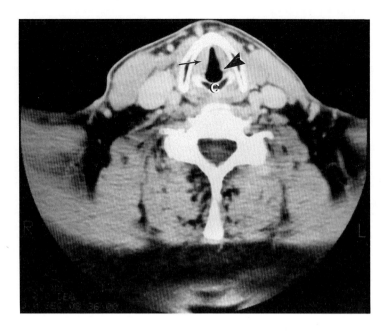

*Figure 2-14.* Axial CT scan through the true cords. The true cord is made up of muscle density (arrow), representing the thyroarytenoid muscle. Note that the cricoid cartilage (C) and the vocal process (arrowhead) of the arytenoid cartilage can be seen at this level. (Reprinted with permission from Curtin [2].)

The thyroid cartilage is the largest of the laryngeal cartilages. It is seen anteriorly at the level of both the true and false cords **(Option (D) is true).** It is normally seen at the level of the true cord, since the vocal ligament is attached to the inner cortex of the thyroid cartilage.

The ventricle is a slitlike space between the true and false cords. A small recess, called the ventricular saccule or appendix, extends superiorly from the ventricle (Figure 2-4). The ventricular appendix is therefore at the level of the false cord and would not be seen at the level of the true cord **(Option (E) is false).**

*Hugh D. Curtin, M.D.*

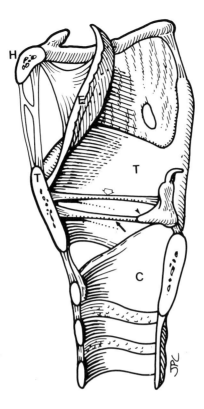

*Figure 2-15.* Schematic sagittal diagram of the larynx showing the relationship of the arytenoid cartilage to the true cord and false cord. The vocal ligament (solid arrow) extends along the free margin of the true cord and attaches to the vocal process of the arytenoid (arrowhead). A less-well-defined ventricular ligament (open arrow) shows the position of the lower part of the false cord. Note that the upper part of the arytenoid is therefore at the level of the false cord. The ventricle would extend between the two indicated ligaments. The cricoid (C) and thyroid (T) cartilages, epiglottis (E), and hyoid bone (H) are also indicated. (Reprinted with permission from Curtin [1].)

SUGGESTED READINGS

1. Curtin HD. Imaging of the larynx: current concepts. Radiology 1989; 173:1–11
2. Curtin HD. The larynx. In: Som PM, Bergeron RT (eds), Head and neck imaging, 2nd ed. Chicago: Mosby-Year Book; 1991:593–692
3. Lawson W, Biller HF. Supraglottic cancer. In: Bailey BJ, Biller HF (eds), Surgery of the larynx. Philadelphia: WB Saunders; 1985:257–278
4. Lawson W, Biller HF, Suen JY. Cancer of the larynx. In: Myers EN, Suen

JY (eds), Cancer of the head and neck. New York: Churchill Livingstone; 1991:533–592

5. Lufkin RB, Hanafee WN, Wortham D, Hoover L. Larynx and hypopharynx: MR imaging with surface coils. Radiology 1986; 158:747–754

*Notes*

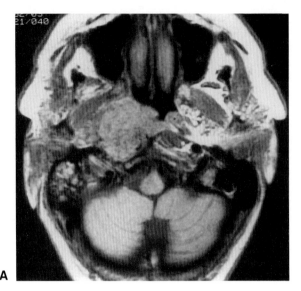

SE 600/20

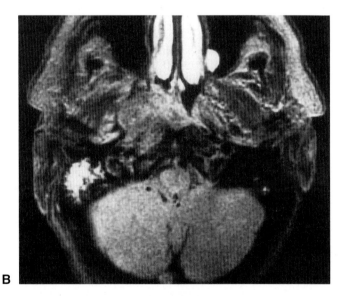

SE 2,800/80

*Figure 3-1.* This 46-year-old man presented with right-sided conductive hearing loss and fifth-nerve dysesthesia. You are shown axial T1-weighted (A) and T2-weighted (B) MR scans and a coronal T1-weighted MR scan (C).

# Case 3:  Carcinoma of the Nasopharynx

## *Question 8*

Which *one* of the following is the MOST likely diagnosis?

(A)  Necrotizing otitis externa
(B)  Adenoidal hypertrophy
(C)  Cellulitis of the retropharyngeal space
(D)  Carcinoma of the nasopharynx
(E)  Rhabdomyosarcoma of the nasopharynx

Figure 3-1A is an axial T1-weighted image through the midnaso-pharynx that demonstrates a soft tissue mass arising from the mucosa of the right nasopharynx (arrows, Figure 3-2A). The mass has a higher signal intensity than surrounding muscle, infiltrates the right preverte-bral muscles, and displaces the right lateral pterygoid muscle (M). On the axial T2-weighted scan (Figure 3-1B), the tumor increases in signal intensity relative to muscle but not to the degree of the serous effusion within the right mastoid air cells (arrows, Figure 3-2B). The coronal T1-weighted image (Figure 3-1C) demonstrates a large tumor (white arrows, Figure 3-2C), which has eroded through the right basisphenoid and extended into the region of the foramen rotundum (open arrows, Figure 3-2C). The findings in this test case are most probably due to carcinoma of the nasopharynx **(Option (D) is correct).**

Necrotizing otitis externa (NOE) (Option (A)) is an aggressive inflam-matory condition of the external ear that predominantly affects elderly diabetic patients and immunocompromised patients. Chronic otorrhea, hearing loss, and cranial neuropathies are common presenting com-plaints. CT typically demonstrates a soft tissue density filling the external canal, with infiltration of the normal tissue planes surrounding the mastoid tip. The infection spreads through fissures within the cartilage at the inferior aspect of the external auditory canal (fissures of Santorini) and into the subperiosteal space of the skull base. Osteomyeli-tis of the temporal and sphenoid bones results, leading to a permeative destruction of these osseous structures best detailed by CT scanning

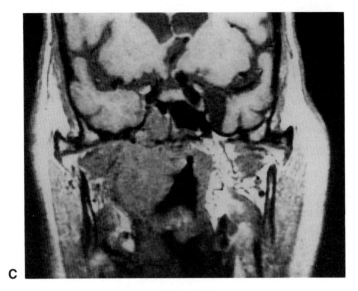

SE 600/20

*Figure 3-1 (Continued)*

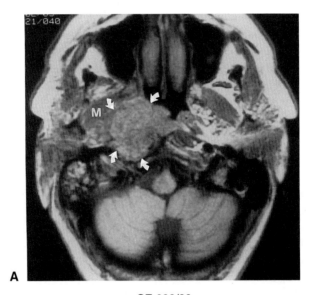

SE 600/20

*Figure 3-2* (Same as Figure 3-1). Nasopharyngeal carcinoma. (A) Axial T1-weighted MR image through the midnasopharynx demonstrates a right soft tissue mass emanating from the mucosa of the nasopharynx with invasion of the right prevertebral musculature (arrows) and displacement of the right lateral pterygoid muscle (M). Note also the serous effusion in the right mastoid air cells. (B) Axial T2-weighted MR image through the same region as panel A. The mass increases in signal intensity but to a lesser degree than does the fluid in the mastoid air cells (arrows). (C) Coronal T1-weighted image through the nasopharynx. The tumor (solid arrows) invades the right basisphenoid and enters the foramen rotundum (open arrows).

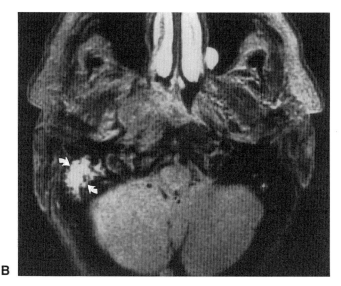

SE 2,800/80

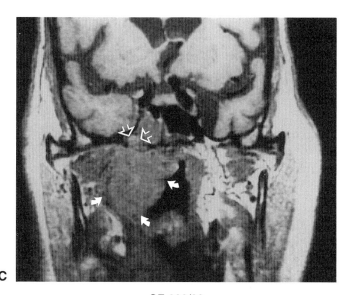

SE 600/20

(Figure 3-3). Extension into the masticator space musculature is not uncommon. T2-weighted MR images demonstrate an increase in signal intensity within the external ear and mastoid air cells, which may extend into the masticator space and the temporomandibular joint. Although some of these features are present in the test images, NOE does not usually include a large localized soft tissue nasopharyngeal mass.

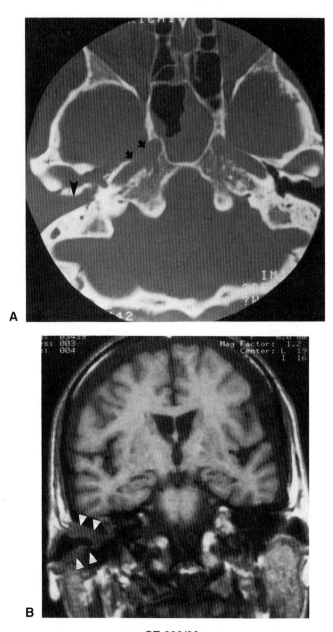

SE 600/20

*Figure 3-3.* Necrotizing otitis externa in a male diabetic patient. (A) Transaxial CT scan demonstrates tissue filling the external ear canal (arrowhead) with destruction of the anterior margin of the carotid canal (arrows) and soft tissue within the sphenoid sinus. (B) Coronal T1-weighted MR image. Soft tissue density fills the external canal and middle ear (arrowheads). (C) T2-weighted transaxial MR image. The right masticator muscle and prevertebral muscles (solid arrows) have high signal intensity. Note also the soft tissue filling the external canal and mastoid (open arrows). The inflammatory component in the right masticator space and prevertebral muscle is typical of the extension of necrotizing otitis externa into the subperiosteal region.

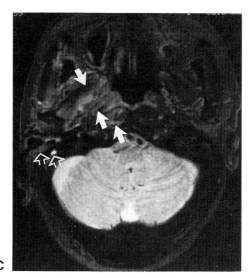

c

SE 2,000/80

Moreover, NOE most commonly occurs in elderly patients and is associated with a history of external auditory canal disease.

Adenoidal hypertrophy (Option (B)) is usually encountered in children, does not result in cranial neuropathies, and appears on MR images as a homogeneous nasopharyngeal mass with signal intensity similar to that of the nasal turbinates on T1- and T2-weighted images. Adenoidal hypertrophy is confined to the mucosal side of the airway and does not infiltrate the soft tissue planes deep to the nasopharyngeal musculature.

Cellulitis of the retropharyngeal space (Option (C)) is also an unlikely diagnosis. The retropharyngeal space is a well-defined space bordered posteriorly by the prevertebral muscles and anteriorly by the posterior pharyngeal mucosa. The lateral margin abuts the carotid space on either side. The mass shown in the test images clearly involves the mucosa of the nasopharynx and invades the right side of the retropharyngeal space. In addition, hearing loss and fifth-nerve palsy would be unusual manifestations of retropharyngeal cellulitis; rather, this disorder usually presents as a septic process with fever, neck pain, and sore throat.

Rhabdomyosarcoma of the nasopharynx (Option (E)) can have an MR appearance similar to that seen in the test images. However, rhabdomyosarcoma is a tumor seen predominantly in patients under the age of 20 years and is therefore not the most likely diagnosis.

# Question 9

Concerning necrotizing otitis externa,

    (A) it is usually caused by *Pseudomonas aeruginosa*
    (B) it generally occurs in diabetic patients
    (C) seventh-nerve palsy is an ominous sign
    (D) cranial neuropathy usually indicates extension into the posterior fossa
    (E) extension into the masticator space usually occurs

NOE is an infection of the external ear canal and surrounding tissues; it is caused almost exclusively by *Pseudomonas aeruginosa* **(Option (A) is true)**. It should be noted, however, that on rare occasions infection with other bacterial or fungal organisms, such as *Aspergillus*, can result in an identical clinical picture. The disease is seen almost exclusively in elderly diabetic patients **(Option (B) is true)**. Other immunosuppressed patients, such as those with leukemia, may develop the disease as well. Some evidence points to an iatrogenic cause, with one study noting that many patients had had external ear lavage performed by their physicians. The disease often begins as a superficial infection of the external auditory canal. It is thought that small-vessel disease (of diabetes) results in an ischemia of the mucosa of the external canal, which inhibits the healing process, leading to an aggressive infection. The infection spreads from the external canal to the subperiosteal compartment of the skull base through the fissures of Santorini in the inferior external auditory canal. This event is often associated with increased ear pain and a fever. If the infection goes unchecked, extension to the stylomastoid foramen and the jugular foramen often occurs, leading to neuropathies of the seventh and of the ninth through twelfth cranial nerves. This event is associated with a poorer prognosis since neurologic complications indicate the potential for permanent neurologic sequelae **(Option (C) is true)**. The cranial neuropathies probably result from vascular thrombosis either within the neural canal or at the skull base. Intracranial spread of external otitis is rare **(Option (D) is false)**. Extension inferiorly into the temporomandibular joint and the masticator space is common **(Option (E) is true)**. NOE is successfully treated today with appropriate anti-*Pseudomonas* antibiotics.

    The diagnosis of NOE is based on findings of both clinical and radiographic examinations. Clinically, the patient with necrotizing externa is typically an elderly, diabetic patient with external otitis, severe otalgia, and evidence of associated mastoiditis, with or without cranial neuropathies. For radiologic evaluation, MRI, CT, and scintigraphy with Tc-99m

MDP and Ga-67 citrate have been used. Gherini et al. found that MRI was superior to CT or Tc-99m MDP and Ga-67 citrate scintigraphy in evaluating the anatomic extent of NOE; however, MRI was not reliable in monitoring the physiological response to therapy. Parisier et al. found that Tc-99m MDP bone scintigraphy was positive in all of 18 patients with osteomyelitis of the temporal bone. However, more recently, Levin et al. have shown that Tc-99m MDP bone scintigraphy may be positive in otherwise healthy patients suffering only from severe external otitis without osteomyelitis. They studied 12 otherwise healthy young adults with severe otitis externa and found that all 12 had positive Tc-99m MDP scintigrams, often appearing similar to those performed in patients with NOE. They concluded that there was no correlation between the severity of clinical presentation and the amount of Tc-99m MDP uptake. Ga-67 scintigraphy has been combined with Tc-99m MDP scintigraphy to monitor the response to therapy. Parisier et al. found that serial gallium imaging was useful in evaluating the effectiveness of therapy since the uptake of Ga-67 citrate decreased with the control of the infection, despite persistent activity on the Tc-99m MDP bone images. Rubin et al. have recently documented the utility of CT in following the regression of soft tissue disease in NOE. They concluded that while remineralization of bone is not common during response to therapy, the reduction in adjacent soft tissue disease is a marker for successful antibiotic therapy. Currently it would seem that a combination of CT and serial Ga-67 citrate imaging may be best in monitoring the response to therapy. MRI may be helpful in excluding other diseases that affect the elderly population, including metastasis and carcinoma of the nasopharynx.

The treatment of choice for NOE is antibiotic therapy, which is associated with a high cure rate if the disease is diagnosed early. Hyperbaric oxygenation and surgical debridement are ancillary therapeutic options.

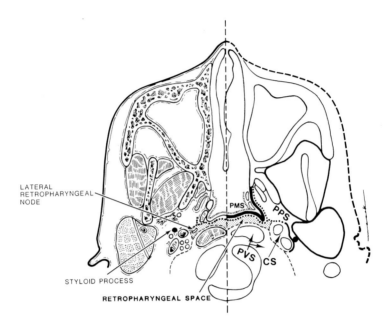

LATERAL
RETROPHARYNGEAL
NODE

STYLOID PROCESS

RETROPHARYNGEAL SPACE

PMS

PPS

PVS    CS

*Figure 3-4.* Schematic diagram of the retropharyngeal space in the upper aerodigestive system. Solid line = pharyngobasilar fascia; dotted line = buccopharyngeal fascia; PVS = prevertebral space; CS = carotid space; PPS = parapharyngeal space; PMS = pharyngeal mucosal space. (Courtesy of H.R. Harnsberger, M.D., University of Utah, Salt Lake City).

## Question 10

Concerning the retropharyngeal space,

(A) it is posterior to the prevertebral space
(B) it contains no lymph nodes
(C) it communicates with the mediastinum
(D) in children, tonsillitis is the most common antecedent illness preceding cellulitis of this space
(E) juvenile angiofibromas usually involve this space

The retropharyngeal space (RPS) is a potential space formed by reflection of the buccopharyngeal fascia and the deep layer of the deep cervical fascia. The mucosas of the nasopharynx and oropharynx lie anterior to the retropharyngeal space (Figure 3-4). The carotid space is lateral to the RPS, whereas the prevertebral space is located posteriorly, in the midline **(Option (A) is false).** Laterally, slips of the fascia making up the RPS also contribute to the carotid sheath. The RPS contains fat, the medial and lateral retropharyngeal lymph nodes, and small penetrating arteries and veins **(Option (B) is false).** The medial retropharyngeal nodes are rarely detected radiographically unless they are pathologically involved. The lateral retropharyngeal nodes are normally 3 to 5 mm in size and are frequently visualized on CT or MR scans of normal patients. This group of nodes is the first-echelon drainage system for the nasopharynx and oropharynx. Enlargement of these nodes (longest diameter, >8 mm) should be considered suspicious for involvement by metastatic tumor.

In adults, cellulitis and abscess of the RPS can result from septic jugular thrombophlebitis, from extension of other deep neck infections, or from endoscopic or surgically related trauma such as occurs with surgical exposure for an anterior cervical diskectomy. It is important to detect such a cellulitis rapidly, as the RPS provides a pathway of direct spread of the infection into the superior mediastinum **(Option (C) is true).** Thompson et al. have shown that in children, tonsillitis is the most frequent antecedent illness preceding retropharyngeal cellulitis and abscess (28% of cases) **(Option (D) is true).** Laryngotracheal bronchitis and otitis media are also frequently associated with RPS abscess. As with infections in other areas of the body, CT or MRI assists in localizing a drainable abscess, as well as in monitoring the resolution of the disease after antibiotic and surgical therapy. Holt et al. examined 22 patients suspected of having deep neck infections with CT. It identified six abscesses, and there were no false-positive or false-negative results. In general, surgical drainage of a retropharyngeal abscess is required if imaging demonstrates a low-density collection within the space or if significant airway compromise exists. Cellulitis without abscess may be treated successfully by antibiotic therapy alone. MRI assists in this determination and demonstrates diffuse enhancement after administration of contrast agent (Figure 3-5).

Neoplasms may also arise within or extend into the RPS. Lipoma, vascular malformations, hemangiomas, and plexiform neurofibromas may all involve the RPS. Lymphoproliferative disorders may affect the medial retropharyngeal lymph nodes within the RPS, and posterior pharyngeal wall squamous cell carcinoma may invade the RPS. However, juvenile angiofibromas, which arise in the upper nasal vault near the sphenopalatine foramen, do not extend into the RPS **(Option (E) is false),** but rather extend through the skull base foramina.

Edema of the RPS occurs with some regularity and must be distinguished from inflammatory disease. Edema commonly occurs in patients after radiation therapy to the head and neck region, with lymphatic

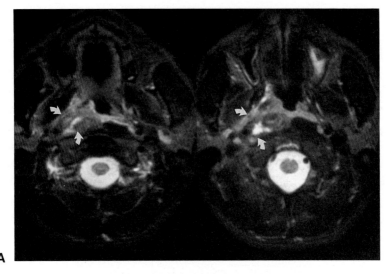

SE 2,800/80

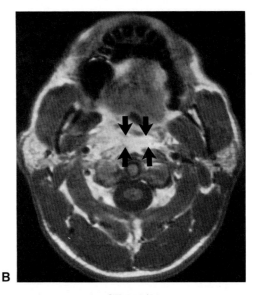

SE 600/20

*Figure 3-5.* Prevertebral and retropharyngeal cellulitis in a young male intravenous drug abuser with acute febrile illness and neck pain. (A) Contiguous T2-weighted MR scan through the mid- and lower nasopharynx. Elevated signal intensity and mass effect (arrows) are seen involving the right parapharyngeal space, prevertebral muscles, and lateral retropharyngeal lymph node. Note, however, that most of the mass is posterior to the mucosa of the nasopharynx. (B) Postcontrast axial T1-weighted MR scan showing diffuse homogeneous enhancement involving the RPS (arrows), as well as the right prevertebral muscles, and right parapharyngeal space. Although this appearance could also be seen with carcinoma, the patient presented with a febrile illness and had gradual improvement following antibiotic therapy. No low-intensity areas are seen to suggest the formation of an abscess.

obstruction due to tumor invasion, and in patients with thrombosis of the internal jugular vein(s). The CT findings usually consist of enlargement of the RPS by a fluid-density mass that conforms to the contour of the space. No focal enhancement occurs, which differentiates this entity from nodal disease and abscess. MRI demonstrates this finding with great clarity on T2-weighted sequences, which show very high-signal-intensity fluid within the RPS without areas of peripheral enhancement or mass effect. Patients with such edema do not usually have the fever, malaise, and other systemic symptoms that are commonly associated with infectious cellulitis or abscess in the RPS.


## Question 11

Concerning nasopharyngeal carcinomas,

- (A) more than 80% are squamous cell carcinomas
- (B) they are not related to cigarette smoking
- (C) most begin in the fossa of Rosenmüller
- (D) nodal metastases are infrequent at presentation
- (E) surgery is the primary treatment of choice

Carcinoma of the nasopharynx is a rare cancer in the United States. However, it it one of the most common cancers in Asia, particularly in the southern provinces of China and in Taiwan. Approximately 80 to 90% of nasopharyngeal carcinomas are squamous cell carcinomas **(Option (A) is true).** Other primary tumors of this region include non-Hodgkin's lymphoma, minor salivary gland tumors such as adenocarcinoma, and, in children and adolescents, rhabdomyosarcoma. Unlike most other squamous cell carcinomas of the head and neck, carcinoma of the nasopharynx is not related to cigarette smoking **(Option (B) is true).** It most often begins in the lateral pharyngeal recess of the nasopharynx, the "fossa of Rosenmüller" **(Option (C) is true).** Because tumor in this area is usually clinically silent, early detection is rare. Nevertheless, even if imaged at this early stage, the lesion may not be easily differentiated from residual adenoidal tissue, which exists in the nasopharynx and can be identified on CT or MRI in adults. Subtle enlargement of the fossa of Rosenmüller may be the only indication of disease on either CT or MRI (Figure 3-6). As the tumor grows, it penetrates the submucosal tissues, invading the deep soft tissues surrounding the nasopharynx. Conductive hearing loss related to eustachian tube dysfunction may be

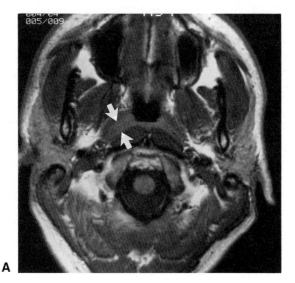

SE 600/20

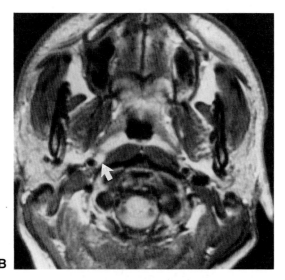

SE 2,800/35

*Figure 3-6.* Right nasopharyngeal carcinoma, stage T1. (A) Axial T1-weighted MR image through the midnasopharynx in a patient with right conductive hearing loss. Enlargement of the right fossa of Rosenmüller is present (arrows). This is the earliest radiographic manifestation of nasopharyngeal carcinoma. (B) Proton-density-weighted MR image demonstrating that the carcinoma increases in signal intensity, as does a small homogeneous retropharyngeal node of Rouvier (arrow).

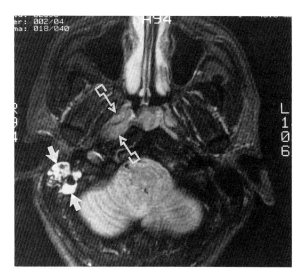

SE 2,800/80

*Figure 3-7.* Right nasopharyngeal carcinoma with serous middle ear effusion. Axial T2-weighted MR scan of an individual with a carcinoma of the nasopharynx (open arrows), larger than that in the patient in Figure 3-6. Also apparent are a right retropharyngeal node and a middle ear effusion (solid arrows), which are related to eustachian tube obstruction.

one of the earliest symptoms. The resultant serous otitis is present in nearly half of all patients with nasopharyngeal tumors (Figure 3-7). The tumor may then extend along the foramen rotundum, pterygoid canal, and foramen ovale to involve the skull base and cavernous sinuses.

The nasopharynx has a rich lymphatic drainage. The primary draining nodal group for the nasopharynx and oropharynx consists of the lateral retropharyngeal nodes, of which the node of Rouvier is the largest and the one seen most often on sectional imaging. This node can be detected only by imaging studies, as it is inaccessible to clinical palpation. Normally the lateral retropharyngeal nodes are less than 8 mm in greatest diameter and are homogeneous in their appearance. With tumor invasion, these nodes may enlarge and develop central necrosis, which appears as a low-intensity center surrounded by peripheral enhancement on contrast CT or T1-weighted MR. Nodal metastases are frequent at the time of initial presentation of nasopharyngeal carcinoma **(Option (D) is false).** The majority of patients will have evidence of abnormal lymphadenopathy in the lateral retropharyngeal nodes, and approximately 60% will have palpable lymph nodes, most of which are located in the

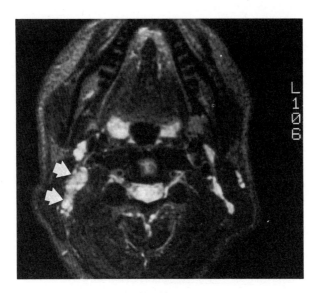

SE 2,800/80

*Figure 3-8.* Spinal accessory adenopathy secondary to nasopharyngeal carcinoma. T2-weighted MR scan showing the presence of metastatic adenopathy of the spinal accessory chain nodes (arrows). This is the second-echelon nodal group involved by cancers of the nasopharynx, but it is the first that can be palpated. The patient also has smaller nodes on the left in the same nodal chain.

second-echelon group called the spinal accessory chain or posterior cervical chain of nodes (Figure 3-8).

The choice of CT or MRI for evaluation of carcinoma of the nasopharynx is controversial. Many prefer MRI for its superior soft tissue contrast capabilities and the use of direct coronal imaging. CT, however, is useful in evaluating adenopathy, is sufficient for the evaluation of most tumors, and is excellent for identifying early bone erosion in the skull base. If MRI is used, intravenous contrast agent administration will improve the specificity for diagnosing malignant adenopathy. Fat-saturated T1-weighted imaging combined with contrast enhancement is probably the optimal technique, as enhancement and central nodal necrosis are better visualized if the adjacent high signal intensity of fat is suppressed (Figure 3-9). Direct coronal scans are required whether one is using CT or MRI to optimize the evaluation of skull base integrity, which is critical in planning treatment.

Carcinoma of the nasopharynx is treated primarily with radiation therapy **(Option (E) is false).** Treatment consists of lateral opposed

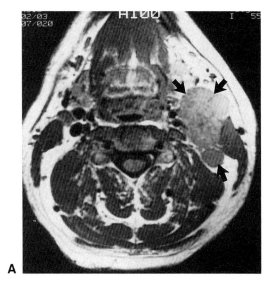

SE 600/20

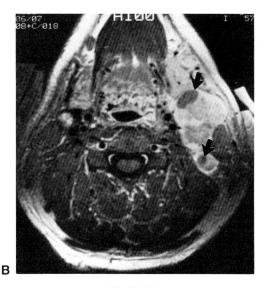

SE 600/20

*Figure 3-9.* Malignant adenopathy shown by enhanced fat-saturated MRI. (A) T1-weighted scan through the base of the tongue and the neck in a patient with squamous cell carcinoma of the left tongue metastatic to the left mid-jugular lymph nodes. A large nodal mass is present with no definite evidence of necrosis (arrows). (B) Fat-saturated axial T1-weighted image after contrast agent administration demonstrates areas of necrosis or tumor in the jugulodigastric nodal chain (arrows). This is optimally demonstrated with the suppression of fat and the administration of contrast material (gadolinium DTPA).

beams delivering 60 to 70 Gy (6,000 to 7,000 rads) to the primary tumor, with an additional 50 Gy (5,000 rads) usually delivered to the node-bearing areas. If the skull base is involved, additional irradiation with high-energy particles, such as helium nuclei, can be given. This therapy requires a cyclotron and is not widely available; however, it has the advantage of delivering a focused tumoricidal dose of radiation while sparing the surrounding central nervous system structures, which cannot tolerate doses of more than 60 Gy (6,000 rads). The current 5-year survival statistics for nasopharyngeal carcinoma still depend on the stage of tumor at diagnosis, the presence of lymphadenopathy, and the newer radiation therapy protocols. Stage T1 disease, which is confined to one side of the nasopharynx, is associated with a 5-year survival rate after treatment of 90%. The larger the primary tumor, the lower the chances of survival. Skull base invasion is associated with the worst prognosis, with fewer than 30% of these patients surviving for 5 years.

*William P. Dillon, M.D.*

## SUGGESTED READINGS

### NASOPHARYNGEAL CARCINOMA

1. Hwang HN. Nasopharyngeal carcinoma in the People's Republic of China: incidence, treatment, and survival rates. Radiology 1983; 149:305–309
2. Lederman M. Cancer of the pharynx. A study based on 2,417 cases with special reference to radiation treatment. J Laryngol Otol 1967; 81:151–172
3. Mancuso AA, Hanafee WN. Computed tomography and magnetic resonance imaging of the head and neck, 2nd ed. Baltimore: Williams & Wilkins; 1985:437–440
4. Mancuso AA, Harnsberger HR, Muraki AS, Stevens MH. Computed tomography of cervical and retropharyngeal lymph nodes: normal anatomy, variants of normal, and applications in staging head and neck cancer. Part II: pathology. Radiology 1983; 148:715–723
5. Schaefer SD, Maravilla KR, Suss RA, et al. Magnetic resonance imaging vs computed tomography. Comparison in imaging oral cavity and pharyngeal carcinomas. Arch Otolaryngol 1985; 111:730–734
6. Smoker WR, Gentry LR. Computed tomography of the nasopharynx and related spaces. Semin US CT MR 1986; 7:107–130

### NECROTIZING OTITIS EXTERNA

7. Benecke JE Jr. Management of osteomyelitis of the skull base. Laryngoscope 1989; 99:1220–1223

8. Cohen D. Borderline cases of malignant external otitis. Am J Otol 1990; 11:209–211

9. Gherini SG, Brackmann DE, Bradley WG. Magnetic resonance imaging and computerized tomography in malignant external otitis. Laryngoscope 1986; 96:542–548

10. Lang R, Goshen S, Kitzes-Cohen R, Sadé J. Successful treatment of malignant external otitis with oral ciprofloxacin: report of experience with 23 patients. J Infect Dis 1990; 161:537–540

11. Levin WJ, Shary JH III, Nichols LT, Lucente FE. Bone scanning in severe external otitis. Laryngoscope 1986; 96:1193–1195

12. Lucente FE, Parisier SC, Som PM. Complications of the treatment of malignant external otitis. Laryngoscope 1983; 93:279–281

13. Parisier SC, Lucente FE, Som PM, Hirschman SZ, Arnold LM, Roffman JD. Nuclear scanning in necrotizing progressive "malignant" external otitis. Laryngoscope 1982; 92:1016–1019

14. Phillips P, Bryce G, Shepherd J, Mintz D. Invasive external otitis caused by *Aspergillus*. Rev Infect Dis 1990; 12:277–281

15. Rubin J, Curtin HD, Yu VL, Kamerer DB. Malignant external otitis: utility of CT in diagnosis and follow-up. Radiology 1990; 174:391–394

16. Rubin J, Yu VL, Kamerer DB, Wagener M. Aural irrigation with water: a potential pathogenic mechanism for inducing malignant external otitis? Ann Otol Rhinol Laryngol 1990; 99:117–119

17. Shupak A, Greenberg E, Hardoff R, Gordon C, Melamed Y, Meyer WS. Hyperbaric oxygenation for necrotizing (malignant) otitis externa. Arch Otolaryngol Head Neck Surg 1989; 115:1470–1475

18. Sobie S, Brodsky L, Stanievich JF. Necrotizing external otitis in children: report of two cases and review of the literature. Laryngoscope 1987; 97:598–601

19. Strashun AM, Nejatheim M, Goldsmith SJ. Malignant external otitis: early scintigraphic detection. Radiology 1984; 150:541–545

20. Wolff LJ. Necrotizing otitis externa during induction therapy for acute lymphoblastic leukemia. Pediatrics 1989; 84:882–885

RETROPHARYNGEAL SPACE

21. Batsakis JG, Sneige N. Parapharyngeal and retropharyngeal space diseases. Ann Otol Rhinol Laryngol 1989; 98:320–321

22. Davis WL, Smoker WR, Harnsberger HR. The normal and diseased retropharyngeal and prevertebral spaces. Semin US CT MR 1990; 11:520–533

23. Dillon WP, Mills CM, Kjos B, DeGroot J, Brant-Zawadzki M. Magnetic resonance imaging of the nasopharynx. Radiology 1984; 152:731–738

24. Holt GR, McManus K, Newman RK, Potter JL, Tinsley PP. Computed tomography in the diagnosis of deep-neck infections. Arch Otolaryngol 1982; 108:693–696

25. Thompson JW, Cohen SR, Reddix P. Retropharyngeal abscess in children: a retrospective and historical analysis. Laryngoscope 1988; 98:589–592

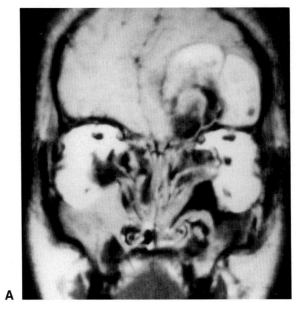

SE 900/30

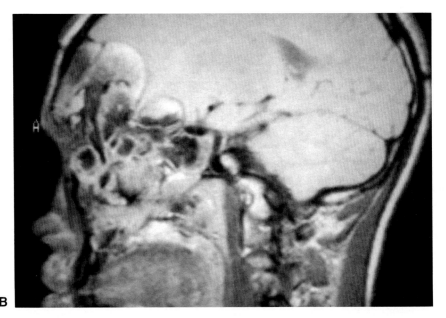

SE 900/30

*Figure 4-1.* This 36-year-old man has nasal obstruction and headache. You are shown sagittal (A) and coronal (B) T1-weighted MR images.

# Case 4: Nasal Polyposis and Mucocele

## Question 12

Which *one* of the following is the MOST likely diagnosis?

(A) Squamous cell carcinoma
(B) Polyposis and mucocele
(C) Melanoma
(D) Esthesioneuroblastoma
(E) Extramedullary plasmacytoma

The coronal and sagittal T1-weighted MR images (Figures 4-1 and 4-2) show a multiseptated or polypoid mass that extends intracranially through the left frontal and ethmoid sinuses and the roof of the sphenoid sinuses. The process does not primarily invade the brain but rather acts as an extra-axial mass. The lesion also fills both ethmoid and sphenoid sinuses, extends laterally into each orbit, and obstructs the right maxillary sinus. Neither orbit is infiltrated by the process. Instead, the lesion pushes or bulges into the orbits. The nasal cavity is filled caudally to the level of the inferior turbinates. The striking MR finding is the variety of signal intensities present in the lesion; there are areas of signal void and of low, intermediate, and high signal intensity. This diversity of signal intensities is characteristic of chronic inflammatory masses and uncharacteristic of cellular tumors. Both the anatomic pattern of the lesion and the variety of signal intensities are most consistent with a combination of polyposis and mucoceles **(Option (B) is correct).**

The diversity of signal intensities reflects the fact that, given time, the obstructed secretions become more concentrated within such a mass of polyps and mucoceles. This occurs because the surrounding mucosa produces and secretes more glycoproteins while slowly reabsorbing any free water within the secretions. Thus, over time, there is a progressive buildup of protein content and a dehydration effect. These two processes occur at different rates, and the factors mediating these processes are poorly understood. The MR signal intensities in different portions of the

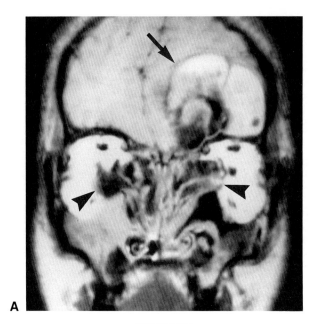

SE 900/30

*Figure 4-2* (Same as Figure 4-1). Polyposis and mucoceles. (A) Coronal T1-weighted MR scan shows a large multiseptated or polypoid mass that extends intracranially (arrow) through the left frontal and ethmoid sinuses. The mass bulges into the medial portion of each orbit (arrow-heads) and fills the majority of the nasal fossae. There is opacification of the right maxillary sinus. Throughout the mass there is a great variety of signal intensities, ranging from high values to signal voids. It is this diversity of signal intensities that differentiates these polyps and mucoceles from cellular tumors (compare with Figure 4-3). (B) Sagittal T1-weighted MR scan shows the multiseptated, polypoid, variable-signal-intensity mass to actually extend intracranially through the sphenoid sinuses as well as the ethmoid and frontal sinuses. The mass does not infiltrate the brain but instead has a sharp interface with it (arrows). (Compare with tumor infiltration of the brain in Figure 4-3.)

lesion reflect these changes occurring over time. Normal secretions are 95% water and therefore have low T1-weighted and high T2-weighted signal intensities. When the protein content is about 20 to 25%, there is significant T1 shortening and the secretions have high T1- and T2-weighted signal intensities. At protein content above 30 to 35%, relaxation times are shortened even further and the T2 effect dominates the T1 signal intensity. Thus the secretions have low T1- and T2-weighted signal intensities. When the protein content exceeds 40 to 45%, the

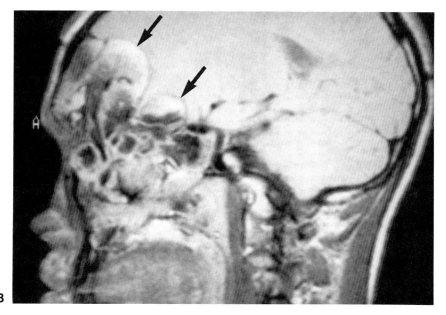

B

SE 900/30

viscous properties of the secretions become dominant. At these high protein contents, the secretions are essentially solids, with ultrashort T1 and T2 relaxation times. These are detected as signal voids on the MR images. Because the effects of these changes in protein content and the degree of dehydration do not occur uniformly within the conglomerate mass of polyps and mucoceles, the wide variation in signal intensities described above often occurs and is characteristic of such chronic inflammatory lesions.

Squamous cell carcinoma (Option (A)) is the most common tumor in the nasal cavity and paranasal sinuses, representing 70 to 80% of all tumors in these sites. Most patients are men between 55 and 65 years of age. There is a wide variation in the degree of cellular differentiation, ranging from well-differentiated squamous cell carcinomas to undifferentiated tumors. However, all of these tumors are cellular lesions with little intercellular stroma and water. There is usually a fairly high mitotic ratio, so that the nuclear-to-cytoplasmic ratio is high, and there is thus little intracellular water. Presumably reflecting these histologic changes, these cellular tumors have low to intermediate T1-weighted signal intensities and usually brighten somewhat on T2-weighted images to an intermediate signal intensity (Figure 4-3).

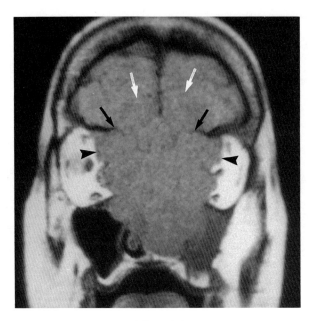

SE 700/30

*Figure 4-3.* Squamous cell carcinoma. Coronal T1-weighted MR scan shows a homogeneous mass of low to intermediate signal intensity that has destroyed the central floor of the anterior cranial fossa (black arrows) and infiltrated the brain (white arrows) and both orbits (arrowheads). The tumor involves all of both nasal fossae and has extended into both maxillary sinuses. This squamous cell carcinoma had only a slightly higher signal intensity on T2-weighted images than on T1-weighted sequences.

On occasion, hemorrhage can occur within these tumors, and such sites are usually identified as localized areas of high signal intensity on both T1- and T2-weighted images, reflecting the presence of methemoglobin (Figure 4-4). Areas of necrosis can also occur; they have low T1- and high T2-weighted signal intensities. These changes are not diffuse and are usually localized to one or two areas of the tumor, which otherwise has an almost monotonously homogeneous appearance. In addition, squamous cell carcinoma is the classic invasive tumor in the head and neck. When it extends intracranially or into the orbit, it infiltrates rather than displaces the brain (Figure 4-5).

Melanomas (Option (C)) represent less than 4% of sinonasal neoplasms. Most occur in the nasal cavity and maxillary sinuses, and the ethmoid sinuses are involved less commonly. The frontal and sphenoid

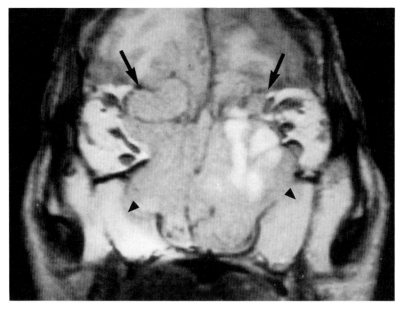

SE 750/30

*Figure 4-4.* Squamous cell carcinoma. Coronal T1-weighted MR scan shows a large mass that has destroyed the central floor of the anterior cranial fossa (area between the arrows) and invaded both orbits, both maxillary sinuses (arrowheads), and the nasal fossae. The remaining portions of both antra are filled with obstructed secretions of slightly higher signal intensity. The tumor itself has an overall homogeneous intermediate signal intensity with several localized areas of high signal intensity that represent hemorrhage.

sinuses are rarely the primary sites of these tumors. Most tumors develop in patients 50 to 70 years of age, and up to one-third of these lesions are amelanotic. Most of these melanomas tend to remodel the surrounding bone, although areas of frank bone erosion may also be present. These are highly cellular tumors, and they can be confused histologically with anaplastic carcinoma, histiocytic lymphoma, embryonal rhabdomyosarcoma, esthesioneuroblastoma, and extramedullary plasmacytoma. Most of these tumors have MR signal intensities similar to those of squamous cell carcinomas, namely fairly homogeneous low to intermediate T1-weighted and slightly higher (intermediate) T2-weighted signal intensities (Figure 4-6). Some of the melanotic melanomas have a uniformly high T1-weighted signal intensity, which appears to be due to the presence of methemoglobin rather than to the paramagnetic effect of melanin. Thus, a melanoma can be present with or without high

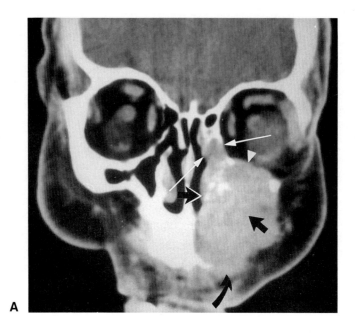

A

*Figure 4-5.* Squamous cell carcinoma. (A) Coronal CT scan shows a destructive mass of the left maxillary sinus. The tumor has destroyed the floor of the left orbit (arrowhead), the lower ethmoid complex (thin arrows), the medial and lateral antral walls (wide arrows), the inferior sinus recess, and the left hard palate and alveolus (curved arrow). The bone is not remodeled (compare with Figure 4-8). (B) Coronal T1-weighted MR scan of another patient shows a homogeneous intermediate-intensity right antral mass that has completely destroyed the walls of the maxillary sinus. This squamous cell carcinoma has invaded the orbit, ethmoid, and nasal fossa. The left maxillary sinus is opacified with inflamed mucosa (open arrow) and centrally entrapped secretions.

T1-weighted signal intensity. In addition, vascular flow voids may be seen on MR images of this highly vascular neoplasm (Figure 4-7).

Esthesioneuroblastoma (Option (D)), or olfactory neuroblastoma, is an uncommon tumor of neural crest origin. It has one incidence peak at 11 to 20 years of age and another at 50 to 60 years of age. It is a soft tumor and can bleed profusely. Most tumors are discovered as unilateral polypoid masses, and only the very large lesions are bilateral. They usually arise in the nasal fossa and extend into the ethmoid and maxillary sinuses; the sphenoid sinuses are rarely involved. Calcifications are present within some of these tumors, and these lesions tend to remodel bone rather than destroy it (Figure 4-8). On MRI, esthesioneuroblastomas are similar in appearance to squamous cell carcinomas, having low to

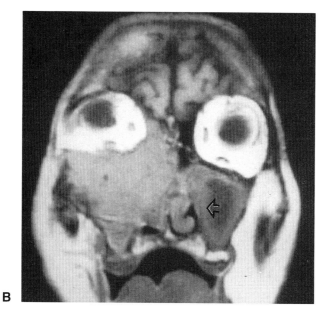

B

SE 700/30

intermediate T1-weighted and higher intermediate T2-weighted signal intensities (Figure 4-9).

Extramedullary plasmacytomas (Option (E)) are rare soft tissue tumors composed of plasma cells. Of these, 80% occur in the head and neck, but only 3 to 4% arise in the sinonasal cavities. Ninety-five percent develop in patients who are over the age of 40 years (mean, 59 years). About 20% of head and neck extramedullary plasmacytomas are initially associated with multiple myeloma, and 35 to 50% of patients with this tumor will eventually develop multiple myeloma. These tumors are usually unilateral polypoid vascular masses and have signal intensities similar to those of squamous cell carcinoma. Thus, they have low to intermediate T1-weighted and higher intermediate T2-weighted signal intensities (Figure 4-10). Vascular flow voids may be seen within the tumor.

Contrast-enhanced MRI will also distinguish the polyposis and mucoceles from the remaining tumors discussed. In the polyps and mucoceles, contrast enhancement occurs in the surrounding mucosa but not within the entrapped secretions (Figure 4-11). In the tumors, the entire lesion (exclusive of areas of necrosis or hemorrhage) enhances (Figure 4-12).

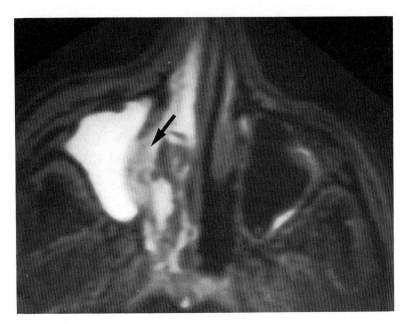

SE 2,000/100

*Figure 4-6.* Melanoma. Axial T2-weighted MR scan shows an intermediate-signal-intensity mass in the right nasal fossa (arrow) that obstructs
the right maxillary sinus, which is filled with high-signal-intensity
secretions. Secretions are also present in the remaining right nasal fossa.
This melanoma is essentially indistinguishable from a carcinoma.

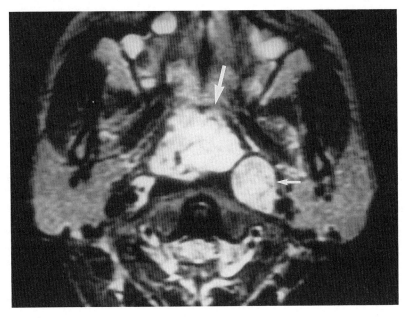

SE 2,000/100

*Figure 4-7.* Melanoma with lymph node metastasis. Axial T2-weighted
MR scan shows a posterior nasal fossae-nasopharyngeal mass (large
arrow) and a left retropharyngeal lymph node (small arrow). Within the
mass and the node are serpiginous areas of signal void that represent
vascular flow within these structures.

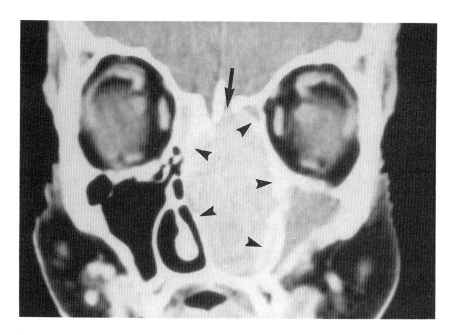

*Figure 4-8.* Esthesioneuroblastoma. Coronal CT scan shows an expansile left nasal fossa mass that has remodeled the nasal vault bones around it (arrowheads). The mass obstructs the left maxillary sinus and has eroded the cribriform plate region (arrow).

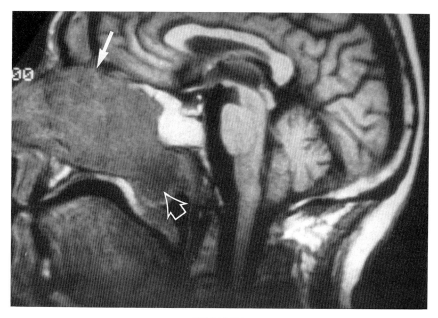

SE 900/30

*Figure 4-9.* Esthesioneuroblastoma. Sagittal T1-weighted MR scan shows a nasoethmoid mass that has broken through the cribriform plate and fovea ethmoidalis region (solid arrow). The mass obstructs the sphenoid sinus, which is filled with high-signal-intensity secretions. The tumor has a necrotic lower-signal-intensity region that hangs down into the nasopharynx (open arrow).

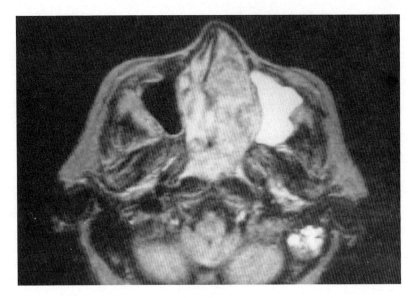

SE 2,000/90

*Figure 4-10.* Extramedullary plasmacytoma. Axial T2-weighted MR scan shows an expansile intermediate-signal-intensity mass in the nasal fossae that obstructs the left maxillary sinus, which is filled with high-signal-intensity secretions. The nasal mass extends back into the naso-pharynx and obstructs the left middle ear and mastoid system, which is filled with high-signal-intensity serous secretions. The mass is primarily expansile.

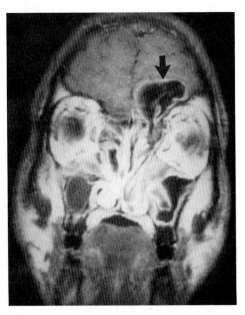

SE 700/30

*Figure 4-11.* Polyps. Coronal T1-weighted postcontrast MR scan shows a low-signal-intensity mass that has broken into the left anterior cranial fossa through the left frontal and ethmoid sinuses. There is enhancement of the surrounding mucosa (arrow). The central secretions do not enhance. Similar masses with peripheral enhancement are seen in both maxillary sinuses and in scattered areas throughout the nasal fossae.

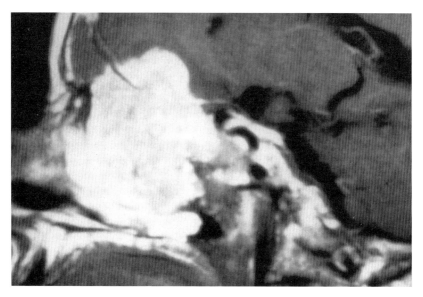

SE 900/30

*Figure 4-12.* Carcinoma. Sagittal T1-weighted postcontrast MR scan shows intense enhancement of a large nasoethmoid mass that has broken through into the floor of the anterior cranial fossa. This diffuse enhancement suggests a solid tumor (compare with Figure 4-11).

## *Question 13*

Concerning nasal polyps,

- (A) they are local upheavals of mucosa
- (B) the major cause of enlargement is an accumulation of extracellular fluid
- (C) most small ones have high signal intensity on T2-weighted MR images
- (D) the coexistence of multiple polyps and mucoceles usually occurs in atopic patients
- (E) about 25% are antrochoanal lesions

Polyps arising in the paranasal sinuses and nasal fossae are local upheavals of mucosa **(Option (A) is true).** Their pathogenesis remains unclear, and allergy, atopy, infection, and vasomotor dysfunction have all been proposed as etiologic factors. The growth of the polyp results primarily from the extracellular accumulation of fluid, which progressively causes further elevation of the mucosa **(Option (B) is true).** The synthesis of collagen within the stroma of the polyp appears to represent an attempt by the stroma to limit the growth of the polyp. Polyps in the paranasal sinuses and nasal fossa are histologically the same; the only difference appears to be that they are located in different places.

The majority of the mass of a polyp is extracellular fluid, and there are surface mucosal secretions covering the polyp. Both these secretions and the extracellular fluid are initially 95% water, and they remain this way in most small polyps. Since water has long T1 and T2 relaxation times, the MR appearance of small polyps is characterized by low T1-weighted and high T2-weighted signal intensities **(Option (C) is true).** As polyps grow, the extracellular fluid can be replaced by collagen and dehydration starts to occur. As a result, the MR signal intensities change as the net protein content rises.

Polyps can directly obstruct the ostia of paranasal sinuses, or the swollen mucosa secondary to the associated inflammation can obstruct these ostia. As a result, it is common to find mucoceles in patients who have polyps. This situation is most often encountered when there are multiple polyps and occurs almost exclusively in atopic patients **(Option (D) is true).**

On occasion, a maxillary sinus or antral polyp can enlarge sufficiently to prolapse through the sinus ostium and present clinically as a nasal polyp. Such antrochoanal polyps represent only 4 to 6% of all nasal polyps **(Option (E) is false).** Most antrochoanal polyps occur in teenagers and are unilateral, and 15 to 40% of patients have a history of allergy.

## Question 14

Concerning sinonasal melanomas,

(A) they account for 10% of melanomas
(B) epistaxis is a common complaint
(C) about 60% are amelanotic
(D) about 95% have high signal intensity on T1-weighted MR images
(E) the 10-year survival rate is about 35%

Sinonasal melanomas arise from melanocytes that have migrated during embryologic development from the neural crest to the mucosa of the nasal fossae and paranasal sinuses. Less than 2.5% of all melanomas occur in the sinonasal cavities **(Option (A) is false).** These melanomas are two to three times more common in the nose than in the paranasal sinuses and frequently arise in the nasal septum or about the inferior and middle turbinates. They are highly vascular tumors, and the most common complaints are nasal obstruction and epistaxis **(Option (B) is true).**

Between 10 and 30% of these sinonasal melanomas are amelanotic **(Option (C) is false).** These tumors have MR imaging characteristics similar to those of squamous cell carcinomas. Thus, they have low to intermediate T1-weighted and slightly higher intermediate T2-weighted signal intensities. Vascular flow voids may be seen; if present, they serve to distinguish melanoma from squamous cell carcinoma on MRI. Only some melanotic melanomas have the high T1-weighted signal intensity that is associated with the presence of the paramagnetic melanin. This appears to reflect the fact that the melanin per se is not the primary cause of this high T1-weighted signal intensity. Rather, the high T1-weighted signal intensity reflects hemorrhage and the presence of methemoglobin within the tumor. Only about half of the melanotic melanomas have such high T1-weighted signal intensity, and when all sinonasal melanomas are considered, fewer than half have this MR appearance **(Option (D) is false).** Thus, the absence of such high T1-weighted signal intensity does not exclude the diagnosis of a melanoma.

Melanomas are among the most lethal tumors arising in the sinonasal cavities; the average survival is only 2 to 3 years. The 10-year survival rate is 0.5% **(Option (E) is false).**


# Question 15

Concerning esthesioneuroblastomas,

(A) most patients are under 20 years of age
(B) intracranial extension demonstrable by CT or MRI is present in most patients
(C) most present as unilateral nasal masses
(D) bone remodeling around the tumor is common
(E) tumoral calcification identifiable by CT is present in most cases

Esthesioneuroblastomas (olfactory neuroblastomas) are uncommon tumors of neural crest origin that arise from the olfactory mucosa. The reported age range is 3 to 88 years. There are two incidence peaks, one at 11 to 20 years of age (16.8% of all tumors) and one at 50 to 60 years of age (22.8% of all tumors) **(Option (A) is false).** At the time of diagnosis, 30% of these tumors are confined to the nasal cavity, 42% are in the nasal cavity and one or more paranasal sinuses, and 28% extend,

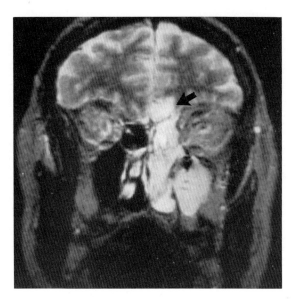

SE 1,800/90

*Figure 4-13.* Esthesioneuroblastoma. Coronal T2-weighted MR scan shows a left nasoethmoid mass that has extended through the cribriform plate and fovea ethmoidalis area into the floor of the anterior cranial fossa (arrow). The left maxillary sinus was obstructed with secretions that had a low T1-weighted signal intensity. The tumor had an intermediate T1-weighted signal intensity.

primarily intracranially, beyond the nasal cavity and paranasal sinuses. Thus, gross intracranial disease demonstrable by CT or MRI occurs in 28% of patients at most (Figure 4-13) **(Option (B) is false).** Microscopic foci of intracranial tumor are probably present in the olfactory bulbs in nearly all patients, but these cannot be seen on CT or MRI.

Most tumors present as unilateral nasal masses, which clinically can appear like an inflammatory polyp **(Option (C) is true).** The diagnosis, which is established by biopsy, is often something of a surprise to the clinician. On sectional imaging, most of these tumors remodel bone around them (Figure 4-8) **(Option (D) is true)** rather than aggressively destroying bone as seen with squamous cell carcinomas. This remodeling often contributes to the false impression that these are benign masses and not malignant neoplasms.

Calcifications are uncommon in sinonasal tumors. The two tumors that have most often been reported to contain calcifications identifiable on CT are inverted papillomas and esthesioneuroblastomas. Although no good statistics are available from large series, such calcifications are uncommon even in these tumors and are not identified in most cases **(Option (E) is false).**

## Question 16

Concerning extramedullary plasmacytomas,

- (A) about 80% occur in the head and neck
- (B) most occur in patients over 40 years of age
- (C) subsequent development of multiple myeloma is rare
- (D) they are highly vascular tumors
- (E) they usually have high signal intensity on T1-weighted images

Extramedullary plasmacytomas are rare soft tissue tumors composed of plasma cells. Some 80% occur in the head and neck region, mainly in the upper respiratory tract and oral cavity **(Option (A) is true).**

About 95% of these tumors occur in patients over the age of 40 years (mean, 59 years) **(Option (B) is true).** There is a 4:1 male predominance, and about 90% of the patients are white.

At initial presentation, about 20% of patients with extramedullary plasmacytomas also have disseminated multiple myeloma. However, 35 to 50% of patients with primary extramedullary plasmacytomas eventually develop disseminated multiple myeloma **(Option (C) is false).**

These tumors are highly vascular lesions **(Option (D) is true),** which enhance intensely on contrast CT scans. They also may have vascular flow voids on MRI. About one-third of patients present with epistaxis, reflecting the highly vascular nature of these tumors.

Extramedullary plasmacytomas are highly cellular tumors with MR signal intensities similar to those of squamous cell carcinomas. Thus, they usually have low to intermediate T1-weighted and slightly higher intermediate T2-weighted signal intensities **(Option (E) is false).** If flow voids are present, there are localized areas of low signal intensity or signal void on routine T1-weighted images.

*Peter M. Som, M.D.*

SUGGESTED READINGS

1. Carter BL. Part II, Paranasal sinuses, nasal cavity, pterygoid fossa, nasopharynx and infratemporal fossa. In: Valvassori GE, Buckingham RA,
   Carter BL, Hanafee WN, Mafee MR (eds), Head and neck imaging. New
   York: Thieme; 1988:174–250
2. Lloyd GA, Lund VJ, Phelps PD, Howard DJ. Magnetic resonance imaging in
   the evaluation of nose and paranasal sinus disease. Br J Radiol 1987;
   6:957–968
3. Som PM. Sinonasal cavity. In: Som PM, Bergeron RT (eds), Head and neck
   imaging, 2nd ed. St. Louis: Mosby-Year Book; 1991:51–276
4. Som PM, Dillon WP, Fullerton GD, Zimmerman RA, Rajagopalan B, Marom
   Z. Chronically obstructed sinonasal secretions: observations on T1 and T2
   shortening. Radiology 1989; 172:515–520
5. Som PM, Dillon WP, Sze G, Lidov M, Biller HF, Lawson W. Benign and
   malignant sinonasal lesions with intracranial extension: differentiation
   with MR imaging. Radiology 1989; 172:763–766
6. Som PM, Shapiro MD, Biller HF, Sasaki C, Lawson W. Sinonasal tumors and
   inflammatory tissues: differentiation with MR imaging. Radiology 1988;
   167:803–808

*Notes*

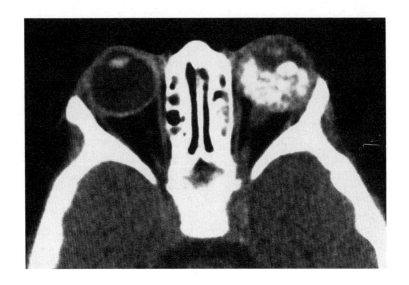

*Figure 5-1*

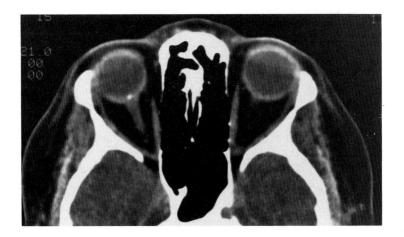

*Figure 5-2*

# Case 5: Calcifications of the Eye

## Questions 17 through 20

For each of the numbered CT scans (Figures 5-1 through 5-4), select the *one* lettered diagnosis (A, B, C, D, or E) that is MOST closely associated with it. Each diagnosis may be used once, more than once, or not at all.

17. Figure 5-1
18. Figure 5-2
19. Figure 5-3
20. Figure 5-4

    (A) Retinoblastoma
    (B) Drusen of the optic nerve head
    (C) Coats's disease
    (D) Colobomatous cyst
    (E) Retinopathy of prematurity

Figure 5-1 is a noncontrast CT scan showing a large calcified mass within the left globe. These CT findings are characteristic of retinoblastoma **(Option (A) is the correct answer to Question 17).** The DNA released from necrotic cells in retinoblastoma has a propensity to form a DNA-calcium complex. In children, any intraocular calcification in a normally developed eye is highly suggestive of retinoblastoma. Retinoblastoma is almost always seen in the fully developed eye. Therefore, calcification in a microphthalmic eye (Options (D) and (E)) is unlikely to be due to retinoblastoma. Calcification is not seen in Coats's disease (Option (C)). With drusen of the optic nerve head (Option (B)), the calcification would be buried within the optic nerve head rather than seen as the extensive intraocular calcification in Figure 5-1. The left optic nerve is enlarged in Figure 5-1. Pathologic examination revealed retinoblastoma. The entire intraorbital segment of the optic nerve was infiltrated by tumor.

Figure 5-2 is a noncontrast CT scan showing a well-defined calcification within the right optic nerve disk. This finding is characteristic of drusen

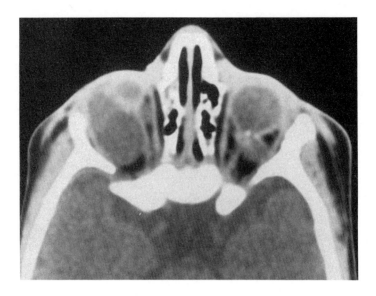

Figure 5-3

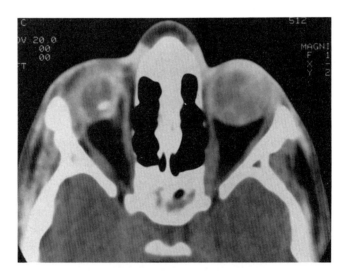

Figure 5-4

of the optic nerve head **(Option (B) is the correct answer to Question 18).** Drusen are laminated, acellular, calcareous bodies within the prelaminar zone of the optic nerve disk of a normally developed eye.

Figure 5-3 is a noncontrast CT scan showing bilateral microphthalmus and funnel-shaped deformity of both posterior globes at the optic disks characteristic of coloboma of the optic disk **(Option (D) is the correct answer to Question 19).** Coloboma of the disk is a congenital anomaly in which a portion of the optic disk is lacking, resulting in funnel-shaped deformity of the disk. The image shows low-density retrobulbar masses compatible with colobomatous cysts, the right being greater that the left. Calcification at the left optic disk is due to dystrophic calcification in abnormal gliotic tissue.

Figure 5-4 is a noncontrast CT scan showing microphthalmic eyes and a dystrophic calcification within the right globe. These findings are characteristic CT features of retinopathy of prematurity **(Option (E) is the correct answer to Question 20).** The image shows increased density of the globes and irregular curvilinear densities within the globes. These changes represent scar tissues as well as proliferative organized retinal tissues in this premature patient who received supplemental oxygen therapy. Retinoblastoma (Option (A)) is extremely rare in microphthalmic eyes. Drusen of the optic nerve head (Option (B)) are seen in the prelaminar zone of the optic nerve disk of a fully developed eye. Coloboma of the optic nerve (Option (D)) results in funnel-shaped deformity of the optic nerve disk. At times, dystrophic calcification of abnormal gliotic tissue may be present at the colobomatous defect, as is noted in Figure 5-3.

## Question 21

Concerning retinoblastoma,

  (A) it arises from the pigmented layer of the retina
  (B) it is the most common intraocular malignant tumor in childhood
  (C) it is bilateral in about 70% of cases
  (D) all patients with bilateral retinoblastoma harbor the retinoblastoma gene

Retinoblastoma is a highly malignant retinal tumor that arises from neuroectodermal cells (nuclear layer of the retina) that are destined to become retinal photoreceptors **(Option (A) is false).** The manner of intraocular and extraocular extension, the patterns of metastasis and recurrence, and the ocular complications and associated malignancies make the diagnosis of retinoblastoma one of the most challenging problems of pediatric ophthalmology and radiology. To ensure appropriate therapy, retinoblastoma must be differentiated from a host of benign lesions that simulate it. This diagnosis must be established rapidly to permit maximum ocular salvage and to minimize tumor-associated mortality. When the disease extends beyond the eye, mortality approaches 100%. With earlier diagnosis, the 5-year survival rate is 92%. Useful vision in the treated eye is attained in 90% of group I patients (see below) and overall in about 75% of eyes that are not enucleated. The classification of retinoblastomas has been established in terms of expected results of therapy. Group I tumors are those with a very favorable prognosis. These are either solitary tumors or multiple tumors of less than 4 disk diameters in size at or behind the equator. Group II also has a favorable prognosis. This group includes one or several tumors measuring between 4 and 10 disk diameters. Group III tumors are anterior to the equator; this group also includes a solitary tumor larger than 10 disk diameters. This group has a doubtful prognosis. Group IV tumors include those that are multiple and extend up to the ora serrata, which is the wavy or serrated ring in the retina, just posterior to the ciliary body, which limits the pars optica or perception portion of the retina. Group V includes tumors that involve half of the retina or those in which there are also vitreous seeds. Patients in groups IV and V have an unfavorable prognosis.

*Pathologic features.* Virchow was the first to recognize that retinoblastoma was of glial origin. He used the term "glioma of the retina" to describe the tumor. Bailey and Cushing, in their classification of tumors of the glial group, divided retinoblastomas into two types: medulloblastomas and neuroepitheliomas. The medulloblastomas were undifferentiated retinoblastomas and, like medulloblastomas of the central nervous system, were derived from the medulloblast, a pluripotential cell of origin. Bailey and Cushing considered both types of retinoblastomas to have a potential for glial differentiation. Verhoeff was the first to give the tumor the name of retinoblastoma, which was prompted by the fact that the majority of cells composing the tumor histologically resemble the cells of the undifferentiated retina of the embryo. It is now well known that retinoblastoma is derived from primitive embryonal retinal cells (either photoreceptor or neuronal retinal cells). The tumor is composed of small round or ovoid cells with scant cytoplasm and relatively large nuclei. There is marked variability in the histologic features of retinoblastoma; some tumors display significant necrosis and prominent foci of calcification, and a few show areas of glial differentiation.

Retinoblastoma is the most common malignant intraocular tumor in childhood **(Option (B) is true).** Its worldwide incidence has been reported to be 1 in 18,000 to 30,000 live births. The tumor is congenital in origin but is usually not recognized at birth. Ocular involvement and metastasis may be present at birth. In the United States, the average age at diagnosis is 13 months. In other countries, the disease is often not detected until the fourth year of life, when it is usually far advanced. More than 90% of all diagnoses are made in children younger than 5 years of age. Sex distribution is equal, and there is no preference for either the right or left eye. The tumor occurs in one eye in 67% to 75% of patients and in both eyes in 25 to 33% **(Option (C) is false).**

Four types of retinoblastomas have been recognized: (1) those that are nonheritable and are presumably due to postzygotic retinoblast mutations; (2) those that are inherited as an autosomal dominant trait; (3) those that are associated with the deletion of band 14 of the long arm of chromosome 13; and (4) bilateral retinoblastoma and pinealoma (trilateral retinoblastoma).

The genetics of retinoblastoma have been the subject of many investigations. When retinoblastoma follows a genetic pattern, it is almost always an autosomal dominant trait with virtually complete penetrance. All patients with bilateral retinoblastoma harbor the germinal mutation **(Option (D) is true).** Fifteen percent of patients with unilateral retinoblastoma also harbor the retinoblastoma gene. A parent with bilateral retinoblastoma has about a 50% chance of passing retinoblastoma to one child. A parent with unilateral retinoblastoma has about a 50% chance of passing retinoblastoma to one child if the tumor is truly multifocal. When the parent's tumor is unifocal, there is about a 15% chance that the children will be affected. Some affected children have an associated deletion of the long arm of chromosome 13 involving band 13q14. The association between retinoblastoma and the deletion of the q14 band of chromosome 13, j(13q14), has been convincingly documented. Esterase D, an electrophoretically polymorphic human enzyme, has also been mapped to chromosomal band 13q14. In several families with hereditary retinoblastoma without apparent chromosomal deletion, the gene for retinoblastoma has been shown to be closely linked to that for esterase D and assigned to chromosomal band 13q14. Compilation of data from recent studies suggests an incidence of approximately 7% of 13q-chromosomal deletion in patients with retinoblastoma. Only a few of the patients with retinoblastoma have a sufficiently large chromosomal deletion to produce systemic dysmorphic features such as microcephaly, genital malformations, ear abnormalities, mental retardation, and toe and finger abnormalities. Karyotype analysis of these children with congenital dysmorphic features may allow detection of a chromosome 13 deletion involving band 13q14, prompting ophthalmic examination and therefore allowing early diagnosis of retinoblastoma.

*Trilateral retinoblastoma.* The occurrence of ectopic nonmetastatic retinoblastoma in the pineal body or in a parasellar region, "trilateral retinoblastoma," stemmed from reports of Jakobiec and Bader in 1977 and 1980, respectively. Bader and coworkers used the term "trilateral retinoblastoma" to describe the syndrome of bilateral retinoblastoma with a solitary midline intracranial tumor. In this communication a case of "tetralateral retinoblastoma" is presented in a child with bilateral retinoblastomas and a midline suprasellar as well as pineal body retinoblastoma (see Figure 5-7). The association of retinoblastoma and pinealoma (trilateral retinoblastoma) suggests that these tumors may be related. In addition to sharing a common neuroectodermal origin with retinal tissue, it is well known that the pineal gland, in lower vertebrates, has photoreceptor function (similar to that seen in their retinas) and endocrine function. It is also well known that the histologic appearances of retinoblastomas and pinealomas may be indistinguishable. It is postulated that, because of their similar origin, the same mutations may be carcinogenic for both retinoblasts and pinealoblasts.

The occurrence of a second cancer arising outside the field of radiation was pointed out by Jensen and Miller and by Abramson. Abramson also demonstrated that patients with heritable retinoblastoma are highly susceptible to the development of other nonocular cancers, usually osteogenic sarcomas and other neoplasms at sites of irradiation. He further demonstrated that of 688 patients who survived therapeutic radiation for retinoblastoma, 89 developed second tumors (62 in the field of radiation and 27 outside the field). Of 23 patients who received no radiation, 5 developed second tumors. The most common tumors were osteosarcoma and soft tissue sarcoma. The incidence of a second tumor is 20% at 10 years, 50% at 20 years, and 90% at 30 years.

*Clinical features.* The diagnosis of retinoblastoma can usually be made as a result of an ophthalmoscopic examination. However, clinical differentiation of retinoblastoma from a host of benign simulating lesions may be difficult. Leukokoria, a pink-white or yellow-white pupillary reflex (cat's eye), is the most common presenting sign of retinoblastoma (60% of patients). Leukokoria in eyes with retinoblastoma represents replacement of the vitreous by a pink-white tumor, total retinal detachment caused by a tumor, or a tumor directly in the macula. Strabismus (deviation of the eye) is the second most common sign. In contrast to congenital strabismus, in which esotropia (eyes crossing in) is more common, in the strabismus associated with retinoblastoma, esotropia and exotropia (eyes crossing out) are equally common. Pain due to secondary glaucoma, often with heterochromia (different colored irides), is the next most common symptom. The ophthalmologic recognition of retinoblastoma is quite reliable. Small lesions are seen as gray-white intraretinal foci. Because of the difference in color from the surrounding retina and choroid, retinoblastomas can be seen ophthalmoscopically when they are as small as 0.02 mm. Other characteristic ophthalmoscopic findings include tumor calcification and vitreous seeding. These seedings are the result of poorly developed vascular and collagenous stroma of the tumor, which allows small portions to break off and float free in the vitreous cavity or subretinal space. Vitreous seeds can grow within the vitreous even though they lack a blood supply. As tumors grow, they often assume a convex configuration and produce three forms of growth patterns. The first is endophytic retinoblastoma, in which the tumor projects anteriorly, breaks through the internal limiting membrane of the retina, and grows into the vitreous. The second is exophytic retinoblastoma, in which the tumor arises intraretinally and subsequently grows into the subretinal space, causing elevation of the retina. A progressive retinal detachment occurs with growth of the tumor, associated exudation, and (rarely) subretinal hemorrhage. Exophytic tumors may simulate a traumatic retinal detachment ophthalmoscopically. The third pattern is diffuse retinoblastoma, in which the tumor grows along the retina, appearing as a placoid mass. This diffuse form represents a perplexing diagnostic difficulty because of its atypical ophthalmoscopic appearance (which simulates inflammatory or hemorrhagic conditions); its characteristic lack of calcification; and its occurrence, usually outside the typical age group.

# Question 22

Concerning imaging of retinoblastoma,

(A) CT demonstrates calcification in about 90% of cases
(B) intense contrast enhancement on CT is characteristic
(C) retinoblastomas are hypointense relative to the vitreous in T1-weighted MR images
(D) the tumor margin is easily differentiated from retinal detachment by CT
(E) extraocular extension of retinoblastoma is reliably detected by both CT and MRI
(F) involvement of Tenon's capsule is characterized as optic nerve enlargement with subarachnoid seeding

Diagnosis of retinoblastoma can usually be made by visual examination alone. The presence of the tumor, as well as calcification within the tumor, can be shown by ultrasonography. The accuracy of ultrasonography for identifying this condition can be as high as 94%. Evaluation of tumor extension to the medial and lateral aspects of the eye and extraocular extension is particularly limited with ultrasonography. Although ophthalmoscopic and ultrasonographic recognition of retinoblastoma is usually reliable, all patients should also be studied by CT or MRI to determine the presence of involvement of Tenon's capsule (Figure 5-5); retrobulbar spread (Figure 5-6); or intracranial, intraspinal, or other distant involvement (Figure 5-7). The disease often extends into Tenon's capsule or spreads along the optic nerve (Figures 5-1 and 5-6). Tenon's capsule is a fibroelastic membrane that envelops the eyeball from the optic nerve to the level of the ciliary muscle. It is separated from the sclera by the potential episcleral space (Tenon's space). Tumor extension into Tenon's space results in a characteristic well-defined semilunar mass behind the globe (Figure 5-5) **(Option (F) is false).**

CT and MRI are also important because these imaging techniques may differentiate retinoblastoma from lesions that simulate retinoblastomas clinically, such as persistent hyperplastic primary vitreous (PHPV) (see Figure 5-16), Coats's disease (see Figure 5-19), retinopathy of prematurity (ROP) (see Figure 5-23), toxocariasis (see Figures 5-13 and 5-14), retinal detachment, organized subretinal hemorrhage, organized vitreous, endophthalmitis, retinal gliosis, myelinated nerve fibers, choroidal hemangioma, coloboma (Figure 5-3), morning glory anomaly, congenital cataract, choroidal osteoma, drusen of the optic nerve head (Figure 5-2), and other so-called pseudogliomas and leukokorias.

High-resolution, thin-section (1.5-mm) CT scanning can detect tumor and calcification within it with a high degree of accuracy. More than 90%

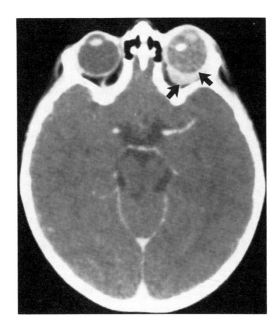

*Figure 5-5.* Retinoblastoma with extension into Tenon's space. Postcontrast CT scan. Note replacement of the left vitreous by a mass with calcification. Tumor extension into Tenon's space (arrows) is visible.

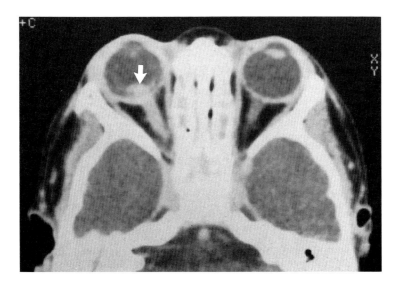

*Figure 5-6.* Retinoblastoma with extension along the optic nerve. Postcontrast CT scan. Note the intraocular tumor (arrow) and marked involvement of the right optic nerve.

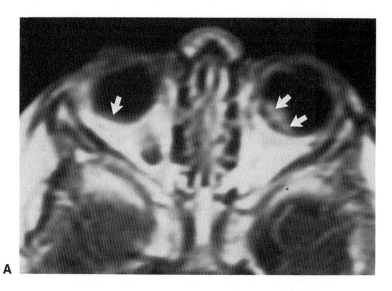

**A**

*Figure 5-7.* "Tetralateral retinoblastoma." (A) T1-weighted MR scan with gadolinium DTPA contrast enhancement shows bilateral enhanced retinoblastoma (arrows). (B) Precontrast proton-weighted MR scan shows a suprasellar mass (arrow) and enlargement of the temporal horns of the lateral ventricles. (C) Postcontrast T1-weighted MR scan shows marked enhancement of the suprasellar mass seen in Figure 5-7B. Notice the marked leptomeningeal enhancement (arrows) due to subarachnoid seeding by tumor. (D) Sagittal T1-weighted MR scan shows a large pineal mass (arrows) and enlargement of the lateral and third ventricles. (E) T2-weighted MR scan shows low signal intensity of the pineal mass (arrows) and enlarged lateral ventricles. (F) Postcontrast T1-weighted MR scan shows marked enhancement of the pineal tumor. (G) Postcontrast sagittal T1-weighted MR scan of the spine shows enlargement and enhancement of the spinal cord (arrows) due to metastasis.

of retinoblastomas show evidence of calcification on CT **(Option (A) is true).** Calcification may be small and single (Figure 5-8), large and single, or multiple and punctate (Figure 5-1), or it may involve a few to several fine speckled foci. The DNA released from necrotic cells in retinoblastoma has a propensity to form a DNA-calcium complex. It is the frequent presence of this calcified complex that allows the intraocular tumor to be identified by funduscopic, ultrasonographic, and CT methods. Calcification is rarely present in the extraocular component of retinoblastoma. The presence of intraocular calcification in children under 3 years of age is highly suggestive of retinoblastoma. None of the lesions (except microphthalmus and colobomatous cyst) (Figure 5-3) that simulate

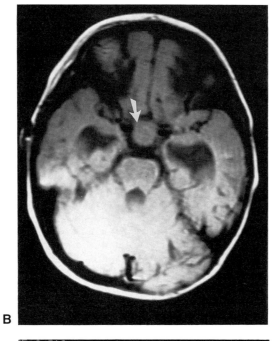

**B**

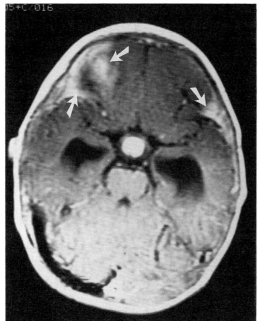

**C**

retinoblastoma contain calcification in children up to 3 years of age. This is the age range in which retinoblastoma is usually diagnosed (98% of cases present prior to age 6 months). In children over 3 years of age,

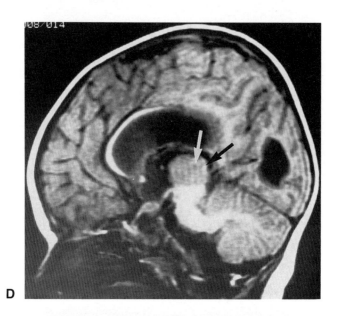

D

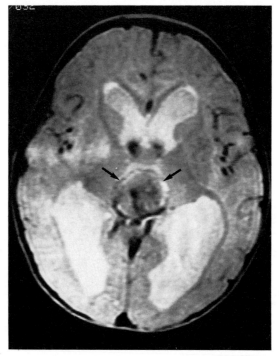

E

F

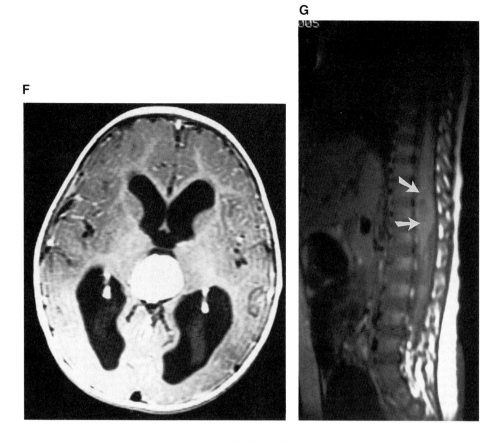

*Figure 5-7 (Continued)*

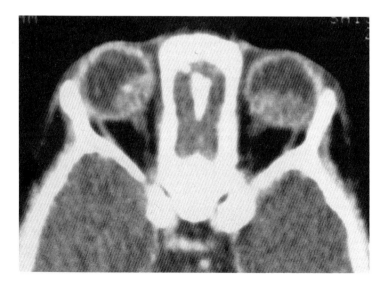

*Figure 5-8.* Bilateral retinoblastoma. Note the large noncalcified intraocular tumor within the left eye and a large mass containing a single calcification in the right eye.

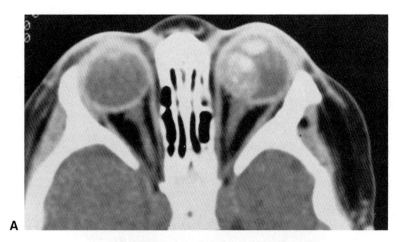

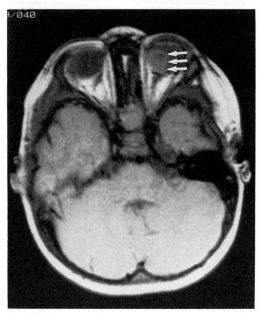

*Figure 5-9.* Retinoblastoma. (A) CT scan shows a large mass containing areas of calcification within the left eye. (B) Proton-weighted MR scan shows that the mass (arrows) is hyperintense in relation to normal vitreous. (C) T2-weighted MR scan shows that the mass (arrows) is hypointense in relation to vitreous.

some of the simulating lesions, including retinal astrocytoma (see Figure 5-19), ROP (Figure 5-4), toxocariasis, and optic nerve head drusen (Figure 5-2), can produce calcification. The diffuse infiltrating form of retinoblastoma is rare and may have no calcification.

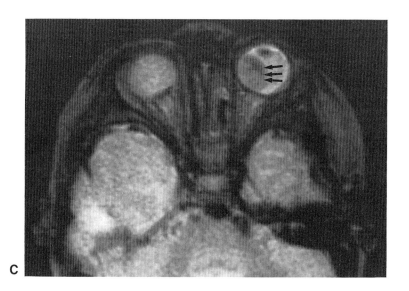

C

Retinoblastomas display a moderate degree of contrast enhancement following intravenous injection of iodinated contrast material. However, intense contrast enhancement is not typical for these tumors **(Option (B) is false).** This is particularly true when the tumor is heavily calcified or contains a large amount of necrosis.

MRI has been used to evaluate retinoblastoma and other lesions that simulate it. In the diagnosis of retinoblastoma, MRI is not as specific as CT scanning as a result of its lack of sensitivity in detecting calcification (Figure 5-9). However, the MR appearance of retinoblastoma may be specific enough to differentiate it from simulating lesions. Retinoblastomas appear slightly or moderately hyperintense in relation to the normal vitreous on T1-weighted and proton-weighted MR images (Figure 5-9B) **(Option (C) is false).** On T2-weighted MR images they appear as areas of markedly to moderately decreased signal intensity (Figure 5-9C). The tumor margin is readily differentiated from associated retinal detachment by MRI but not by CT **(Option (D) is false).** This reflects the fact that on MR the tumor is hypointense while the subretinal fluid (exudate) is hyperintense on T2-weighted images. By comparison on CT both the tumor and the subretinal fluid are dense and thus tumor conspicuity is less. Tumors elevated 3 to 4 mm may not be definitely identified on MR scans. Lesions elevated less than 3 mm are not recognized by present MR technology. Calcifications may be seen as varied degrees of hypointensity in all pulse sequences on MR scans. In contrast to CT scanning, which is highly specific for calcification, MRI may be nonspecific. In many cases a calcification may not be recognized on MR scans. Accord-

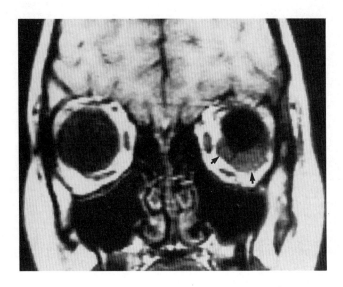

*Figure 5-10.* Recurrence of retinoblastoma. Coronal T1-weighted MR scan shows marked tumor recurrence (arrows) around the left eye, which is a false eye.

ingly, in the diagnosis of retinoblastoma, CT is the study of choice because of its superior sensitivity for detecting calcifications. Calcifications as small as 2 mm can be reliably detected by CT scan. MRI, however, has superior contrast resolution and provides more information for differentiation of leukokoric eyes. Pre- and postcontrast CT scans or MRI (including gadolinium DTPA contrast enhancement) is highly sensitive for detecting optic nerve involvement (Figures 5-1 and 5-6), subarachnoid seeding and central nervous system involvement (Figure 5-7), recurrence (Figure 5-10), and secondary tumor development (Figure 5-11) **(Option (E) is true).**

In an MR study by Mafee et al. of 27 patients with leukokoria, a mass was present in all patients with retinoblastoma (17 cases). These masses had relatively short T1 and T2 relaxation-time characteristics on MR images (Figure 5-9B and C). All retinoblastomas were seen as mildly to moderately hyperintense lesions on T1-weighted and proton-weighted MR scans; they became hypointense on T2-weighted MR scans. This appearance is very similar to the MR characteristics of uveal melanoma (Figure 5-12). None of the patients with PHPV, ROP, Coats's disease, or toxocariasis demonstrated MR characteristics similar to those found with retinoblastoma. Gadolinium DTPA contrast enhancement increases the sensitivity of MRI in detecting retinoblastoma. Most tumors demonstrate

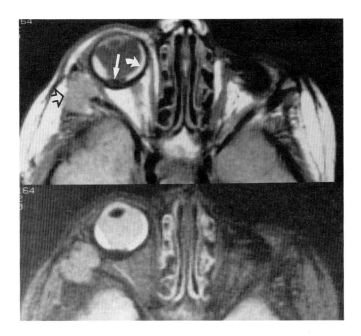

*Figure 5-11.* Regressed retinoblastoma and presumed secondary sarcoma. Proton-weighted (top) and T2-weighted (bottom) MR scans showing a regressed retinoblastoma (straight arrow) and associated subretinal fluid (curved arrow). Notice a large destructive mass (open arrow) arising within the field of radiation. The left eye is a false eye.

moderate to marked enhancement. Gadolinium contrast enhancement also increases the sensitivity of MRI for detecting extraocular metastases, as well as intracranial and intraspinal metastases (Figure 5-7).

When examining a child with leukokoria, the major diagnostic considerations are retinoblastoma, PHPV, ROP, congenital cataract, Coats's disease, toxocariasis, total retinal detachment, ocular hamartoma, and a variety of other nonspecific causes. Howard and coworkers studied 500 consecutive patients in whom the diagnostic possibility of retinoblastoma was raised. Of these 500 patients, diagnoses other than retinoblastoma were made in 265 cases (53%). Of 27 different conditions, the most common was PHPV, followed in frequency by ROP, posterior cataract, coloboma of the choroid or optic disk, uveitis, and larval granulomatosis. Identification of the cause of the leukokoria is critical to ensure prompt recognition and appropriate treatment. Diagnostic accuracy is particularly important since retinoblastoma is one of the few human cancers in which definitive treatment is carried out without a confirmed histopathologic diagnosis.

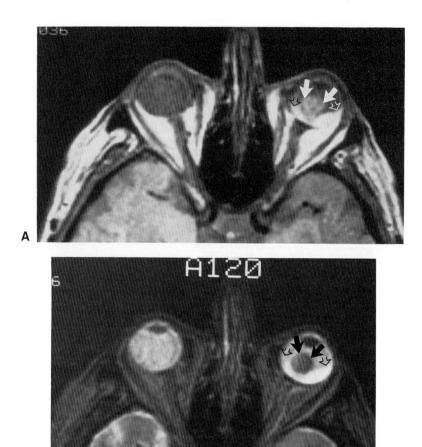

*Figure 5-12.* Uveal melanoma. Proton-weighted (A) and T2-weighted (B) MR scans showing a large intraocular mass (solid arrows) and associated subretinal exudate (open arrows). The tumor is hyperintense in proton-weighted MR scans and hypointense in T2-weighted MR scans. The subretinal exudate appears hyperintense in proton-weighted and T2-weighted images.

As indicated above, ocular toxocariasis (nematode endophthalmitis, sclerosing endophthalmitis) is one of the important conditions that must be considered in the differential diagnosis of retinoblastoma. The granuloma of *Toxocara canis* is actually an eosinophilic abscess with the second-stage *Toxocara* larva within the abscess. The infection results from ingestion of eggs of the nematode *T. canis*. In these patients, death of the larva results in a wide spectrum of intraocular inflammatory reactions, the most severe of which has a characteristic pathologic appearance. In most but not all instances, the anterior segment is uninvolved. A funnel-shaped retinal detachment is typically associated with organized vitreous. The histologic changes of the globe are characterized by an infiltration with lymphocytes, plasma cells, eosinophils, and giant cells. Retinal, subretinal, and vitreous hemorrhages may be frequent. Remnants of the secondary larval stage of *T. canis* are often difficult to find. The larva was present in 24 of 46 cases originally reported by Wilder. In the remaining 22 cases, however, larvae were not identified. In many cases, the diagnosis of ocular nematode infection is presumptive based on the characteristic histopathologic features of sclerosing endophthalmitis. An enzyme-linked immunosorbent assay (ELISA) for *T. canis* is available with sufficient specificity and sensitivity.

Margo et al. reported the CT findings in three cases of histopathologically proven sclerosing endophthalmitis. These findings consisted of a homogeneous intravitreal density that corresponded to detached retina, organized vitreous, and inflammatory subretinal exudate. These investigators concluded that the findings are similar to those seen in Coats's disease and noncalcified retinoblastoma. Mafee et al. reported on three young adults with toxocariasis that appeared on CT scans as a localized or diffuse ill-defined mass with no significant enhancement. Clinical examination in such patients frequently shows vitreous, retinal, or choroidal signs of previous inflammation. This inflammatory process (chronic abscess) is seen on CT as an irregularity of the uveoscleral coat (Figure 5-13). This CT appearance is usually indicative of *T. canis* or other granulomatous disease of the globe and is due to diffuse inflammatory infiltration of the choroid and sclera.

In the appropriate clinical setting, the CT findings of the granuloma of *T. canis* should be relied upon to establish a presumptive diagnosis of ocular toxocariasis. MRI has been reported to be able to detect the site of the larval granuloma. MR images of a patient with a presumptive diagnosis of toxocariasis are shown in Figure 5-14. In general, the proteinaceous subretinal exudate produced by the inflammatory response to larval infiltration is seen as a variable hyperintense image on T1-, proton-, and T2-weighted MR scans. These MR characteristics were found in two of our patients with suspected toxocariasis. Further studies are needed to establish the spectrum of MR characteristics of this relatively uncommon ocular disease. It should be noted that the MR as well as the CT appearance of chronic retinal detachment and organized vitreous may

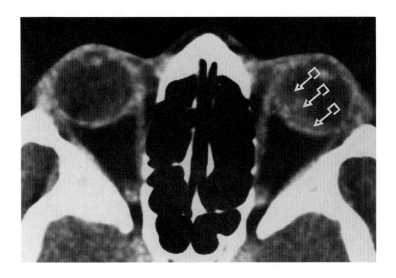

*Figure 5-13.* *Toxocara canis* granuloma. Postcontrast CT scan shows an irregular mass (arrows) in the posterior left globe.

make it very difficult to differentiate between *Toxocara* granuloma, Coats's disease, and even ROP and PHPV, as well as retinoblastoma.

Although retinoblastoma constitutes the major life-threatening cause of leukokoria in children, a host of other simulating conditions (pseudogliomas) can cause diagnostic confusion. In some cases of leukokoria, it is exceedingly difficult to exclude the possibility of retinoblastoma without having to resort to enucleation. Retinal astrocytomas are rare tumors that are seen in patients with tuberous sclerosis and neurofibromatosis or as an isolated finding. Early retinal astrocytoma (astrocytic hamartoma) may look exactly like early retinoblastoma and may be present before any neurologic or dermatologic manifestations of tuberous sclerosis appear. These tumors may appear in the retina or in the optic nerve. The usual appearance is that of a single nodule or multiple nodules elevated 1 or 2 mm above the surface of the retina. At this stage, CT and MRI cannot visualize the lesions. Tumors elevated more than 3 mm can be demonstrated by CT and MRI. The CT appearance of astrocytic hamartoma is similar to that of retinoblastoma (Figure 5-15). If typical tuberous sclerosis is not present, the differentiation between astrocytic hamartoma and other ocular lesions may be very difficult. The CT appearance of myelinated nerve fiber also is identical to that of retinoblastoma. MRI, however, may prove valuable in differentiating these

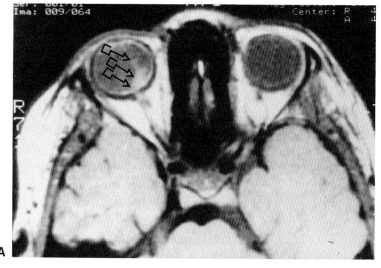

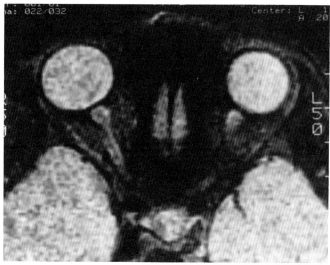

*Figure 5-14. Toxocara canis* granuloma. Proton-weighted (A) and T2-weighted (B) MR scans showing an irregular lesion (arrows, panel A) in the nasal aspect of the right globe. Unlike the retinoblastoma, the lesion is isointense with vitreous on the T2-weighted MR scan.

lesions from retinoblastoma, provided the lesion is visualized (it is more than 2 to 3 mm thick).

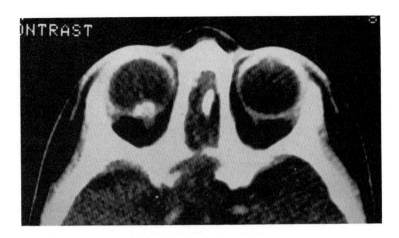

*Figure 5-15.* Astrocytic hamartoma. Postcontrast CT scan shows an enhancing mass in the right eye. (Courtesy of B.G. Haik, M.D., Tulane University, New Orleans.)

## Question 23

Concerning persistent hyperplastic primary vitreous,

    (A) it occurs when the embryonic hyaloid vascular system (primary vitreous) fails to regress

    (B) it presents clinically as leukokoria

    (C) calcification is rare

    (D) it often presents as a dense globe on CT

PHPV is caused by the failure of the embryonic hyaloid vascular system to regress normally **(Option (A) is true).** The basic lesion is caused by persistence of various portions of the primary vitreous and tunica vasculosa lentis, with hyperplasia and extensive proliferation of the associated embryonic connective tissue. The nosology of PHPV is extremely complex. The ocular malformation can reflect either an isolated congenital defect or a manifestation of more-extensive ocular or systemic involvement. The term PHPV, therefore, is a marked oversimplification that offers no etiologic precision and only the grossest of prognostic implications. The embryonic intraocular vascular system may be divided into two components: an anterior system in the region of the iris and a posterior (retrolental) component within the vitreous. The anterior system is composed of the pupillary membrane, which is formed by small vascular buds that grow inwardly to vascularize the iris mesoderm anterior to the lens. The posterior system includes the main hyaloid artery, vasa hyaloidea propria, and tunica vasculosa lentis. The hyaloid artery branches from the dorsal ophthalmic artery during the third gestational week and grows anteriorly toward the lens, where its terminal branches (vascular tunics of the lens) drain into the annular vessels. Besides branching from the vessels supplying the lens and vitreous, the hyaloid artery also supplies the developing optic nerve. The hyaloid artery continues to function as an important source of intraocular nutrition until the beginning of the eighth month of gestation. The vasa hyaloidea propria are small capillary branches that extend throughout the vitreous. The posterior tunica vasculosa lentis is formed by terminal branches of the main trunk of the hyaloid artery. The hyaloid vascular system normally begins to show signs of regression even before some of its components have reached their height of development. The first vessels to undergo regression are the vasa hyaloidea propria, followed by the tunica vasculosa lentis and eventually the hyaloid artery. During the first month of gestation, the space between the lens and the retina contains the primary vitreous. It consists of two parts: mesodermally derived tissue, including the hyaloid vessel and its branches; and a fibrillar meshwork that is of ectodermal origin. In the second month of embryonic development, collagen fibers and a ground substance or gel component consisting of hyaluronic acid are produced. They form the secondary vitreous and begin to replace the vascular elements of the primary vitreous. By week 14, the secondary vitreous begins to fill the vitreous cavity. By the fifth to the sixth month of development, the cavity of the eye is filled primarily with the secondary or adult vitreous. The primary vitreous is thus reduced to a small central space, Cloquet's canal, which runs in an S-shaped course between the optic nerve head and the posterior surface of the lens.

Diagnosis of PHPV is often made difficult by its extremely broad array of clinical manifestations, etiologic heterogeneity, and frequently opaque ocular media. Complete inspection of the interior of the eye may be precluded not only by cataract but also by vitreous hemorrhage or opaque retrolental fibrovascular tissue. This condition usually manifests clinically as unilateral leukokoria in a microphthalmic eye **(Option (B) is true)**. At birth, the lens is clear with a white to pinkish fibrovascular mass behind it; later the lens usually becomes swollen and cataractous. In the natural course of untreated PHPV, the eye often develops glaucoma and eventually buphthalmos or phthisis bulbi, sometimes leading to loss of the globe. The clinical presentation of PHPV is variable. Its main features include a unilateral (rarely bilateral) presentation, usually with leukokoria, microphthalmus, lens opacity, retinal detachment, and vitreous hemorrhage. In severe form, elongated ciliary processes, elongated radial iris vessels, shallow anterior chamber, and phthisis bulbi may occur. The diagnosis of the different types or causes of PHPV can sometimes be inferred from the family and birth histories, as well as from the details of the clinical examination. Direct visualization of remnants of the fetal hyaloid vascular system offers the best evidence. However, direct visualization by ophthalmoscopy or microscopy is sometimes impossible because of the opaque media. In these circumstances, indirect visualization by CT and MRI can be diagnostically useful. The CT characteristics of PHPV were first reported by Mafee in 1982. Maximum information was derived from CT when intravenous contrast medium was used and also when scanning was repeated in the lateral decubitus position. The CT findings include the following: (1) microphthalmus is usually detectable, although it may be minimal or absent; other deformities in the globe configuration are also demonstrable even when undetectable by physical examination or ultrasonography; (2) calcification is absent within or around the globe **(Option (C) is true)**; (3) generalized increased density of the entire vitreous chamber may be visible **(Option (D) is true),** although minimally affected cases may show normal attenuation values in the vitreous chambers; (4) enhancement of the CT image of abnormal intravitreal tissue may be seen after intravenous administration of contrast agent; (5) tubular, cylindrical, triangular, or other discrete intravitreal densities suggest the persistence of fetal tissue in Cloquet's canal or congenital nonattachment of the retina (Figure 5-16); (6) decubitus positioning may show a gravitational effect on a fluid level within the vitreous chamber, reflecting a serosanguineous fluid in either the subhyaloid space or subretinal space (Figure 5-16B); and (7) the lens may be small and irregular, and the anterior chamber may be shallow.

The MR appearance of different types of PHPV may be different. Early experience with MRI in patients with PHPV has revealed microphthalmus and hyperintense vitreous chambers on all pulse sequences. In a patient with bilateral PHPV caused by Warburg's syndrome, MR scanning revealed bilateral retinal detachment with hyperintensity of the subretinal fluid and layered blood in the vitreous chamber (Figure 5-17). The MR appearance of eyes with ROP may be identical to that of PHPV. The appearance of retinal detachment in PHPV has two forms: (1) retinal elevation into the vitreous from the optic nerve, resembling acquired forms of retinal detachment, and (2) retinal elevation from a point in the wall of the eye that is eccentric to the optic nerve, suggesting a falciform fold or congenital nonattachment of the retina. The ocular malformation

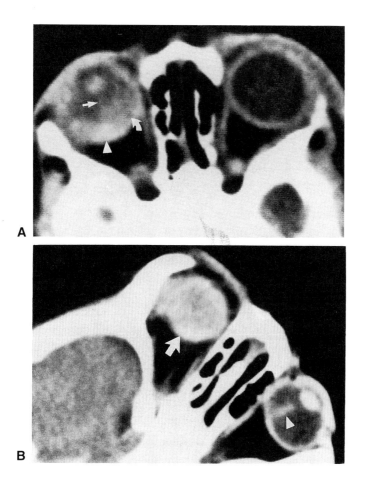

*Figure 5-16.* Persistent hyperplastic primary vitreous. (A) Postinfusion CT scan shows marked posterior intravitreal soft tissue enhancement (curved arrow). There is a retrolental band of soft tissue (straight arrow) that extends along Cloquet's canal. There is layering of high-density fluid in the vitreous (arrowhead). This is due to serosanguineous fluid in the subhyaloid or subretinal space. (B) CT scan of another patient with PHPV obtained with the patient in the lateral decubitus position. The right globe has increased density, and there is shifting fluid (straight arrow) in the right vitreous. There is soft tissue along the left Cloquet canal (arrowhead) corresponding to congenitally nonattached retina observed ophthalmoscopically.

usually reflects a manifestation of more-extensive disease including Warburg's syndrome (Figure 5-17), Norrie's disease (Figure 5-18), primary vitreoretinal dysplasia, and other congenital defects. Warburg's syndrome is an autosomal recessive oculocerebral disorder consisting of congenital malformation of the central nervous system and retinal

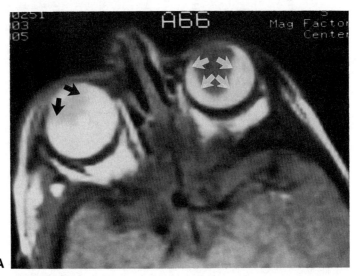

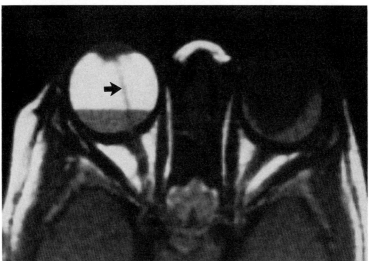

*Figure 5-17.* Bilateral PHPV in a patient with Warburg's syndrome. (A) T1-weighted MR scan showing bilateral retinal detachment (arrows). The hyperintensity of subretinal fluid is due to chronic hemorrhage. (B) T1-weighted MR scan of the same patient obtained 4 months later showing fluid-fluid level in the right globe as a result of recent hemorrhage, which appears hypointense. The tubular structure (arrow) is thought to be a congenitally nonattached retina. There is retinal detachment in the left eye.

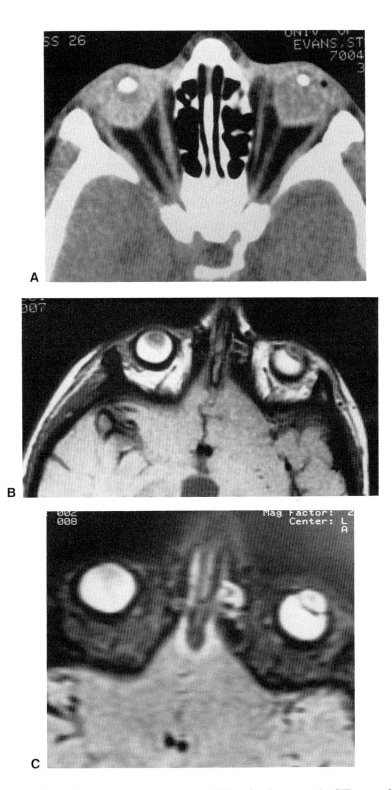

*Figure 5-18.* Norrie's disease with PHPV in both eyes. (A) CT scan shows bilaterally dense vitreous bodies and small eyes. Proton-weighted (B) and T2-weighted (C) MRI scans showing hyperintense vitreous chambers. This is due to proteinaceous fluid or chronic hemorrhage in the subhyaloid or subretinal space.

dysplasia. Norrie's disease, or congenital progressive oculo-acoustico-cerebral degeneration, is a rare X-linked recessive syndrome of retinal malformation, deafness, and mental retardation and/or deterioration. Nonetheless, the clinical or imaging detection of PHPV alerts the clinician to the appropriate diagnostic and prognostic possibilities. CT and MR scanning are certainly not indicated if the diagnosis and management of PHPV can be determined easily by conventional techniques. On the other hand, any procedure, such as CT or MRI, that aids in the complex diagnostic and therapeutic decision-making that is often required for such affected children should be considered clinically useful and should be employed in these selected circumstances. Goldberg and Mafee performed a CT study of eight children referred with several diagnoses, including retinoblastoma, congenital cataract, and microphthalmus. PHPV, which was not the initial diagnosis in any case, proved to be the most acceptable diagnosis for all patients after collation of data from clinical examinations of patients under anesthesia and from CT. MRI provides even more information in the diagnosis of PHPV. In our patients with PHPV we were unable to visualize T1 hyperintensity and T2 hypointensity of a mass within the vitreous chamber that is characteristic of retinoblastoma. However, differentiation of a retinoblastoma from PHPV is not always easy by CT.

## Question 24

Concerning Coats's disease,

(A) it is more common in boys than in girls
(B) it is a congenital telangiectasia of the retina
(C) MRI is superior to CT for the diagnosis
(D) calcification is a common finding on CT

Coats's disease is a primary vascular anomaly of the retina characterized by idiopathic congenital retinal telangiectasis and exudative retinal detachment (exudative retinopathy) **(Option (B) is true).** The condition occurs more frequently in boys than in girls **(Option (A) is true).** It is also seen in adults and is almost always unilateral. The formation of retinal telangiectasia and the breakdown in the blood-retina barrier at the telangiectasia are the essential underlying causes of changes that occur in Coats's disease. The breakdown in the blood-retina barrier causes the leakage of the lipoproteinaceous exudate that accounts for the pathologic changes of Coats's disease. The primary cause of the telangiectasia and of the leakage of serum and lipid and eventual closure of the retinal vessels in the area of the telangiectasia is unknown. The degree of lipoproteinaceous subretinal exudation in Coats's disease appears to be proportional to the extent of the retinal telangiectasia. Intraretinal or subretinal exudation, hemorrhages, and lipid and ultimately glial- and fibrous-tissue organization of the retina form the spectrum of pathologic changes in Coats's disease. The vascular anomaly of Coats's disease, although present at birth, usually does not cause symptoms until the retina detaches and central vision is lost. The ophthalmoscopic findings in Coats's disease vary with the stages of progression. The telangiectasia can be observed in the early stages. In the later stages, when the retina is filled with, and detached by, a mass of cholesterol exudate (total bullous exudative retinal detachment), the telangiectasia can be seen only on fluorescent angiography. In the early stage of the disease, when the retinal disease is not too extensive and the retinal detachment is shallow, photocoagulation or cryotherapy usually obliterates the telangiectatic vessels and reduces or eliminates the exudative retinal detachment. When there is extensive retinal telangiectasia and a total bullous exudative retinal detachment, cryotherapy and photocoagulation may not be sufficient to obliterate leaking vessels. The ocular disease in this condition commonly progresses to secondary angle closure or iris neovascularization, and the eyes become blind and painful as a result of acute congestive (neovascular) glaucoma.

The ophthalmoscopic and biomicroscopic features of eyes with advanced Coats's disease may closely resemble findings in eyes with exophytic retinoblastoma and leukokoria. It is important to distinguish retinoblastoma from Coats's disease. Many eyes with advanced Coats's disease have been enucleated because retinoblastoma could not be excluded. In a study of 62 eyes satisfying the histologic diagnostic parameters of Coats's disease, Chang et al. found that 52 (79%) were enucleated with the diagnosis of retinoblastoma or suspected retinoblastoma. Coats's disease is almost always unilateral, and it usually appears in boys slightly older (4 to 8 years) than those who have retinoblastoma. Many diagnostic techniques including ultrasonography, CT, and MRI are available that enable the ophthalmologist to diagnose clinical conditions. CT and MRI are extremely valuable in the diagnosis of Coats's disease.

The CT and MRI findings in Coats's disease vary with the stages of progression of the disease. At early stages, both techniques may yield little information. In the later stages, retinal detachment accounts for all the pathologic findings in CT and MRI. Sherman et al. reported two children with Coats's disease and concluded that CT could not differentiate between Coats's disease—which, as noted previously, does not cause calcification **(Option (D) is false)**—and unilateral noncalcifying retinoblastoma. Haik et al. reported their CT findings in 14 patients with Coats's disease; they routinely saw a total retinal detachment in advanced Coats's disease. Our experiences with CT in patients with Coats's disease agree with those of Haik et al. MRI is superior to CT in differentiating Coats's disease from retinoblastoma and other leukokoric eyes **(Option (C) is true)**. The subretinal exudation of Coats's disease is usually seen as increased density of the globe on CT scans (Figure 5-19A). On MRI, it is usually seen as a hyperintense mass T1-, proton-, and T2-weighted MR scans (Figure 5-19B and C). MRI of retinoblastomas characteristically shows a mass that can easily be differentiated from associated subretinal exudate. The retinoblastoma is relatively hyperintense on T1- and proton-weighted MR images and becomes hypointense on T2-weighted images (Figure 5-9B and C). The subretinal fluid of associated retinal detachment will be seen as various degrees of hyperintensity in all pulse sequences (Figure 5-11). Although Coats's disease can theoretically produce a subretinal mass resembling retinoblastoma, the mass in Coats's disease is caused by cholesterol, organized hemorrhage, and fibrosis and is therefore presumed to be inhomogeneous in signal character. In our study of four patients with Coats's disease, the MR findings were compatible with retinal detachment without the presence of an intraocular mass (Figure 5-19B and C). The MR findings in some of these patients with early stages of the disease were normal.

In general, if an ophthalmologist suspects advanced Coats's disease but is uncertain of the correct clinical diagnosis and unable to rule out retinoblastoma conclusively, he or she should request a diagnostic imaging study. When retinoblastoma presents with what appears to be total retinal detachment, there are basically three diagnoses to consider: PHPV, Coats's disease, and ROP. In the appropriate clinical setting, the MR and CT findings of Coats's disease should help establish a correct diagnosis (Figure 5-19).

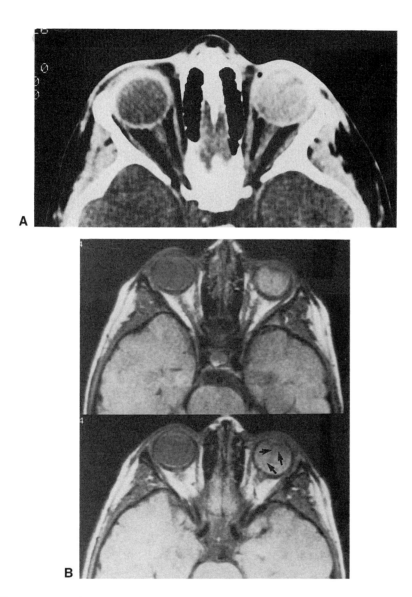

*Figure 5-19.* Coats's disease. (A) CT scan shows increased density of the left globe as a result of total retinal detachment. Proton-weighted (B) and T2-weighted (C) MR scans show retinal detachment without evidence of any intraocular mass. Notice the leaves of the detached retina (arrows).

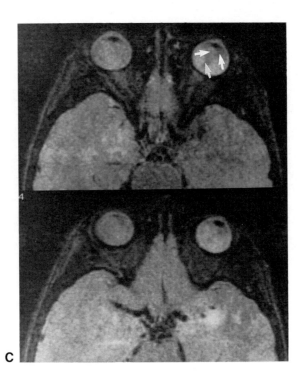

C

## Question 25

Drusen of the optic nerve head:

(A) occur in the intraocular portion of the optic nerve
(B) are usually bilateral
(C) are rarely detected by CT in early childhood
(D) simulate papilledema on clinical examination
(E) appear on CT as a well-defined calcification beneath the surface of the optic disk

Disk drusen or hyaline bodies are spherical, acellular, laminated concretions from an unknown source, often partially calcified and possibly related to accumulation of axoplasmic derivatives of degenerating retinal nerve fibers. Drusen are buried within the substance of the nerve head, usually anterior to the lamina scleralis **(Option (A) is true).** They are covered by axonal and glial tissue, together with the vascular supply of the nerve head. Therefore, drusen of the optic nerve head are recognizable because of characteristic distortion in the shape of the nerve head. Drusen of the optic nerve head are usually bilateral **(Option (B) is true).**

Clinically, the term drusen is more frequently applied to the very common multiple small, round, discrete punctate subretinal nodules (drusen of the pigmented retinal epithelium) at the posterior pole. From the standpoint of pathology, drusen of the optic disk should not be confused with drusen of the pigmented retinal epithelium, which are deposits of basement membrane material between the pigment epithelium of the retina and Bruch's membrane. Bruch's membrane is a tough, acellular, amorphous, bilamellar structure, situated between the outer layer of the retina, the so-called retinal pigment epithelium (RPE), and the choroid. Microscopically, Bruch's membrane consists of five layers: (1) basement membrane of the RPE, (2) inner collagenous zone, (3) elastic layer, (4) outer collagenous zone, and (5) basement membrane of the choriocapillaris. Retinal pigment epithelial drusen are extracellular deposits that lie between the basement membrane of the RPE and the inner collagenous zone of Bruch's membrane. It has been suggested that apoptosis, a process by which cells cast off a part of their cytoplasm, may lead to formation of drusen. The RPE drusen are believed to develop by the shedding of basal cytoplasm of RPE through its basement membrane. With time, RPE and optic disk drusen change in size, shape, and consistency and may become calcified. Drusen contain sialic acid, cerebrosides, calcium, carbohydrate, mucopolysaccharides, and iron. Optic disk drusen vary in size (50 to 750 μm in diameter) and number; often, smaller drusen appear to coalesce to form larger aggregates. Once their calcified component is more than 1 to 1.5 mm they should be recognized on thin-section (1- to 1.5-mm) CT scans. The RPE drusen are not large enough to be visible on CT scans. Although optic disk drusen are rarely seen in early childhood, most drusen are believed to be present at birth. They become more apparent in later life as they enlarge and approach the disk surface, becoming ophthalmologically visible as "hyaline" or "colloid" bodies. Drusen are rarely detected by CT scanning in early childhood **(Option (C) is true).** Optic disk drusen have been reported in 20 to 24 per 1,000 patients at autopsy and are bilateral in 73% of cases. When drusen are located well beneath the surface of the disk, they may blur the disk margin and may lead to misdiagnosis of papilledema **(Option (D) is true).** Clinically, drusen are usually asymptomatic, but arcuate field defects (arcuate scotomas) or peripheral field constrictions may be present. These field defects are usually not apparent until adulthood, which further emphasizes the slowly progressive nature of drusen. There also appears to be an association between drusen of the optic disk and retinal hemorrhages. On CT, drusen appear as discrete, rounded, high-density or calcified bodies that are confined to the optic disk surface and are found at any level within the prelaminar zone of the optic nerve (Figure 5-2) **(Option (E) is true)**. Optic nerve drusen are difficult to visualize by MRI. In our experience with five patients with drusen visualized by CT, none of the drusen were detected on MR scans.

## Question 26

Concerning optic nerve coloboma and colobomatous cyst,

(A) optic nerve coloboma arises from failure of closure of the embryonic fissure
(B) isolated coloboma of the optic nerve is a common congenital disorder
(C) microphthalmus with colobomatous cyst is an anomaly seen in an eye with a retinochoroidal coloboma
(D) optic nerve coloboma characteristically appears on CT and MRI as an area of excavation of the disk
(E) calcification commonly occurs within a colobomatous cyst

A coloboma is a notch, gap, hole, or fissure that is congenital or acquired and in which a tissue or portion of a tissue is lacking. When examining a child with leukokoria, the major diagnostic considerations are retinoblastoma, PHPV, congenital cataract, Coats's disease, and a variety of other nonspecific causes, including coloboma of the choroid or optic disk. There are three types of optic nerve colobomas: isolated coloboma of the optic nerve, retinochoroidal coloboma, and Fuchs' coloboma. The congenital optic pit has also been considered by some to be a coloboma of the optic nerve, as has the morning glory disk anomaly. A variety of ocular and systemic abnormalities may be seen with an optic nerve coloboma. Fuchs' coloboma (tilted-disk syndrome, nasal fundus ectasia syndrome) is a form of coloboma in which there is a congenital, inferiorly tilted optic disk in conjunction with an inferonasal crescent or conus along the border of the disk in the direction of the tilt. Myopia and astigmatism accompany these changes.

Ophthalmoscopically, optic nerve colobomas characteristically show enlargement of the papillary areas, with partial or total excavation of the disk (Figure 5-20). A brief review of the embryonic derivation of the posterior ocular structures is important to the understanding of the origin of optic nerve colobomas (Figure 5-21). By the third week of gestation, two indentations appear, one on each side of the optic vesicles, which can be viewed externally in the 4-mm embryo (less than 4 weeks of gestation) as two lateral diverticula, one on each side of the forebrain. The distal parts of the optic vesicles expand, whereas the proximal parts of the optic

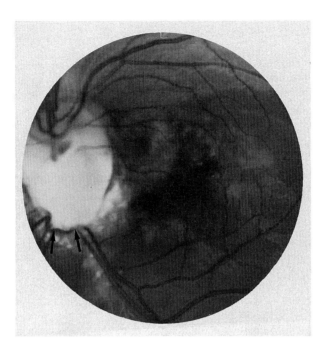

*Figure 5-20.* Isolated optic disk coloboma. The disk is enlarged, with an inferior defect (arrows). Pigmentary changes are present as a result of a macular detachment.

vesicles become the tubular optic stalks. At the 5-mm embryonic stage (4 weeks of gestation), the external surface of each optic vesicle invaginates. The concavity created by the invagination is known as the optic cup. The inner wall of the optic cup (the former outer wall of the optic vessels) gives rise to the sensory retina, and the outer wall of the cup is the forerunner of the retinal pigment epithelium. During the invagination of the optic vesicle, a groove remains open for some distance along the optic stalk at the inferior and slightly nasal aspect of the optic cup. This groove is the embryonic fissure, or cleft, through which mesenchyme extends into the optic stalk and cup, carrying the hyaloid artery with it. As growth proceeds, the edges of the fissure become approximated, and they close during the fifth week. Failure of the tissue to fuse properly results in some of the congenital colobomatous defects discussed below **(Option (A) is true).** At the 7.5-mm stage, the area in the optic cup where the optic nerve head will develop can be identified. It is referred to as the primitive epithelial papilla and is located at the superior end of the embryonic fissure.

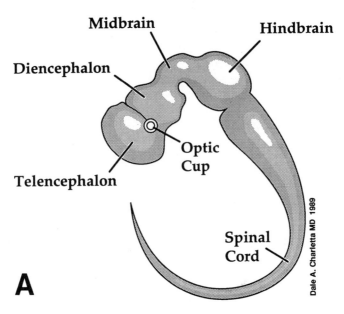

Midbrain

Hindbrain

Diencephalon

Optic
Cup

Telencephalon

Spinal
Cord

Dale A. Charletta MD 1989

**A**

*Figure 5-21.* Developing human embryo. (A) By the third week of gestation, two indentations appear, one on each side of the neural groove. These are the optic pits, and they deepen to form the optic vesicles, one on each side of the forebrain. The optic vesicles give rise to an optic cup on each side. (B) In the 4-mm embryo, lateral diverticulae on each side of the forebrain (F) have given rise to two optic vesicles. (C) At the 5-mm stage, the external surface of each optic vesicle invaginates to form the optic cup. Note the embryonic fissure, through which mesenchyme extends into the optic stalk and cup. L = lens. (Reprinted with permission from Mafee et al. [18].)

 

Isolated optic nerve colobomas arise from failure of closure of only the most superior end of the embryonic fissure. Failure of closure of other parts of the fissure causes iridic, lenticular, ciliary body, or retinochoroidal colobomas. Isolated coloboma of the optic nerve is an uncommon congenital disorder **(Option (B) is false).** The visual acuity in eyes with optic nerve colobomas is variable and may range from normal to no light perception. Nonrhegmatogenous or rhegmatogenous retinal detachment (retinal detachment resulting from a hole or tear in the retina is referred to as rhegmatogenous detachment) has been well described in association with optic nerve coloboma. Optic nerve colobomas have been observed in association with other abnormalities including congenital optic pit, cyst of the optic nerve sheath, posterior lenticonus, and remnants of the hyaloid artery. Systemic abnormalities, including cardiac defects, dysplastic ears, facial palsy, and transsphenoidal encephalocele, have

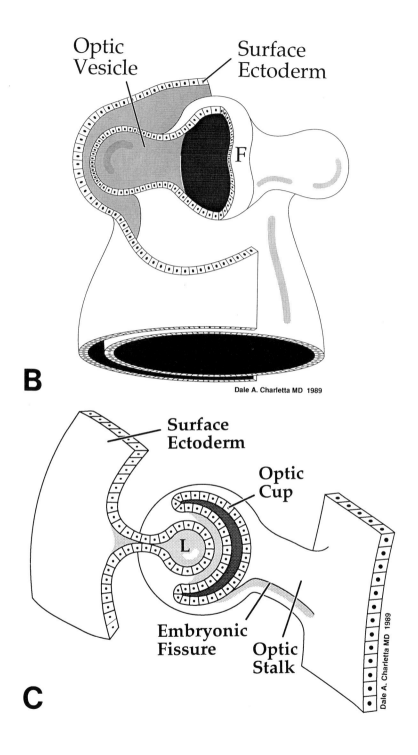

Optic Vesicle

Surface Ectoderm

F

B

Dale A. Charletta MD 1989

Surface Ectoderm

Optic Cup

L

Embryonic Fissure

Optic Stalk

Dale A. Charletta MD 1989

C

also been reported in these patients. Microphthalmus with cyst is an anomaly in which an eye with a retinochoroidal coloboma also has a cyst, which is usually attached to the inferior aspect of the globe **(Option (C) is true)**.

Morning glory disk anomaly was first characterized by Kindler in 1970. He described a unilateral congenital anomaly of the optic nerve head in 10 patients. Because of the similarity in appearance between the nerve head and a morning glory flower, he referred to the anomaly as the morning glory syndrome. Ophthalmoscopically, the abnormal nerve head has several characteristic features. The disk is enlarged and excavated, has a central core of white tissue, and is surrounded by an elevated annulus of light and variably pigmented subretinal tissue.

The CT and MR appearance of optic disk coloboma includes posterior global defect with optic disk excavation **(Option (D) is true).** The CT and MR appearance of the morning glory anomaly is quite characteristic, corresponding to its clinical appearance as a large funnel-shaped disk. The colobomatous cyst associated with coloboma of the optic cyst can be easily identified on CT and MR scans. Dystrophic calcification is occasionally seen on CT scans at the colobomatous defect. This calcification is probably within the abnormal glial tissue at the site of the coloboma **(Option (E) is false).** Any retroglobal cyst associated with a microphthalmic eye should be suspected to be a colobomatous cyst (Figures 5-3 and 5-22). These patients may have associated congenital anomaly of the brain.

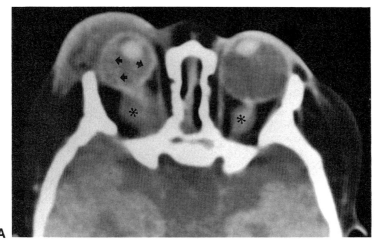

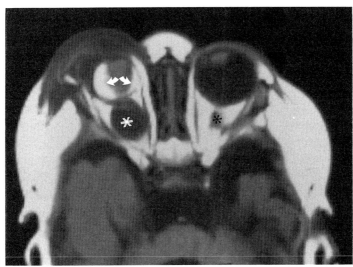

*Figure 5-22.* Bilateral coloboma and colobomatous cysts. (A) CT scan shows retinal detachment of the right globe (arrows) and bilateral colobomatous cysts (*). (B and C) T1-weighted (B) and T2-weighted (C) MR images show the retinal detachment of the right eye (arrows) and colobomatous cysts (*).

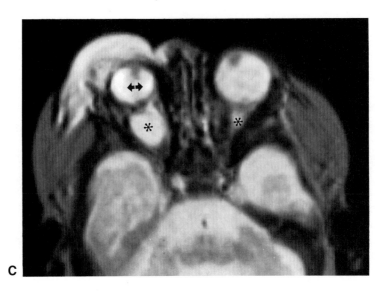

C

## Question 27

Concerning retinopathy of prematurity,

    (A) it usually develops as a response to prolonged supplemental oxygen therapy
    (B) pathologically, there is retinal neovascularization
    (C) both retinal detachment and vitreous hemorrhage are common
    (D) calcification is common

    In about 1940, pediatricians began to treat premature infants with supplemental oxygen to alleviate their respiratory distress and to improve their survival. In 1942, Terry published his report and alluded to "extreme prematurity and fibroplastic overgrowth of persistent vascular sheath behind each crystalline lens." This was the first report of the condition that was termed in later reports "retrolental fibroplasia" and that is now generally referred to as retinopathy of prematurity (ROP). Clinical and pathologic reports began to appear after Terry's study, but it was not until 1952 that the remarkable experimental work of Ashton et al. and Patz et al., combined with the clinical study of Kinsey and Hemphill, showed the association between the use of supplemental oxygen and the development of ROP **(Option (A) is true).** These landmark studies ended the first epidemic of ROP in the mid-1950s. Following the awareness of the exclusive role of supplemental oxygen in this condition, ROP was not eliminated, but it was seen with much less frequency. We are now in the midst of a second ROP epidemic, in which the exclusive role of supplemental oxygen is being questioned. It has been stated that prematurity per se may be responsible for many of the current cases, in contrast to the overuse of oxygen, which was the major cause earlier. Ashton has stated that "despite the many current speculations which seem feasible to some and not to others, no certain opinions can at present be expressed as the cause or causes of the second epidemic of ROP." The essential feature of ROP appears to be prematurity. The smaller the infant, the greater the risk of developing this disease. ROP usually develops in response to prolonged exposure to supplemental oxygen therapy. It is possible that excessive oxygen plays only a secondary role in the development of ROP. Eller et al. noticed that 14 patients had an associated persistent hyaloid vascular system. A massive persistent hyaloid vascular system was found in seven of their patients. The authors concluded that ROP may be related to a combination of developmental and environmental factors that prevent normal retinal vasculogenesis outside the womb.

*Ophthalmoscopic appearance.* The ophthalmoscopic findings of ROP have been divided into active, regressive, and cicatricial phases. The initial active phase is characterized by arteriolar narrowing due to a spastic response of the vessels to hyperoxia. The vessels then start to dilate and become tortuous. A subsequent sign is the presence of fine delicate neovascularization in the periphery **(Option (B) is true).** These changes are most marked in the temporal periphery because this is the region where the retinal vascularization develops last. Commonly, as long as premature infants are in oxygen therapy there is no vascular dilatation or tortuosity, both of which occur 24 to 48 hours after the infants are removed rapidly from the oxygen incubator. Gradually, strands containing new vessels pass into the vitreous from the retina. There may be vitreous hemorrhage, and the retina may become detached **(Option (C) is true).** Detachment may become complete, and occasionally the vitreous hemorrhage is massive.

A characteristic of ROP is a tendency, during the early stage, toward spontaneous regression with disappearance of the neovascularization and even toward a general detachment of the retina. This is known as the regressive phase. The detached retina, however, may not always reattach. About 85 to 90% of cases show spontaneous regression.

Finally, a dense membrane or a gray-white vascularized mass will be left as permanent evidence of the active phase. This is the cicatricial phase. The lens always remains clear. The retina is detached with associated retinal scars. Growth of the eye is often inhibited with microphthalmus as the final outcome.

*Pathogenesis.* The earliest histologic changes in ROP are patchy proliferations of the capillary endothelium in the nerve fiber layer of the retina. This is associated with glial overgrowth. There is abundant evidence that this vascular change is associated with the abnormal oxygen environment in which the premature infants have been placed.

Patz et al. have shown specific vasoconstriction as a response to hyperoxia in their animal experimentation. They demonstrated the production of the microscopic changes of retrolental fibroplasia in experimental animals. The electron-microscopic examinations have shown that vasoconstriction as a response to hyperoxia results in selective damage of the capillary endothelium. The endothelial disturbance, with the increased capillary permeability following the vasoconstriction, is probably the initial change in the capillaropathy stage of the disease and leads to the reaction stage with its neovascularization. In the reaction stage, hemorrhages and transudations are developed in relation to abnormal vessels, which now extend through the internal limiting membrane of the retina to spread on the surface of the retina or to ramify into the vitreous chamber. The ensuing retinal detachment results in part from the transudation and in part from the fibrosis of the vascular strands in the vitreous.

*CT and MRI.* The early stage of ROP may have no specific CT or MRI findings, except that the eyes may be microphthalmic. In more-advanced cases, the differential CT and MRI diagnosis between ROP, PHPV, retinoblastoma, endophthalmitis, and a number of pathologic conditions in which retinal detachment is a common feature may be difficult. The history of incubator treatment, birth weight, bilaterality, and the ophthalmoscopic, ultrasonographic, CT, and MRI findings are usually sufficient to establish the diagnosis. Calcification is rare in ROP **(Option (D) is false);** however, it may be present in the more advanced stages (Figure 5-4). In the most advanced stage, both eyes are microphthalmic with very shallow anterior chambers (Figure 5-23). Calcification in a microphthalmic eye is less characteristic of retinoblastoma, although retinoblastoma has seldom been reported in microphthalmic eyes in the presence and absence of ROP or PHPV. ROP may on occasion present as unilateral leukokoria; however, in the majority of cases it presents as bilateral but often markedly asymmetric disease (Figure 5-23). A persistent hyaloid vascular system may be an associated finding in patients with ROP. Recognition of a massive persistent hyaloid vascular system on clinical, MR, CT, or ultrasonographic examination is of prognostic importance.

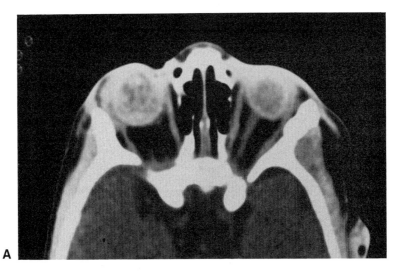

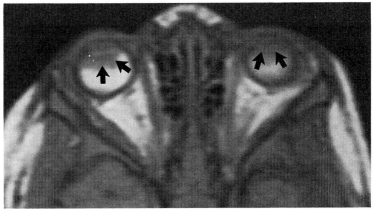

*Figure 5-23.* Retinopathy of prematurity. (A) Axial CT scan. The density of both globes is increased. Both eyes are microphthalmic. (B) Proton-weighted MR scan. The hyperintensity of both globes presumably results from subretinal hemorrhage. There are abnormal retrolental tissues bilaterally (arrows). (C) T2-weighted MR scan. Hyperintensity of the globes, the retrolental fibrotic scar tissue (solid arrows), and layering of acute hemorrhage in the subretinal space (open arrows) are clearly shown.

In these cases, surgical dissection of the retrolental membrane in the presence of a persistent hyaloid vascular system is more difficult because these vessels tend to bleed and the retrolental membrane is tightly adherent to the detached retina.

*Mahmood F. Mafee, M.D.*

*Case 5* / 113

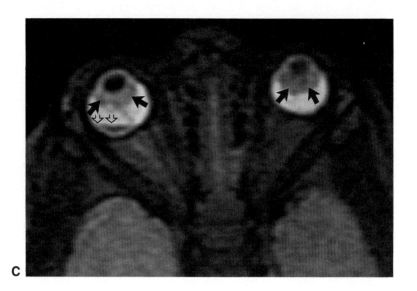

C

*SUGGESTED READINGS*

RETINOBLASTOMA

1. Abramson DH. Retinoblastoma: diagnosis and management. CA 1982; 32:130–140
2. Abramson DH, Ellsworth RM, Kitchin FD, Tung G. Second nonocular tumors in retinoblastoma survivors. Are they radiation-induced? Ophthalmology 1984; 91:1351–1355
3. Bader JL, Miller RW, Meadows AT, Zimmerman LE, Champion LA, Voute PA. Trilateral retinoblastoma. Lancet 1980; 2:582–583
4. Haik BG, Saint Louis L, Smith ME, et al. Magnetic resonance imaging in the evaluation of leukocoria. Ophthalmology 1985; 92:1143–1152
5. Howard GM, Ellsworth RM. Differential diagnosis of retinoblastoma. A statistical survey of 500 children. I. Relative frequency of the lesions which simulate retinoblastoma. Am J Ophthalmol 1965; 60:610–618
6. Jakobiec FA, Tso MO, Zimmerman LE, Danis P. Retinoblastoma and intracranial malignancy. Cancer 1977; 39:2048–2058
7. Jensen RD, Miller RW. Retinoblastoma: epidemiologic characteristics. N Engl J Med 1971; 285:307–311
8. Mafee MF. Magnetic resonance imaging: ocular pathology. In: Newton TH, Bilaniuk LT (eds), Modern neuroradiology, vol 4. Radiology of the eye and orbit. New York: Clavadel Press/Raven Press; 1990:3.1–3.5
9. Mafee MF. The orbit. In: Som PM, Bergeron RT (eds), Head and neck imaging. St. Louis: CV Mosby; 1991:693–813
10. Mafee MF, Goldberg MF, Cohen SB, et al. Magnetic resonance imaging versus computed tomography of leukokoric eyes and use of in vitro proton magnetic

resonance spectroscopy of retinoblastoma. Ophthalmology 1989; 96:965–976

11. Mafee MF, Goldberg MF, Greenwald MJ, Schulman J, Malmed A, Flanders AE. Retinoblastoma and simulating lesions: role of CT and MR imaging. Radiol Clin North Am 1987; 25:667–682

12. Poujol J, Varene B. Contribution of echography to the diagnosis of retinoblastoma: a homogeneous B-scan study. US Med Biol 1985; 11:171–175

## DRUSEN

13. Friedman AM, Henkind P, Gartner S. Drusen of the optic disk. A histopathological study. Trans Ophthalmol Soc UK 1975; 95:4–9

14. Glaser JS. Topical diagnosis: prechiasmal visual pathways. In: Tasman W, Jaeger EA (eds), Duane's clinical ophthalmology. Philadelphia: JB Lippincott; 1989; 2; 5:1–85

15. Lorentzen SE. Drusen of the optic disk. A clinical and genetic study. Acta Ophthalmol (Copenh) 1966; Suppl 90:1–180

## COLOBOMA

16. Brown G, Tasman W (eds). Congenital anomalies of the optic disc. New York: Grune & Stratton; 1983:97–191

17. Kindler P. Morning glory syndrome: unusual congenital optic disk anomaly. Am J Ophthalmol 1970; 69:376–384

18. Mafee MF, Jampol LM, Langer BG, Tso M. Computed tomography of optic nerve colobomas, morning glory anomaly, and colobomatous cyst. Radiol Clin North Am 1987; 25:693–699

19. Makley TA Jr, Battles M. Microphthalmos with cyst. Report of two cases in the same family. Surv Ophthalmol 1969; 13:200–206

20. Mann IC. On the morphology of certain developmental structures associated with the upper end of the choroidal fissure. Br J Ophthalmol 1922; 6:145–163

## RETINOPATHY OF PREMATURITY

21. Ashton N, Ward B, Sperpell G. Role of oxygen in the genesis of retrolental fibroplasia: a preliminary report. Br J Ophthalmology 1953; 37:513–520

22. Eller AW, Jabbour NM, Hirose T, Schepens CL. Retinopathy of prematurity. The association of a persistent hyaloid artery. Ophthalmology 1987; 94:44–448

23. Kinsey VR, Hemphill FM. Etiology of retrolental fibroplasia and preliminary report of cooperative study of retrolental fibroplasia. Trans Am Acad Ophthalmol Otolaryngol 1955; 59:15–24

24. Michaelson IC. Retrolental fibroplasia. In: Michaelson IC (ed), Textbook of the fundus of the eye. New York: Churchill Livingstone; 1980:303–315

25. Patz A, Easthman A, Higgenbotham DH, Kleh T. Oxygen studies in retrolental fibroplasia. II. The production of the microscopic changes of retrolental fibroplasia in experimental animals. Am J Ophthalmol 1953; 36:1511–1522

26. Terry TL. Extreme prematurity and fibroplastic overgrowth of persistent vascular sheath behind each crystalline lens. I. Preliminary report. Am J Ophthalmol 1942; 25:203–204

COATS'S DISEASE

27. Chang MM, McLean IW, Merritt JC. Coats' disease: a study of 62 histologically confirmed cases. J Pediatr Ophthalmol Strabismus 1984; 21:163–168
28. Coats G. Forms of retinal disease with massive exudation. R Lond Ophthalmol Hosp Rep 1908; 17:440–525
29. Sherman JL, McLean IW, Brallier DR. Coats' disease: CT-pathologic correlation in two cases. Radiology 1983; 146:77–78

PERSISTENT HYPERPLASTIC PRIMARY VITREOUS

30. Goldberg MF, Mafee M. Computed tomography for diagnosis of persistent hyperplastic primary vitreous (PHPV). Ophthalmology 1983; 90:442–451
31. Howard GM, Ellsworth RM. Differential diagnosis of retinoblastoma. A statistical survey of 500 children. I. Relative frequency of the lesions which simulate retinoblastoma. Am J Ophthalmol 1965; 60:610–618
32. Mafee MF, Goldberg MF. Persistent hyperplastic primary vitreous (PHPV): role of computed tomography and magnetic resonance. Radiol Clin North Am 1987; 25:683–692
33. Mafee MF, Goldberg MF, Valvassori GE, Capek V. Computed tomography in the evaluation of patients with persistent hyperplastic primary vitreous (PHPV). Radiology 1982; 145:713–717
34. Warburg M. Doyne Memorial Lecture, 1979. Retinal malformations: aetiological heterogeneity and morphological similarity in congenital retinal non-attachment and falciform folds. Trans Ophthalmol Soc UK 1979; 99:272–283

OCULAR TOXOCARIASIS

35. Margo CE, Katz NN, Wertz FD, Dorwart RH. Sclerosing endophthalmitis in children: computed tomography with histopathologic correlation. J Pediatr Ophthalmol Strabismus 1983; 20:180–184
36. Wilder HC. Nematode endophthalmitis. Trans Am Acad Ophthalmol Otolaryngol 1950; 55:99–104

*Notes*

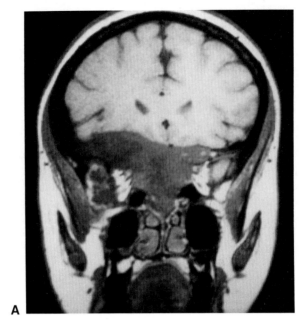

SE 600/20

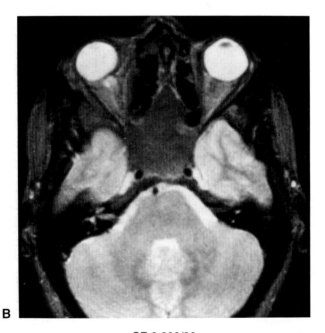

B

SE 2,200/80

*Figure 6-1.* This 23-year-old woman presented with progressively worsening episodes of decreased acuity in her left eye. You are shown coronal T1-weighted (A), adjacent axial T2-weighted (B and C), and coronal post-contrast T1-weighted (D) MR scans.

# Case 6: Fibrous Dysplasia

## Question 28

Which *one* of the following is the MOST likely diagnosis?

(A) Fibrous dysplasia
(B) Mucocele of the sphenoid sinus
(C) Langerhans cell histiocytosis
(D) Mucormycosis
(E) Meningioma

The MR scans (Figure 6-1) demonstrate an expansile process involving the anterior skull base including the planum sphenoidale and greater wings of the sphenoid bone. A coronal T1-weighted MR image through the anterior skull base (Figure 6-1A) demonstrates a low-intensity osseous mass (arrows, Figure 6-2A), which has a sharp margin with the brain, clearly indicating its extra-axial nature. On T2-weighted axial scans (Figure 6-1B and C), the signal intensity of the expansile mass remains low and the optic nerves within the optic canals are seen to be compressed (Figure 6-2B and C). A T1-weighted sequence following the intravenous administration of gadolinium DTPA (Figure 6-1D) demonstrates diffuse homogeneous enhancement of the mass, which replaces the sphenoid sinus and expands the anterior clinoid processes (solid arrows, Figure 6-2D). The expanded anterior clinoid processes encroach upon the optic nerves (open arrows). An expansile osseous process with a low signal intensity on both T1- and T2-weighted sequences and diffuse enhancement is most consistent with a diagnosis of fibrous dysplasia **(Option (A) is correct).**

A mucocele of the sphenoid sinus (Option (B)) can cause an expansile mass of the sphenoid bone, but the lesion is centered in the lumen of the sphenoid sinus; it does not involve the entire sphenoid bone. In addition, most mucoceles of the sphenoid sinus demonstrate high signal intensity on T2-weighted images and often on T1-weighted images as well, and the contents of the mucocele do not enhance with MR contrast. Sphenoid mucoceles also become desiccated and give signal voids on MRI (Figure

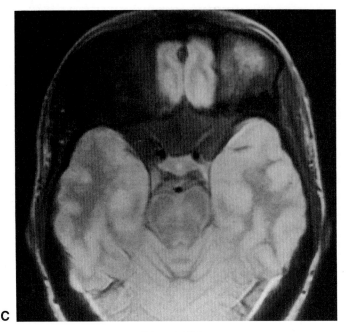

C

SE 2,200/80

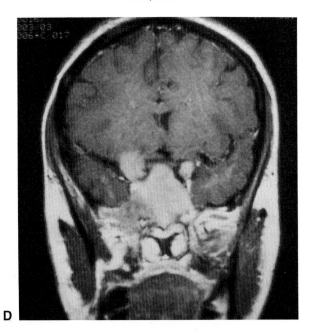

D

SE 600/20

*Figure 6-1 (Continued)*

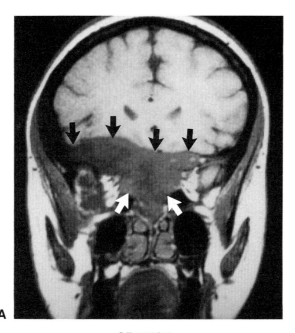

SE 600/20

*Figure 6-2* (Same as Figure 6-1). Fibrous dysplasia of the sphenoid bone. (A) Coronal T1-weighted scan through the anterior skull base demonstrates expansion and diffuse low signal intensity of the planum sphenoidale (black arrows). The mass extends into the upper ethmoid sinuses (white arrows). Note that the mass is extra-axial and displaces the frontal lobes. (B and C) Axial T2-weighted MR scans through the region of the sphenoid sinus (B) and optic nerves (C). The sphenoid sinus has been replaced by a mass of low signal intensity (arrows, panel B). In panel C, compression of the optic nerves (white arrows) by the expanded anterior clinoid processes (black arrows) is evident. (D) Coronal T1-weighted post-contrast MR scan through the region of the sphenoid sinus and anterior clinoid processes. The osseous abnormality expands the sphenoid sinus and anterior clinoid processes (black arrows), which also enhance. Note the relationship of the optic nerves (open arrows) to the expanded anterior clinoid processes. The dura adjacent to the osseous lesion does not enhance, distinguishing fibrous dysplasia from most cases of hyperostosis secondary to meningioma, in which case the involved dura and tumor usually enhance.


6-3). Sphenoid mucoceles occasionally occur secondary to an obstructing mass, such as a polyp or tumor, located at the sphenoethmoidal recess; no such mass is identified in the test images.

Langerhans cell histiocytosis (LCH) (Option (C)) may also result in skull lesions; however, their typical radiographic pattern is that of a

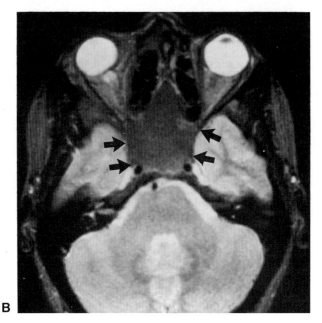

SE 2,200/80

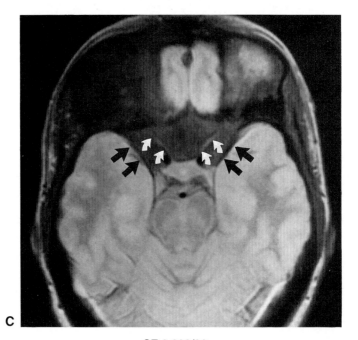

SE 2,200/80

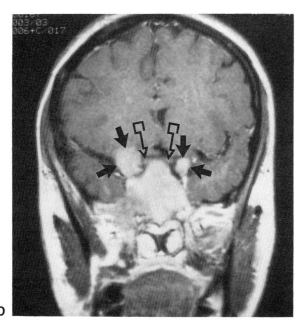

D

SE 600/20

nonsclerotic osteolytic lesion with sharp margins involving a flat bone with or without involvement of the surrounding soft tissues. The osseous lesion usually presents as a gradually enlarging, focally destructive mass. However, the bone itself is not expanded. The test images demonstrate an infiltrative expansile process of an entire bone, without evidence of a nonhomogeneous or lytic site. MRI experience in LCH is limited, but most lesions appear as areas of marrow replacement (decreased signal intensity on T1-weighted scans and increased signal intensity on T2-weighted scans, as well as enhancement on postcontrast images). The T2-weighted signal intensity of the test lesion is decreased. Thus, LCH is an unlikely diagnosis.

Mucormycosis (Option (D)), an opportunistic fungal infection occurring almost exclusively in immunosuppressed or diabetic patients, may involve the anterior skull base and intracranial compartment. The organism initially infects the paranasal sinuses by spread from the nasal cavity. Invasion of arterioles results in thrombosis, with subsequent necrotic infarction of tissues. Extension is primarily via the orbital vessels, which pass through the inferior orbital fissure, and provides entry into the intracranial compartment, leading to cavernous sinus thrombosis.

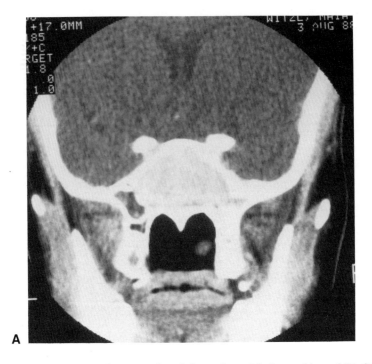

**A**

*Figure 6-3.* Desiccated mucocele of the sphenoid sinus. (A and B) Coronal CT scan photographed at a soft tissue window (A) and bone window (B) demonstrates an opacified, expanded sphenoid sinus with a high density indicative of high protein content. (C) Transaxial T2-weighted MR image through the sphenoid sinus mucocele (arrows). Although the signal intensity of the contents of the mucocele appears to be equal to that of air, this sinus is actually opacified with highly proteinaceous, desiccated material having a very short T2 relaxation time. Therefore at the acquired TE (80 msec), the signal has decayed within this solid desiccated material so that no signal intensity is registered on the image. Therefore, the opacified sinus actually appears mistakenly aerated on MR. Expansion of the sinus is a clue that a mucocele is present.

The radiographic findings of mucormycosis are often quite subtle. Sinusitis without bone destruction is common in the early stages of disease. Proptosis and orbital inflammation followed by carotid artery thrombosis precede the intracranial spread of disease. MR scanning may demonstrate some of these changes earlier than CT; however, it is generally agreed that CT should be the initial choice for imaging inflammatory paranasal sinus disease. In the test images the abnormality is centered entirely in the sphenoid bone, with no evidence of intraorbital, paranasal sinus, or nasal fossa inflammatory disease. Therefore, mucormycosis is unlikely.

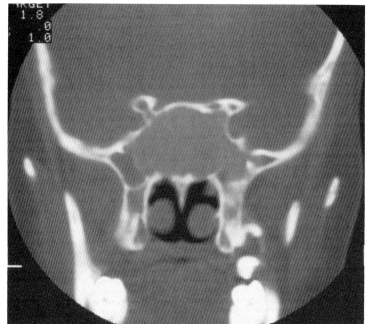

**B**

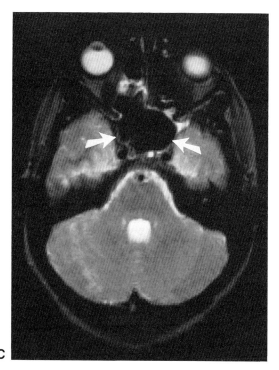

**C**

SE 2,000/80

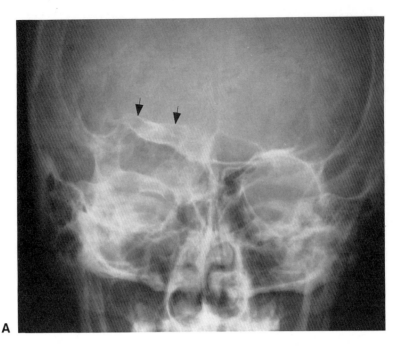

**A**

*Figure 6-4.* Tuberculum sella meningioma. (A) This anteroposterior radiograph of the skull demonstrates hyperostosis overlying the planum sphenoidale and tuberculum sellae (arrows). (B) A lateral radiograph of the skull demonstrates a hyperostosis of the planum sphenoidale (arrows). This is a typical response to meningioma. (C) This sagittal reformatted CT scan following contrast administration demonstrates hyperostosis of the planum sphenoidale and tuberculum sellae. The enhancing meningioma (arrows) is also seen. (D) A sagittal view photographed with bone windows demonstrates the midline hyperostotic tuberculum sellae (arrows).

Meningioma (Option (E)) may involve the anterior skull base and compress the optic nerves. Meningioma is a benign tumor of the meninges and, as such, usually presents as an enhancing extra-axial mass between the brain and the calvarium. Adjacent hyperostosis or sclerosis of bone is frequently present and reflects either osseous invasion by the tumor or adjacent bone reaction to the tumor (Figure 6-4). On MR images, hyperostosis results in an expanded bone with low signal on both T1- and T2-weighted sequences, similar to the test images. However, the pattern of contrast enhancement shown in the test images is different from that expected for meningioma. With en plaque meningioma, the tumor enhances adjacent to the hyperostotic bone. Enhancement of the bone itself would be unusual. Meningioma may develop entirely within bone (intra-

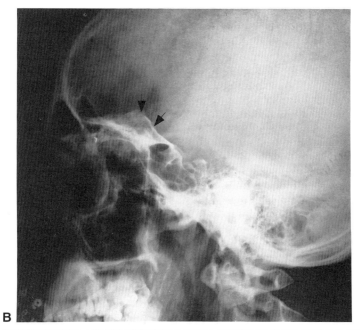

B

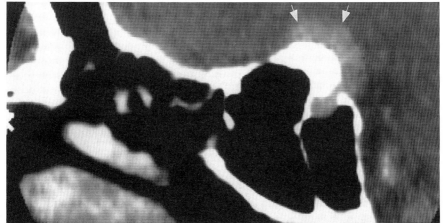

C

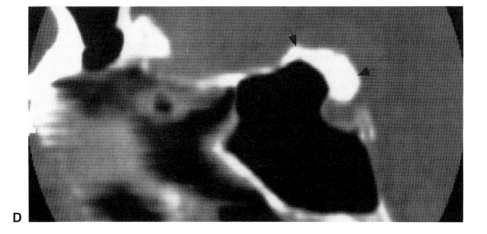

D

127

osseous meningioma); however, this is exceedingly rare, and it would be unusual for such a large area of bone to be involved without an adjacent soft tissue component. Thus the lesion in the test images is not likely to be an intraosseous meningioma.


## Question 29

Concerning fibrous dysplasia,

(A) the calvarium is involved in about 50% of patients with the monostotic form of the disease
(B) fewer than 20% of patients with the polyostotic form of the disease have involvement of the skull and facial bones
(C) the temporal bone is the most commonly involved skull bone
(D) involvement of the base of the skull is usually sclerotic
(E) enhancement after administration of gadolinium DTPA is a typical MR finding

Fibrous dysplasia is a skeletal anomaly in which osteoblasts fail to undergo normal morphologic differentiation and maturation. The process is of unknown etiology and may affect one bone (monostotic fibrous dysplasia) or multiple bones (polyostotic fibrous dysplasia). The polyostotic type may be associated with precocious sexual development and cutaneous pigmentation in females; this is known as the McCune-Albright syndrome. In addition to skeletal lesions, abnormal cutaneous pigmentation may be seen in up to one-half of the individuals with polyostotic disease. This consists of café-au-lait spots and pigmented macules related to increased amounts of melanin. These are often located near the midline of the body, overlying the region of the lower spine, sacrum, buttocks, and upper back.

Skeletal abnormality is a primary feature of fibrous dysplasia. Approximately 70 to 80% of affected patients have monostotic fibrous dysplasia; this variety most frequently involves the ribs, femur, tibia, and mandible and less frequently involves the calvarium and humerus. Polyostotic fibrous dysplasia more frequently involves the skull, facial bones, pelvis, spine, and shoulder girdle. Polyostotic fibrous dysplasia may be either unilateral or bilateral in distribution, affecting several bones of a single limb or multiple bones bilaterally.

Involvement of the skull and facial bones is noted in approximately 10 to 25% of patients with monostotic fibrous dysplasia **(Option (A) is false)** and in up to 50% of patients with polyostotic fibrous dysplasia **(Option (B) is false).** Frequently involved anatomic regions include the sphenoid, frontal, maxillary, and ethmoid bones. The occipital and temporal bones are involved less commonly than the other skull bones **(Option (C) is false).** As in the test case, associated findings result primarily from the mass effect of the expanded abnormal bone and include proptosis and exophthalmos with visual impairment, hearing loss with tinnitus or vestibular dysfunction related to narrowing of the internal or external auditory canal, and hyposmia or anosmia with involvement of the cribriform plate.

Monostotic fibrous dysplasia is most frequently recognized in the second and third decades of life; however, it may remain completely asymptomatic. Deformities or enlargement of a bone may compress critical structures such as the cranial nerves, resulting in neurologic deficits. Polyostotic fibrous dysplasia is usually diagnosed in younger patients than is monostotic disease. Up to 85% of patients with polyostotic fibrous dysplasia sustain pathologic fractures, and the resultant skeletal pain is a frequent presenting feature.

Fibrous dysplasia has a variable radiographic appearance, from osteolytic to sclerotic patterns of bone expansion. Characteristically, it produces extensive sclerosis and osseous enlargement (Figure 6-5A), but occasionally the osteolytic features predominate. Involvement of the skull base and facial bones is usually manifested as sclerosis **(Option (D) is true),** while involvement of the calvarium is mixed osteolytic and sclerotic. The sclerotic form of fibrous dysplasia may be radiologically difficult to differentiate from Paget's disease or hyperostosis secondary to meningioma. Involvement of the facial bones and the external occipital protuberance is more common with fibrous dysplasia than with Paget's disease or meningioma. Fibrous dysplasia is also associated with widening of the diploic space and convex outward expansion of the outer table of the cranial vault. Paget's disease, on the other hand, generally maintains the contour of the inner and outer tables despite enlargement of the diploic space; it usually occurs in older patients than does fibrous dysplasia. On MRI, fibrous dysplasia usually results in diffuse low signal intensity on both short-TR/short-TE (T1-weighted) and long-TR/long-TE (T2-weighted) sequences (Figure 6-5B and C).

Spontaneous and recurrent hemorrhage is a documented complication of fibrous dysplasia since the dysplastic tissue is most often hypervascular. This last feature accounts for the enhancement of areas of fibrous dysplasia on CT and MR scans (Figure 6-2D) **(Option (E) is true).**

The natural history of fibrous dysplasia depends on the degree of skeletal involvement. Monostotic disease is usually limited to the initial bone involved (by definition) and generally does not evolve into the

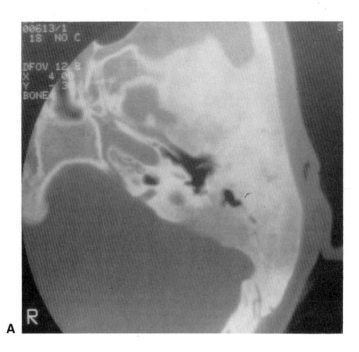

*Figure 6-5.* Fibrous dysplasia of the temporal bone. (A) Axial CT scan through the left temporal bone demonstrates diffuse enlargement of the bone, which encroaches upon the mastoid air cells and middle ear. The bone is of diffuse "ground-glass" density, typical of fibrous dysplasia. Axial T1-weighted (B) and T2-weighted (C) MR scans through the level of the temporal bone are also shown. Note that the left temporal bone has a relatively low signal intensity on both T1- and T2-weighted images (arrows), characteristic of fibrous dysplasia. (Courtesy of H. Ric Harnsberger, University of Utah, Salt Lake City.)

polyostotic form of the disease. Both forms of fibrous dysplasia often become quiescent at puberty and remain dormant during life; however, in rare cases progressive deformity may ensue. Prognosis is poor in these unusual cases, with intervening fractures and persistent symptoms. Hormonal regulation of fibrous dysplasia has been documented, with increased activity noted during pregnancy and exogenous estrogen therapy.

Malignant transformation of fibrous dysplastic lesions is a rare complication, with an estimated frequency of up to 1%. The most common cancers to evolve from fibrous dysplasia are osteogenic sarcoma and fibrosarcoma. Chondrosarcoma occurs less frequently. Prior irradiation of the involved bones may also result in sarcomatous changes. Malignant transformation in patients with monostotic fibrous dysplasia has been

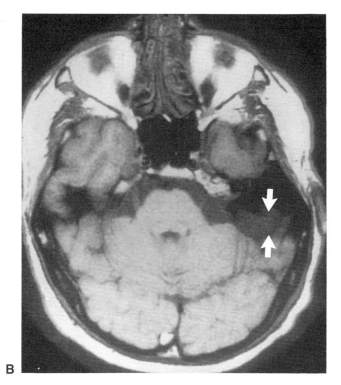

SE 600/20

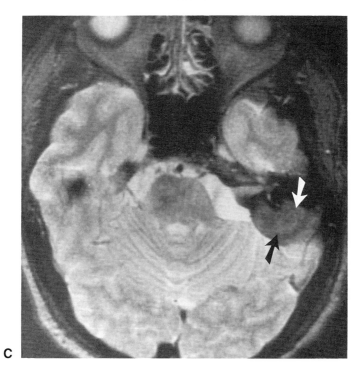

SE 2,800/80

131

noted most often in the skull and facial bones, whereas the femur and facial bones are affected most frequently in the polyostotic variety. Recurrent pain and swelling accompanied by progressive radiographic changes of osteolysis should raise the possibility of intervening malignant transformation.

## Question 30

Concerning mucoceles,

(A) the sphenoid sinus is the most commonly involved sinus
(B) an air-fluid level is usually present
(C) expansion of the sinus is characteristic
(D) they occasionally arise within the middle turbinate
(E) their signal intensity on T1-weighted images is variable

A mucocele of a paranasal sinus most often results from obstruction of the sinus ostium, which results in the replacement of the normal sinus air by sinus secretions. A progressive increase in intraluminal pressure gradually results in sinus cavity expansion. Thus a mucocele is by definition a completely opacified sinus under pressure. The etiologies of sinus obstruction are diverse and include mechanical obstruction by benign or malignant neoplasms, inflammatory mucosal thickening or polyps, and deformities secondary to trauma or surgical manipulation. If the sinus is not surgically aerated, continued secretion of mucus and resorption of water by the sinus mucosa result in a gradual increase in protein content and pressure within the sinus.

Mucoceles most frequently form in the paranasal sinuses that have the narrowest or longest ostia. Therefore the frontal and ethmoidal sinuses are more commonly involved by a mucocele than are the maxillary and sphenoid sinuses (Figure 6-6) **(Option (A) is false).** As mentioned above, the definition of a mucocele is an airless sinus, and therefore in the vast majority of cases an air-fluid level, by definition, does not occur **(Option (B) is false).** If the wall of a mucocele is broken, some fluid can drain out, and infection can occur in the otherwise sterile mucocele. Thus, if a rare air-fluid level is seen on imaging studies, it indicates the presence of a mucopyocele and this most often occurs in the ethmoid sinus. Modeling and expansion of the sinus cavity occur with gradual increases in pressure; these findings are characteristic of mucoceles **(Option (C) is true).**

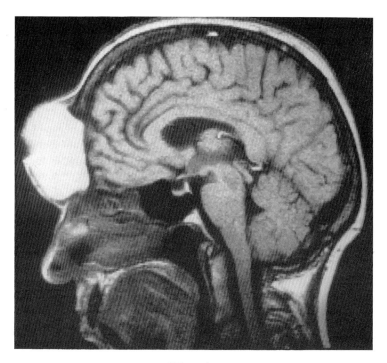

SE 600/20

*Figure 6-6.* Mucocele of the frontal sinus. Sagittal T1-weighted MR image through the left frontal sinus shows an expanded sinus filled with a mucocele that demonstrates a relatively high signal intensity on T1-weighted images, characteristic of T1 shortening due to a high protein content.

Any aerated area of the skull can become obstructed and develop a mucocele. Most commonly, this process involves the main sinus cavities; however, a mucocele may occur in any previously aerated bone such as the pterygoid plate(s) and the anterior clinoid processes. Another unusual site of mucocele formation is a pneumatized middle turbinate (concha bullosa) (Figure 6-7) **(Option (D) is true).**

The presentation of mucoceles depends primarily on the sinuses involved. Frontal or ethmoidal mucoceles enlarge steadily and eventually block the nasofrontal duct. Erosion of the superior medial wall of the orbit with inferolateral displacement of the globe is the classic presentation of a frontal mucocele, whereas lateral displacement of the globe usually occurs with an ethmoid mucocele. Visual loss may occur as a result of compression of the optic nerve within its canal or from extension of inflammatory disease, and this occurs most often with posterior ethmoid

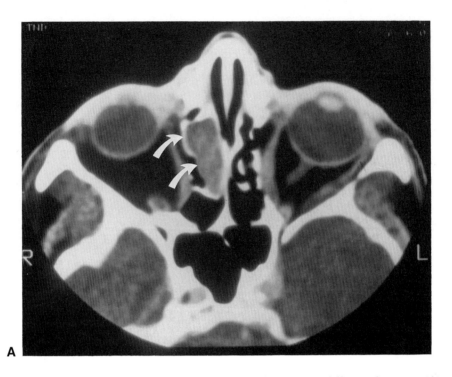

A

*Figure 6-7.* Mucocele of the right ethmoid and middle turbinate. (A) Axial CT scan through the region of the nasal vault demonstrates an expansile soft tissue-density mass (arrows) surrounded by bone. (B) Coronal reformation demonstrates a mucocele (arrows) of the ethmoid sinuses and middle turbinate.

and sphenoid mucoceles. In the maxillary sinus, symptoms or signs of mucocele include a slowly expansile mass in the region of the cheek, unilateral obstruction of the nasal vault, and proptosis with orbital displacement. Mucocele of the sphenoid sinus is a rare entity that can occur alone or in conjunction with an ethmoid mucocele. Sinusitis and polyposis are common underlying processes. A myriad of presentations is possible because of the presence of important contiguous neurologic and vascular structures. These include cavernous sinus syndromes such as diplopia, orbital apex syndrome, and blindness. Sphenoid sinus mucocele may also masquerade clinically as a tumor of the skull base. MRI is usually diagnostic in that such a mucocele generally contains secretions that have an increased signal intensity on T1-weighted images.

The appearance of a mucocele on CT and MRI depends on the protein concentration within the sinus secretions. Initially the secretions are

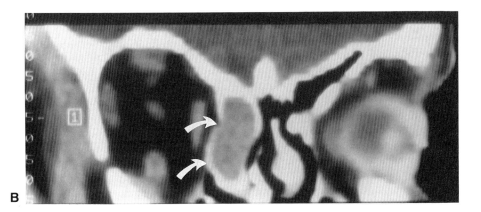

B

predominantly water, and the mucocele therefore has a low attenuation value (0 to 25 HU) on noncontrast CT studies (Figure 6-7). At this point, when the mucocele contains watery secretions, prolonged T1 and T2 relaxation times are seen on MRI, reflecting this high free-water content. Postcontrast scans may demonstrate peripheral mucosal enhancement, but the internal secretions of the mucocele show no enhancement. Over time the sinus secretions gradually inspissate, increasing the protein concentration. This results in increased CT attenuation values as the protein concentration exceeds 25%; the attenuation value may approach that of blood. At this point, the T1 relaxation time begins to shorten and an increased signal intensity on T1-weighted images is observed (Figure 6-6). This is probably the most common MR appearance of mucoceles. The T2-weighted image usually demonstrates high signal intensity as well, reflecting the free-water component of the mucosal secretion. Over time, with gradual inspissation of the secretions, the T2 relaxation time also shortens and low signal intensity may be seen on T2-weighted sequences. With very inspissated mucous secretions, the T2 relaxation time may be so short that no signal intensity is elicited on routine T2- or T1-weighted images. Thus, the obstructed sinus has signal voids and simulates an aerated sinus on T1- and T2-weighted MR scans (Figure 6-3) **(Option (E) is true).** For this reason, the patient with a suspected mucocele is best evaluated radiographically by CT scanning.

The treatment of mucoceles is straightforward. The obstructing lesion must be removed, and a drainage pathway must be established. If this cannot be accomplished, the sinus mucosa must be removed and the sinus must be completely obliterated.

# Question 31

Concerning Langerhans cell histiocytosis,

(A) the chronic recurring (Hand-Schüller-Christian) variety is characterized by monostotic osseous lesions
(B) the osseous lesions are characteristically sclerotic
(C) the temporal bone is involved in about 30% of cases
(D) enlargement of the pituitary infundibulum is an associated finding
(E) diabetes insipidus is most commonly associated with the localized (eosinophilic granuloma) form of the disease

Langerhans cell histiocytosis (LCH), previously referred to as histiocytosis X, is a systemic disease characterized by a proliferation of histiocytic cells in various tissues and organs. The various clinical syndromes, once thought to be separate diseases, are now considered to represent a spectrum of the same disease process. The clinical manifestations vary substantially, ranging from isolated osseous lesions (the localized or eosinophilic granuloma form) to the often fatal multisystem involvement with the fulminant form, previously known as Letterer-Siwe disease. Also within the disease spectrum is another form now called the chronic recurring form and previously referred to as Hand-Schüller-Christian disease, which is characterized by proptosis, diabetes insipidus (DI), and multifocal bone lesions **(Options (A) and (E) are false).**

The etiology of LCH remains uncertain. Currently it is thought that Langerhans cells contribute to the immune response, which suggests that this disease is a manifestation of an immunologic disturbance.

The majority of patients are young and manifest head and neck abnormalities. Therefore, the otolaryngologist and head and neck radiologist will often see the patient at presentation. In one study by DiNardo and Wetmore, 63% of 100 patients aged 6 months to 22 years presented with complaints referable to the head and neck. Osseous lesions of the calvarium occurred most frequently (44%), followed by cutaneous rash, mandibular lesions, cervical adenopathy, and gingival disruption. Of the initial complaints in the head and neck, 50% of the lesions were unifocal, 31% were multifocal, and 19% were diffuse. A slight male predominance has been reported by most investigators. Isolated lesions of the skull were most often noted in the parietal or occipital areas. Classically, the osseous lesions appear as nonsclerotic, lytic foci surrounded by a sharp scalloped or beveled margin (Figure 6-8) **(Option (B) is false).** A soft tissue mass is occasionally the prominent clinical feature of the disease.

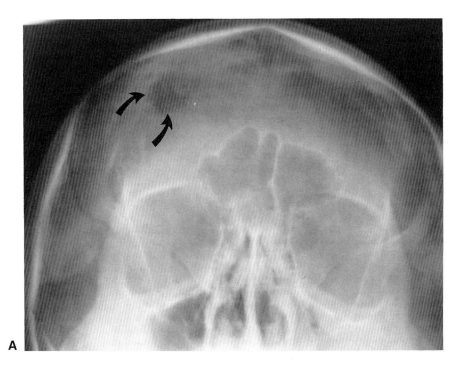

A

*Figure 6-8.* LCH of the calvarium (localized form or eosinophilic granuloma) in a 23-year-old man who had a tender enlarging mass on his skull
for several weeks. (A and B) Waters view (A) and lateral soft tissue view
(B) of the skull demonstrate a nonsclerotic lytic defect (arrows) in the left
frontal bone. The margins of the bone appear beveled on both views. (C)
Bone scintigraphy demonstrates increased uptake in the right frontal
lesion (arrow). (D) Axial CT scan demonstrates the well-circumscribed
lytic lesion centered in the diploic space. Note the oblique margins of
bone destruction that cause the beveled appearance on radiographs.

In the study by DiNardo and Wetmore, no patients with isolated bone
lesions have developed disseminated disease or died.

A cephalic rash was the second most frequent presentation of LCH; it
was seen in 16% of patients in the study of DiNardo and Wetmore. This
more commonly occurs in young, Caucasian, male patients. It represents
the only manifestation of disease in 10% of patients, and it is associated
with multifocal disease in 20% of cases of LCH. Importantly, the
mortality rate in those presenting with cephalic rash is 40%, but it occurs
exclusively in patients with disseminated disease.

An osseous lesion of the mandible occurs in 10 to 15% of patients. Temporal bone involvement with LCH occurs in 11% of cases at presentation.

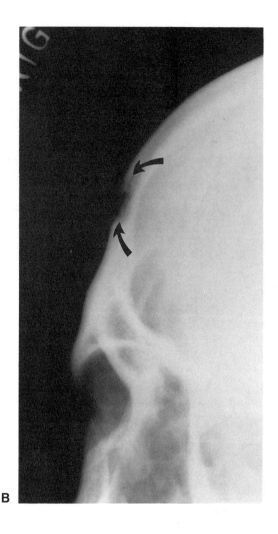

**B**

Many of these patients are younger than 2 years old. Overall, however, aural disease occurs in 20 to 30% of patients **(Option (C) is true).** These patients often present with manifestations of otorrhea and are thought initially to have chronic otitis media. Therefore it is most important to consider the diagnosis of LCH in children under the age of 3 years who have unilateral "chronic otitis media." CT scanning may assist in this determination, because lytic bone destruction is more typical of LCH than it is of chronic otitis media.

Patients presenting with cervical adenopathy as the primary manifestation of LCH are usually boys. Most of these patients have disseminated disease, and up to 20% of them die.

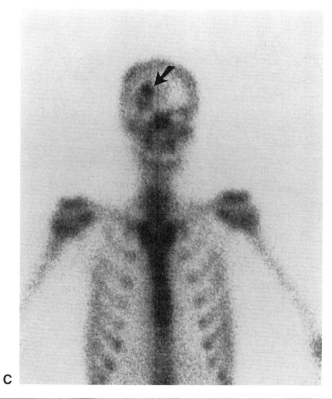

C

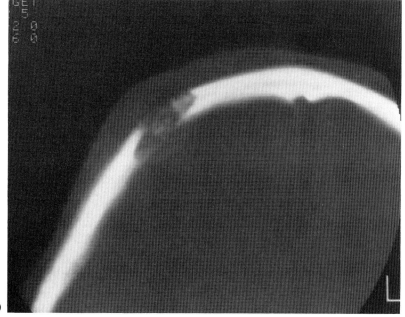

D

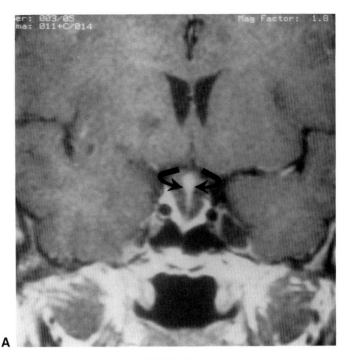

SE 600/20

*Figure 6-9.* LCH involving the pituitary infundibulum. (A) Coronal postcontrast T1-weighted MR image demonstrates an enhancing mass involving the pituitary infundibulum and tuber cinereum (arrows). Enhancement of the infundibulum is normal; however, the bulbous enlargement of the infundibulum in the region of the tuber cinereum is abnormal. (B) Sagittal T1-weighted MR image following administration of contrast material also demonstrates abnormal enhancement near the hypothalamus (arrows). It is this feature that is typical of involvement of the tuber cinereum by LCH. These patients invariably suffer from DI.

DI occurs in 5% of patients at the time of presentation and in approximately 25% of patients with LCH overall. Dunger et al. have suggested that DI results from infiltration of the posterior pituitary or hypothalamus by Langerhans cells, which causes local tissue damage, possibly through excessive production of prostaglandin $E_2$ or interleukin-1. This syndrome is generally associated with an enhancing mass lesion of the pituitary infundibulum **(Option (D) is true).** Contrast-enhanced MR scanning best detects this process (Figure 6-9). Concurrent lesions are diverse and involve the skull, skin, cervical nodes, and gingiva. In the study by Dunger et al., the cumulative risk for developing DI during

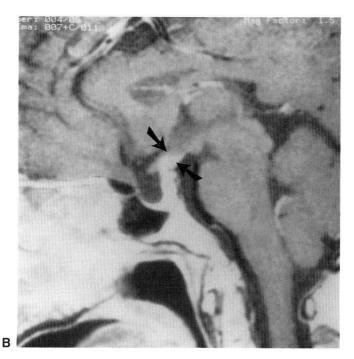

SE 600/20

the first 4 years after presentation and diagnosis of LCH was 42%. DI was most common among young children with multisystem disease, and associated proptosis was common; 47% of the 15 children with DI in the series of Dunger et al. also had proptosis. Subacute deficiency of posterior pituitary gland function may also be more common than previously suspected; 24% of children with LCH had abnormal responses to water deprivation tests, even though none of them had symptoms of DI. Of the five children with abnormal water deprivation responses, two subsequently developed symptomatic DI.

The MR features of children manifesting DI secondary to LCH include absence of the high-intensity signal in the posterior pituitary lobe and an enhancing mass involving the pituitary infundibulum or hypothalamus. The absence of the high-intensity signal within the posterior pituitary lobe reflects the paucity of neurosecretory granules associated with the production of vasopressin. These granules are believed to provide a relaxation sink, shortening the T1 relaxation time.

Radiographically, temporal bone involvement with LCH usually appears as an osteolytic defect without surrounding sclerosis and may demonstrate destructive features similar to those of cholesteatoma.

Mucopurulent otorrhea is the most common presenting symptom, along with bloody otorrhea and painful post-aural swelling. External auditory canal masses are often present, usually in conjunction with erosion of the posterior canal wall. Tympanic membrane perforation is common; however, facial nerve palsy, sensorineural hearing loss, and other manifestations of inner ear disease are infrequent.

LCH is uncommon, and so biopsy of suspicious lesions is imperative for diagnosis. Comprehensive evaluation is required to assess for systemic disease. This would include chest radiograph, skeletal survey, and, if DI is suspected, a water deprivation test and MR scanning of the pituitary gland before and after administration of gadolinium DTPA. Bone marrow evaluation is necessary if there are abnormalities of peripheral blood analysis. On MRI, the temporal bone should be evaluated whenever abnormal enhancement of the pituitary infundibulum is detected, because it may be a preferred area from which to obtain histologic material.

A staging system for LCH based on the age of the patient at presentation, the number of organs involved, and the presence or absence of organ dysfunction has been proposed. In a child under the age of 2 years, involvement of more than four organs in the presence of organ dysfunction indicates the worst prognosis.

Treatment of LCH is tailored to the extent and severity of the disease. Isolated osseous lesions (eosinophilic granuloma) are usually initially treated with either surgical curettage or local irradiation of up to 10 Gy. Multifocal disease is generally treated with chemotherapy. Disseminated LCH still has a very poor prognosis.

*William F. Dillon, M.D.*

SUGGESTED READINGS

FIBROUS DYSPLASIA

1. Feldman F. Tuberous sclerosis, neurofibromatosis, and fibrous dysplasia. In: Resnick D, Niwayama G (eds), Diagnosis of bone and joint disorders, 2nd ed. Philadelphia: WB Saunders; 1988:4033–4072
2. Harris WH, Dudy HR, Barry RJ. The natural history of fibrous dysplasia. J Bone Joint Surg (Am) 1962; 44:207
3. Leeds N, Seaman WB. Fibrous dysplasia of the skull and its differential diagnosis. A clinical and pathologic study of 46 cases. Radiology 1962; 78:570–582

4. Lin JP, Goodkin R, Chase NE, Kricheff II. The angiographic features of fibrous dysplasia of the skull. Radiology 1969; 92:1275–1280
5. Osguthorpe JD, Gudeman SK. Orbital complications of fibrous dysplasia. Otolaryngol Head Neck Surg 1987; 97:403–405
6. Riddell BH. Malignant change in fibrous dysplasia. J Bone Joint Surg (Br) 1964; 46:251

MUCOCELE

7. Avery G, Tang RA, Close LG. Ophthalmic manifestations of mucoceles. Ann Ophthalmol 1983; 15:734–737
8. Dillon WP, Som PM, Fullerton GD. Hypointense MR signal in chronically inspissated sinonasal secretions. Radiology 1990; 174:73–78
9. Hashim AS, Asakura T, Awa H, Yamashita K, Takasaki K, Yuhi F. Giant mucocele of paranasal sinuses. Surg Neurol 1985; 23:69–74
10. Ohnishi T, Ashikawa R, Shirahata Y, Asano Y. Fronto-ethmoidal mucocele—observation of its mode of enlargement. Rhinology 1982; 20:213–221
11. Som PM, Dillon WP, Fullerton GD, Zimmerman RA, Rajagopalan B, Marom Z. Chronically obstructed sinonasal secretions: observations of T1 and T2 shortening. Radiology 1989; 172:515–520
12. Stankiewicz JA. Sphenoid sinus mucocele. Arch Otolaryngol Head Neck Surg 1989; 115:735–740
13. Van Tassel P, Lee YY, Jing BS, De Pena CA. Mucoceles of the paranasal sinuses: MR imaging with CT correlation. AJR 1989; 153:407–412

LANGERHANS CELL HISTIOCYTOSIS

14. Anonsen CK, Donaldson SS. Langerhans' cell histiocytosis of the head and neck. Laryngoscope 1987; 97:537–542
15. DiNardo LJ, Wetmore RF. Head and neck manifestations of histiocytosis-X in children. Laryngoscope 1989; 99:721–724
16. Dunger DB, Broadbent V, Yeoman E, et al. The frequency and natural history of diabetes insipidus in children with Langerhans'-cell histiocytosis. N Engl J Med 1989; 321:1157–1162
17. Jones RO, Pillsbury HC. Histiocytosis X of the head and neck. Laryngoscope 1984; 94:1031–1035
18. Smith RJ, Evans JN. Head and neck manifestations of histiocytosis-X. Laryngoscope 1984; 94:395–399
19. Stoll MA, Kransdorf MJ, Devaney KO. Langerhans cell histiocytosis of bone. RadioGraphics 1992; 12:801:–823

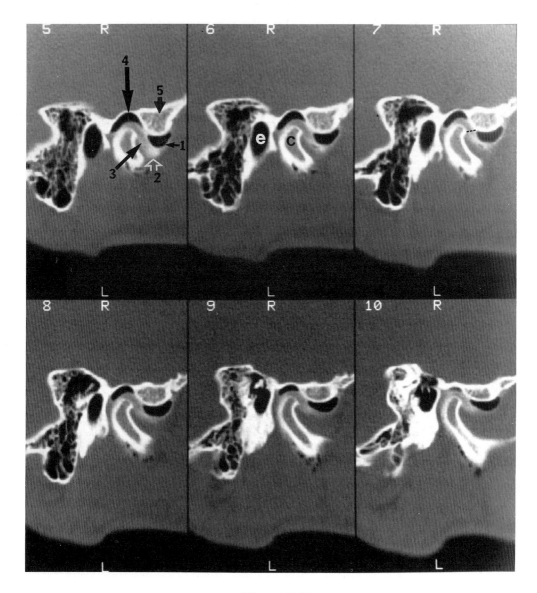

*Figure 7-1*

# Case 7: Temporomandibular Joint Anatomy

## Questions 32 through 36

You are shown a series of direct sagittal CT images from an air-positive contrast arthrogram of a normal left temporomandibular joint (Figure 7-1). For each numbered arrow (Questions 32 through 36), select the *one* lettered part of the anatomy (A, B, C, D, or E) that is MOST closely associated with it.

32. Arrow 1
33. Arrow 2
34. Arrow 3
35. Arrow 4
36. Arrow 5

   (A)  Meniscus
   (B)  Anterior recess of superior joint space
   (C)  Articular eminence
   (D)  Posterior recess of superior joint space
   (E)  Anterior recess of inferior joint space

Figure 7-1 represents a consecutive series of double-contrast (air and iodinated contrast agent) direct sagittal images (extending medially from the section labeled number 5 to that labeled number 10) of a normal left temporomandibular joint (TMJ) in the closed-mouth position. The images demonstrate the external auditory canal (e), mandibular condyle (c), air in the anterior and posterior recesses (arrows 1 and 4) of the superior TMJ space **(Options (B) and (D) are the correct answers to Questions 32 and 35, respectively),** the articular eminence (arrow 5) **(Option (C) is the correct answer to Question 36),** and iodinated contrast material in the anterior recess of the inferior joint space (arrow 2) **(Option (E) is the correct answer to Question 33).** Arrow 3 indicates the meniscus **(Option (A) is the correct answer to Question 34)** outlined by air and iodinated contrast in the superior and inferior joint spaces, respectively. The posterior band of the meniscus (disk) is at the top of the condyle. The anterior band is shown by arrow 3. The intermediate zone of the meniscus is located between the anterior and posterior bands. A disk is said to be in the normal position when the posterior band is at the anterior portion of the superior surface of the condyle, the so-called 11 to 12 o'clock or 12 to 1 o'clock position of the condyle, depending upon the orientation of the condyle. Alternatively, a line can be drawn from a point at the junction between the anterior and superior surfaces of the condyle to a point along the most inferior margin of the posterior slope of the articular eminence (dashed line in section 7). A disk is considered normal when this line passes through the intermediate zone of the meniscus. On the more medial scans (sections 9 and 10), through the middle ear cavity, the malleus (anterior) and incus posterior to the malleus are delineated.

## Question 37

Concerning the temporomandibular joint meniscus,

- (A) it is a fibrous articular disk
- (B) it divides the joint into superior and inferior compartments
- (C) the fibrous joint capsule is attached to its medial and lateral margins
- (D) the tendon of the superior head of the lateral pterygoid muscle inserts into it
- (E) the tendon of the inferior head of the lateral pterygoid muscle inserts into it
- (F) the posterior band is thinner than the anterior band

The TMJ is a diarthrodial synovial joint capable of both translation and rotation. The head of the mandible articulates with the glenoid fossa and articular eminence of the temporal bone. The anterior and superior aspects of the joint are formed by the articular eminence of the temporal bone. The posterior and superior aspects of the joint are bounded by the glenoid fossa and the tympanic portion of the temporal bone. The inferior aspect of the joint is bounded by the superior and anterior surfaces of the mandibular condyle (Figures 7-1 through 7-3).

The glenoid fossa, anterior articular eminence, and mandibular condyle surfaces are lined with fibrous connective tissue. Beneath this layer of fibrous connective tissue lies hyaline cartilage. Interposed between these osseous boundaries is the articular disk or meniscus, composed of fibrous connective tissue **(Option (A) is true),** attaching anteriorly and posteriorly in a vascular plexus. These attachments are termed the

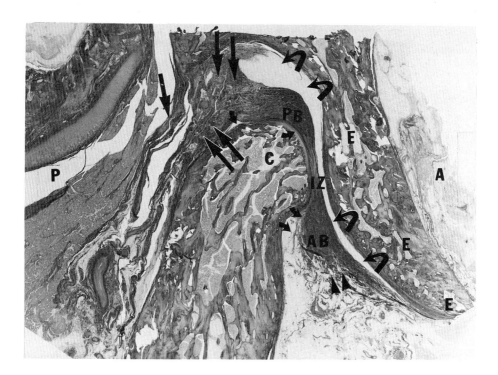

*Figure 7-2.* Sagittal microscopic section through the TMJ. The fibrous disk separates the joint into two separate compartments, the superior (long curved arrows) and inferior (short curved arrows) joint spaces. The surfaces of the glenoid fossa, articular eminence (E), and condyle (C) are lined with fibrous connective tissue, beneath which lies hyaline cartilage. A vascular plexus is found posterior (straight arrows) and anterior (arrowheads) to the disk. The anterior vascular plexus is called the anterior attachment (arrowheads). The portion of the retrodiscal tissue that inserts into the posterior edge of the disk is called the posterior attachment. Notice the parts of the disk that are clearly visible: posterior band (PB), intermediate zone (IZ), and anterior band (AB). A = anterior; P = posterior. (Figure courtesy of Leslie Heffez, D.M.D., University of Illinois, Chicago.)

anterior attachment and retrodiscal tissue. The portion of the retrodiscal tissue that inserts into the posterior edge of the disk is called the posterior attachment (Figure 7-2). There is a general progression of vascular to less vascular to fibrous connective tissue posteroanteriorly, so that there is no clear delineation between retrodiscal tissue and the disk. The disk divides the joint cavity into two separate synovial compartments or spaces, the superior and inferior joint spaces **(Option (B) is true).** These two joint spaces do not normally communicate. A fibrous capsule surrounding the joint is attached to the medial and lateral margins of the

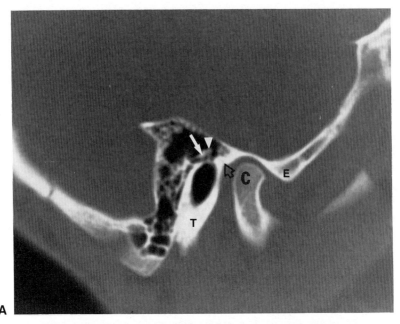

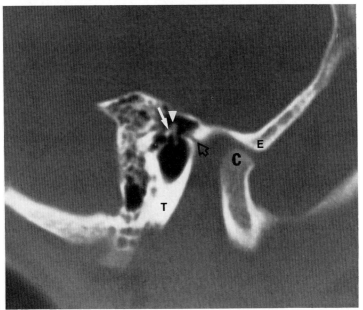

*Figure 7-3.* Sagittal CT scans show a central section of the TMJ in the closed-mouth (A) and open-mouth (B) positions. The relationship between the normal condyle (C), glenoid fossa, and anterior articular eminence (E) is clearly seen. Notice the tympanic bone (T), incus (long arrow), malleus (arrowhead), and squamotympanic fissure (open arrow).

disk **(Option (C) is true),** the perimeter of the glenoid fossa, and the head of the condyle. Anteriorly the disk is attached to the capsule via the anterior attachment; anteromedially, the tendon of the superior head of the lateral pterygoid muscle inserts into the meniscus, while the inferior head of the lateral pterygoid muscle inserts into the mandibular condyle **(Option (D) is true; Option (E) is false).** Thus, the meniscus is secured posteriorly by the retrodiscal tissue (bilaminar zone) and joint capsule. The bilaminar zone is composed of two layers of elastic tissue separated by a highly vascular zone containing the branches of the auriculotemporal, masseteric, and posterior deep temporal nerves. The meniscus has an elongated biconcave, "bow tie" configuration with a moderately thick anterior band, a thicker posterior band **(Option (F) is false),** and a thin intermediate zone. Its undersurface is concave to conform to the shape of the mandibular condyle, and the upper surface of the posterior band is relatively convex to match the convexity of the articular fossa of the temporal bone. The head of the mandible does not merely rotate in the articular (glenoid) fossa; it moves forward into and under the articular eminence of the temporal bone, taking the articular disk with it. Closed-mouth articulation occurs between the condyle and both the posterior articular eminence and glenoid fossa, anterior to the squamo-tympanic fissure (Figure 7-3A). Open-mouth articulation occurs along the inferior and posterior aspect of the articular eminence (Figure 7-3B).

The normal relationship of the disk and the condyle is nearly the same at rest and during opening. The retrodiscal fibroelastic and areolar tissues expand and contract in the opening and resting positions (Figure 7-4). On opening, there will be some change in the shape of the meniscus as compared with that at rest. On mandibular opening, the retromandibular vascular zone engorges with blood, partially filling the space vacated by the mandibular condyle.

A disk is said to be in the normal position when its intermediate zone lies at a location connecting the anterosuperior surface of the condyle and the posteroinferior slope of the articular eminence (Figures 7-2, 7-5, and 7-6). Alternatively, one can look for the position of the posterior band above the condyle, in the so-called 11 to 12 or 12 to 1 o'clock position relative to the position and orientation of the condylar head. This definition is rather subjective and therefore does not allow for complete discrimination between a normal meniscus and a slightly subluxed meniscus. In equivocal cases, one should rely on the position of the meniscus on both the closed- and open-mouth views (Figure 7-7). This allows better evaluation of the position of the meniscus.

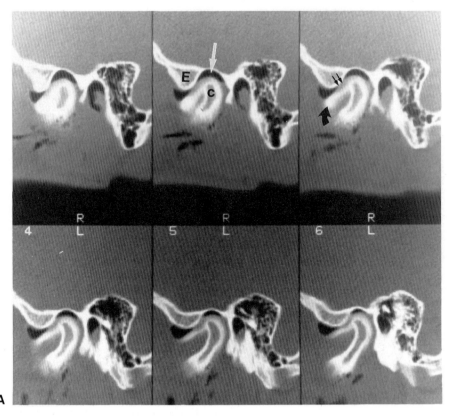

*Figure 7-4.* (A) Series of sagittal double-contrast CT images (extending from lateral to medial) of the right TMJ in the closed-mouth position demonstrating the normal condyle (c), disk (black arrows), and articular eminence (E). Note the air (white arrow) in the superior joint space and contrast (curved arrow) in the inferior joint space. (B) Series of sagittal double-contrast CT images (extending from lateral to medial) of the right TMJ in the open-mouth position. The relationship between the normal condyle (c), disk (straight black arrows), and articular eminence (E) is seen. There is stretching of the retrodiscal tissue (arrowheads). There is air (white arrow) in the superior joint spaces and contrast (curved arrows) in the inferior joint spaces. Note the altered shape of the meniscus from the closed-mouth (A) to the open-mouth (B) position.

Several imaging techniques exist for evaluating condyle-disk-glenoid fossa and condyle-disk-articular eminence relationships. The technique of TMJ arthrography was pioneered by Norgaard in 1944 and has since been modified by several investigators. The disk and the posterior attachment cannot be seen on conventional radiographs and are demonstrated only on conventional or CT-contrast arthrography or MRI (Fig-

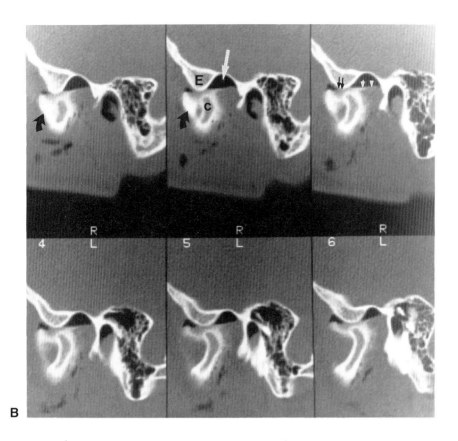

B

ures 7-1 and 7-5). Direct sagittal CT images can be obtained by using a sagittal head holder. MRI provides better information on meniscal anatomy and pathologic alterations than does CT (Figure 7-5). Straight or oblique sagittal MR sections perpendicular to the long axis of the condyles satisfactorily depict the normal meniscus and its anterior or posterior dislocated position. Lateral or medial displacement of the meniscus is better assessed on coronal MR scans. All MR scans presented in this discussion were performed with a 1.5-T superconductive MR imager, using the body coil as the transmitter and a 7.5-cm-diameter circular surface coil as the receiver. Most images were obtained with a 256 × 256 matrix, four excitations, a section thickness of 3 mm, and a field of view of 12 or 16 cm, with the jaw at rest. A spin-echo multislice technique with a TR of 600 to 1,000 msec and a TE of 20 to 30 msec was used to obtain T1-weighted images. For an open-mouth position, a 256 × 128 matrix was used with the other factors the same as for the

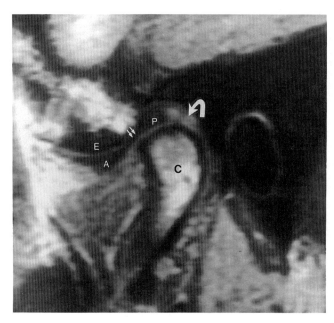

SE 700/20

*Figure 7-5.* T1-weighted central sagittal section of the TMJ in the closed-mouth position. The relationship between the normal condyle (C) and the articular eminence (E) is seen. Note the disk anatomy represented by a low signal intensity: posterior band (P), intermediate zone (straight arrows), and anterior band (A). The intermediate zone is positioned between the posterior slope of the eminence and the anterior surface of the condyle. The retrodiscal tissue is represented by a heterogeneous intermediate signal intensity (curved arrow). The compact bony covering of the condyle is smooth. Compare the anatomy demonstrated here with that of the sagittal microscopic section in Figure 7-6.

closed-mouth position. A disposable mouth prop was used to obtain open-mouth MR images. Proton-weighted and T2-weighted images, with a long TR (2,000 msec) for both, a short TE (30 msec) for proton-weighted images, and a long TE (80 msec) for T2-weighted images, were used to evaluate fluid within the joint and/or inflammatory changes of the TMJ. A low-flip-angle, fast-scanning technique, or gradient-echo or gradient-recalled acquisition in the steady state (GRASS), was used to decrease the imaging time and, in particular, to evaluate joint effusion as well as increased vascularity of the retrodiscal tissues.

Although diverse pathologic conditions can affect the TMJ, the most common is the internal derangement, which represents an abnormal internal structural and functional change of the meniscus, as well as an

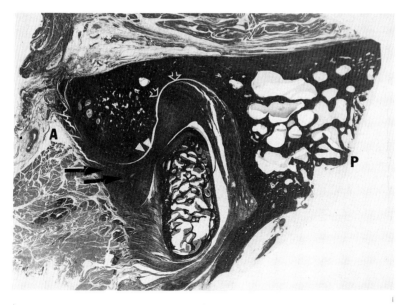

*Figure 7-6.* Sagittal microscopic section of a normal TMJ demonstrating the posterior band (open arrows), intermediate zone (arrowheads), and anterior band (black arrows). A = anterior; P = posterior. (Figure courtesy of Leslie Heffez, D.M.D.)

abnormal relationship of the meniscus to the condyle, fossa, and articular eminence when the teeth are in the closed-mouth position. This includes disk perforation, fragmentation, and dislocation. The disk is usually displaced anteriorly (Figure 7-8), and it is frequently associated with perforation of the posterior disk attachment. The pathophysiology of internal derangement of the TMJ is believed to be related to loss of the ability of the posterior meniscal attachment to counteract the pulling forces of the lateral pterygoid muscle. When this phenomenon occurs, the meniscus remains anterior to the condyle during closure and the condyle impinges directly upon the posterior neurovascular zone (Figure 7-8). McCarty and Farrar reported that more than 70% of patients with TMJ problems have some form of meniscal displacement. Internal derangement of the TMJ is usually divided into subluxation and dislocation. Anterior disk displacement may result in symptomatic abnormal TMJ function. The ability of the condyle to negotiate around the displaced disk is termed "reduction." Anterior meniscal displacement with reduction on opening (referred to by some authors as subluxation) (Figure 7-9) is often accompanied by audible clicking noises. This is because a reducing disk

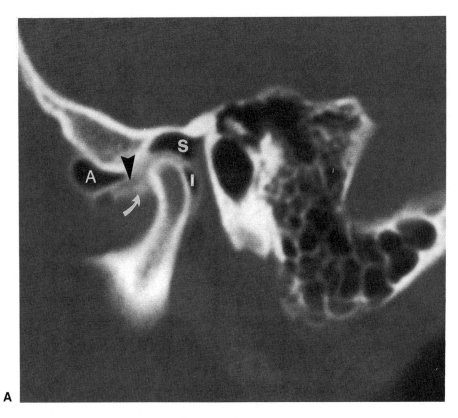

**A**

*Figure 7-7.* Anterior dislocation without reduction. A sagittal CT air-contrast arthrogram in the closed-mouth position, with a dislocated right meniscus (arrowhead), is shown. There is air in the superior (S) and inferior (I) joint spaces. Air is also present in the anterior recess (A) of the superior joint space, and iodinated contrast is present in the anterior recess of the inferior joint space (arrow). (B) Sagittal CT air-contrast arthrogram in the open-mouth position, showing the nonreduced meniscus (arrowhead) being displaced anteriorly. There is stretching of the retrodiscal tissue (curved arrow).

displacement is characterized by a reciprocal clicking as the condyle jumps around the displaced disk upon opening and then slips off the posterior edge of the disk upon closing. Anterior meniscal displacement without reduction on jaw opening (referred to by some authors as dislocation) implies that the condyle is unable to negotiate past the displaced disk (Figure 7-10). This represents a more severe stage of internal derangement of the TMJ and is often accompanied by chronic pain and limitation of opening (closed lock). Clinically, the condyle may

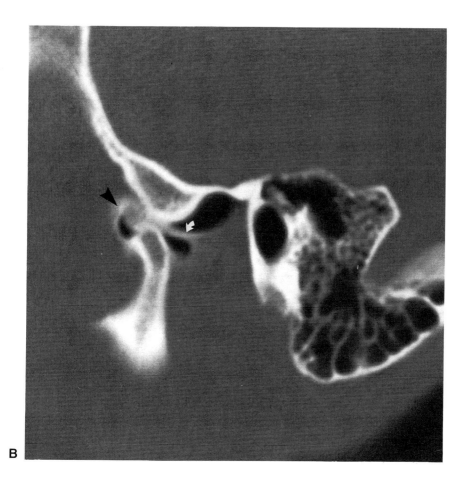

B

demonstrate limited translation; however, this is not always the case. In internal derangements, the disk often becomes displaced forward and usually medially. The posterior attachment undergoes a remodeling process. Compression and friction, possibly secondary to deterioration of the synovial tissue, elicit compensatory changes involving decreased vascularity, fibrosis, and the presence of cartilage cells.

In some cases a distinct posterior band, intermediate zone, and anterior band are no longer discernible (Figure 7-11). As the disk is progressively displaced forward, the retrodiscal tissue is stretched forward over the condyle surface. This tissue then undergoes progressive remodeling. With advanced remodeling, this tissue can resemble the disk (Figure 7-12).

*Text continues on page 161*

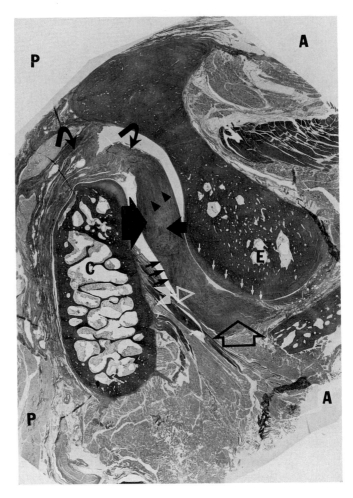

*Figure 7-8.* Sagittal microscopic section of internal derangement. In internal derangements the disk becomes displaced forward and usually medially. The posterior band (large black arrows) of the disk undergoes deformation. In some cases the posterior band, intermediate zone, and anterior band are no longer distinct. The anatomy of the disk illustrated here is still preserved, and the posterior band, intermediate zone (small black arrows), and anterior band (open black arrow and open white arrow) are all present. As the disc is progressively displaced forward, the retro-discal tissue (curved arrows) is stretched forward over the condyle surface. This tissue then undergoes progressive remodeling. With advanced remodeling, this tissue can resemble the disk because it is devoid of vascularity. The approximate delineation between the deformed posterior band and remodeled retrodiscal tissue is indicated (black arrow-heads). There is thickening of the fibrous connective tissue lining the eminence (series of small white arrows). A = anterior; C = condyle; E = eminence; P = posterior. (Figure courtesy of Leslie Heffez, D.M.D.)

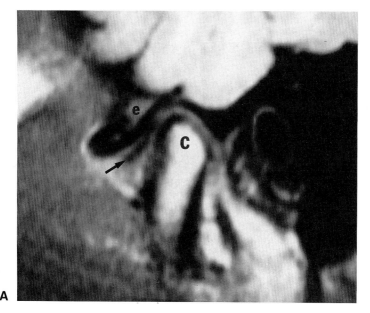

SE 700/20

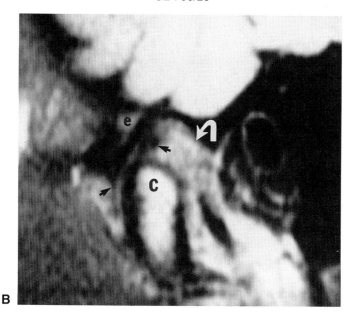

SE 600/20

*Figure 7-9.* Anterior disk displacement with reduction. A central-section, sagittal T1-weighted image of the TMJ in the closed-mouth position is shown. There is slight anterior displacement with reduction (see panel B). The disk is straight (arrow) with no clear delineation of the posterior band, intermediate zone, and anterior band. The remodeled retrodiscal tissue (intermediate signal intensity) lies above the condyle. The cortical bone of the condyle (C), glenoid fossa, and eminence (e) is smooth. (B) Open-mouth position. With slight translation and rotation of the condyle (C), the disk appears to be positioned normally (arrows). The disk shape in the open- and closed-mouth positions may be a factor in deformation. In the closed-mouth position the disk shape was not clear, and in the open-mouth position the disk shape is irregular with poor delineation of its intermediate zone. Note the intermediate signal intensity of the retro-discal tissue (curved arrow) enveloping the posterior band. e = eminence.

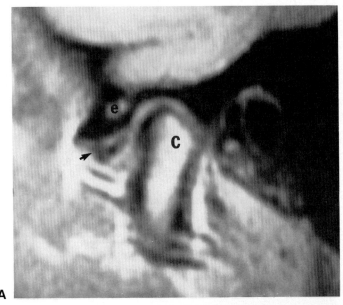

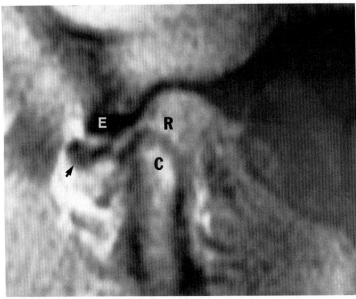

*Figure 7-10.* Anterior disk displacement without reduction. A central-section T1-weighted MR scan of the TMJ in the closed-mouth position is shown. Note the displaced meniscus (arrow) anterior to the condyle (C) and inferior to the eminence (e). The retrodiscal tissues covering the glenoid fossa and eminence are represented by the thin intermediate-intensity material over the condyle. (B) A central T1-weighted MR section of the TMJ in the open-mouth position. There is marked anterior disk displacement without reduction (arrow). The thickened part of the disk has been displaced anterior to the eminence (E). Note the expanded retrodiscal tissue (R) represented by the intermediate-intensity material. C = condyle.

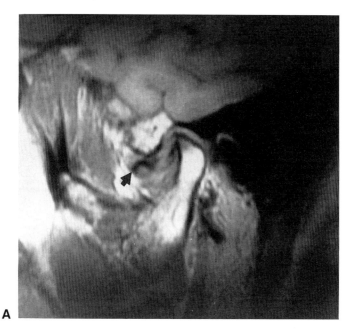

SE 900/20

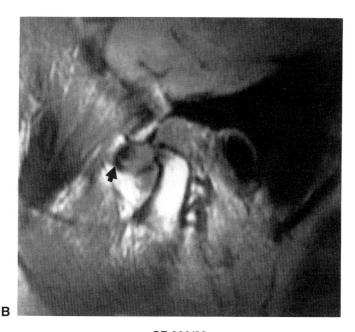

SE 900/20

*Figure 7-11.* Anterior disk displacement without reduction. A central-section T1-weighted scan of the TMJ in the closed-mouth (A) and open-mouth (B) positions, with a deformed buckled disk (arrow) that is displaced anteriorly, is shown.

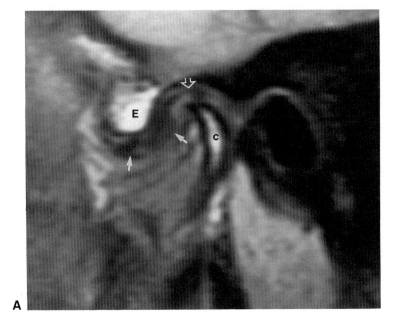

SE 700/20

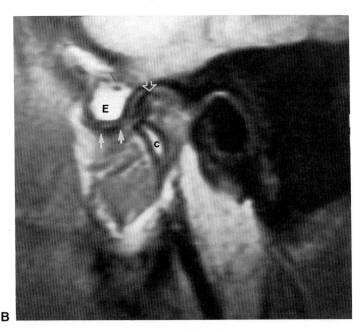

SE 600/20

*Figure 7-12.* Anterior disk displacement with remodeling of retrodiscal tissue. A central-section T1-weighted scan of the TMJ in the closed-mouth (A) and open-mouth (B) positions, with a buckled, anteriorly displaced meniscus (solid arrows), is shown. The low-intensity signal at the top of the condyle (open arrow) is due to remodeled and fibrotic retrodiscal tissue. C = condyle; E = eminence.

*Text continued from page 155*

TMJ dysfunction due to internal derangement is reportedly a fairly common abnormality. The clinical symptoms and signs consist of headache, periauricular pain, joint clicking, limitation of jaw movement, and tightness of the facial musculature. The etiology of internal derangement of the TMJ apparently involves a spectrum of traumatic conditions, including microtrauma (intubation, prolonged dental procedures, bruxism, masticatory muscle spasm, and malocclusion) and macrotrauma (fracture, dislocation, and hemarthrosis), as well as degenerative and inflammatory joint diseases (e.g., osteoarthritis, rheumatoid arthritis, and psoriatic arthritis). Trauma to the TMJ may cause injury to the articular tissues, resulting in condylar fractures and traumatic arthritis. Ankylosis, fibrous adhesions, and limitation or deviation of jaw opening can follow a traumatic event. In 1948, Wakeley described anteromedial displacement of the articular disk as a result of trauma to the mandible. He speculated that the pull of the lateral pterygoid muscle, along with the traumatic force, causes a stretching of the posterior attachment of the meniscus. Weinberg and Lapointe suggested that cervical extension-flexion (whiplash) injury may lead to internal derangement. They postulated that the force applied to the condylar neck could be transmitted to the TMJ and might result in stretching, crushing, tearing, or perforation of the posterior attachment tissue.

It is not clear whether there is absolute progression from an early stage of internal derangement with slight deformation of the posterior band to a late stage with severe resorption of the posterior band, bony remodeling, and perforation of the posterior attachment. The phenomenon of internal derangement has recently been the subject of some scrutiny. Symptoms such as preauricular pain, inability to open the mouth (closed lock), and stiffness or tightness of the facial musculature do not seem to correlate with the severity of the internal derangement (displacement and deformation). Clinicians have long recognized that the presence of a disk displacement per se is not an indication for surgical treatment. The sole indication remains moderate to severe pain and dysfunction that is refractory to a reasonable course of nonsurgical therapy and that significantly interferes with the patient's daily routine. CT and MR findings simply assist the surgeon in the appropriate evaluation of the TMJ disorders. Studies of the clinical relevance of the changes in signal intensity of the disk, posterior attachment, and extracapsular tissues are pending. CT is an excellent means of evaluating pre- and postoperative ankylosis. Sagittal and coronal images help the clinician determine the optimum level for arthroplasty (condyle, condylar neck, ramus, or angle). The position of proplast-Teflon laminated implants may best be followed by using direct sagittal CT. Although most clinicians have now abandoned these alloplasts, many patients have good functional results with these implants. The post-diskectomy bony remodeling changes may be similarly monitored by CT scanning.

In general, imaging of the TMJ by CT and MRI has enhanced the clinician's and radiologist's understanding of the pathogenesis of internal derangements. The radiologist and clinician may derive information on disk displacement and deformation. CT and MRI allow excellent evaluation of traumatic, neoplastic, developmental, and congenital deformities of the TMJ.

*Mahmood M. Mafee, M.D.*

## SUGGESTED READINGS

1. Beltran J, Schoenberg N. MRI of the TMJ: static and kinematic studies. Appl Radiol 1991; 12:40–43
2. Helms CA, Kaban LB, McNeill C, Dodson T. Temporomandibular joint: morphology and signal intensity characteristics of the disk at MR imaging. Radiology 1989; 172:817–820
3. Katzberg RW. Temporomandibular joint imaging. Radiology 1989; 170:297–307
4. Katzberg RW, Bessette RW, Tallents RH, et al. Normal and abnormal temporomandibular joint: MR imaging with surface coil. Radiology 1986; 158:183–189
5. Mafee MF, Heffez L, Campos M, et al. Temporomandibular joint: role of direct sagittal CT air-contrast arthrogram and MRI. Otolaryngol Clin North Am 1988; 21:575–588
6. Mafee MF, Kumar A, Tahmoressi CN, et al. Direct sagittal CT in the evaluation of temporal bone disease. AJR 1988; 150:1403–1410
7. McCarty WL, Farrar WB. Surgery for internal derangements of the temporomandibular joint. J Prosthet Dent 1979; 42:191–196
8. Norgaard F. Arthrography of the temporomandibular joint. Acta Radiol 1944; 25:679–685
9. Rao VM, Farole A, Karasick D. Temporomandibular joint dysfunction: correlation of MR imaging, arthrography, and arthroscopy. Radiology 1990; 174:663–667
10. Scapino RP. The posterior attachment: its structure, function and appearance in TMJ imaging studies. Part II. J Craniomandib Disord Facial Oral Pain 1991; 5:155–166
11. Toller PA. Opaque arthrography of the temporomandibular joint. Int J Oral Surg 1974; 3:17–28
12. Wakeley C. The mandibular joint. Ann R Coll Surg 1948; 2:111–120
13. Weinberg S, Lapointe H. Cervical extension-flexion injury (whiplash) and

internal derangement of the temporomandibular joint. J Oral Maxillofac Surg 1987; 45:653–656

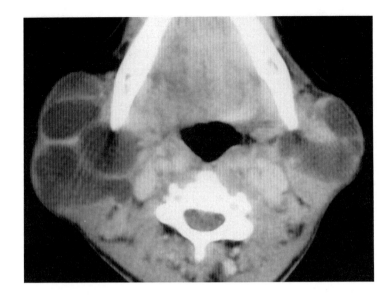

*Figure 8-1*

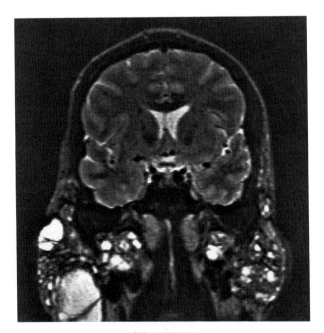

SE 2,000/90

*Figure 8-2*

*Figures 8-1 and 8-2.* You are shown an axial postcontrast CT scan of a 32-year-old man with multiple palpable cervical lymph nodes and bilateral parotid gland enlargement (Figure 8-1). You are also shown a coronal T2-weighted MR scan of another patient, a 28-year-old man with the same clinical findings (Figure 8-2).

# Case 8:  Lymphoepithelial Parotid Cysts

## Question 38

Which *one* of the following is the MOST likely diagnosis in these two patients?

(A) Sarcoidosis
(B) Lymphoepithelial parotid cysts
(C) Warthin's tumors (papillary cystadenoma lymphomatosum)
(D) Non-Hodgkin's lymphoma
(E) Abscesses

The test images (Figures 8-1 and 8-2) show diffuse bilateral parotid gland enlargement. The CT scan of the first patient (Figure 8-1) shows multiple smoothly marginated cystic areas in both parotid glands. The T2-weighted MR image of the second patient shows multiple areas of high signal intensity involving both the superficial and deep portions of each gland. These areas are also consistent with the cysts seen in Figure 8-1. The cysts vary from a few millimeters to a few centimeters in diameter. There is also diffuse prominence of the lymphoid tissue (adenoids) in the nasopharynx (Figure 8-3). In male patients, these findings, along with the multiple palpable cervical lymph nodes, strongly suggest the diagnosis of multiple lymphoepithelial parotid cysts **(Option (B) is correct)** in association with human immunodeficiency virus (HIV) infection. The etiology of the cysts is unclear. They may represent an obstructive phenomenon at the distal ducts secondary to a lymphoid infiltration of the parotid interstitial tissues, they may be cystically degenerated intraparotid lymph nodes, or, most probably, they may be secondary to a combination of these etiologies. Not all cases of parotid enlargement in HIV-infected patients show these characteristic cysts; instead, some show solid masses or both cystic and solid lesions. Rarely, only unilateral parotid involvement is apparent clinically and by imaging in an HIV-infected patient. However, in such cases there usually are microscopic lesions bilaterally.

Sarcoidosis (Option (A)) is a multisystem granulomatous disease of unknown etiology. The disease most commonly involves the lymph nodes,

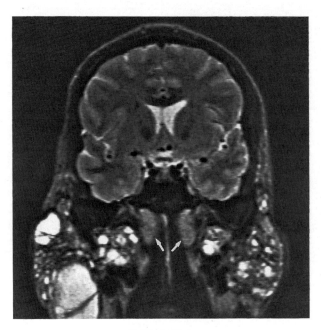

SE 2,000/90

*Figure 8-3* (Same as Figure 8-2). Lymphoepithelial parotid cysts. Coronal T2-weighted MR scan of the second test patient shows diffuse bilateral parotid gland enlargement. The parotid glands contain multiple cysts of high signal intensity that vary in diameter from a few millimeters to a few centimeters. There is also hypertrophy of the visible lymphoid tissue in the nasopharynx (arrows).

lungs, skin, liver, spleen, eyes, and parotid glands. In some cases, parotid gland involvement is the only manifestation of sarcoidosis, but there most often is evidence of the disease elsewhere in the body, especially in the mediastinum or lungs.

Clinically detectable parotid gland involvement occurs in up to 30% of patients with systemic sarcoidosis. The typical clinical manifestation of parotid involvement is diffuse, painless swelling that may or may not be nodular, and there is bilateral (although usually asymmetric) involvement in up to 80% of cases.

On CT or MRI, parotid gland sarcoidosis appears as mild diffuse enlargement of the parotid gland(s), with or without discrete parotid masses of variable size (Figure 8-4). These masses are sharply marginated and represent granulomas either in the intraparotid lymph nodes or within the parotid parenchyma. Typically, these lesions have a homogeneous or a fine, honeycombed (foamy) appearance on CT or MRI. The multiple

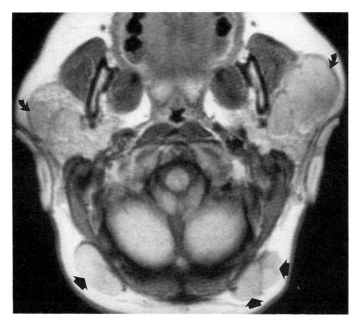

SE 700/20

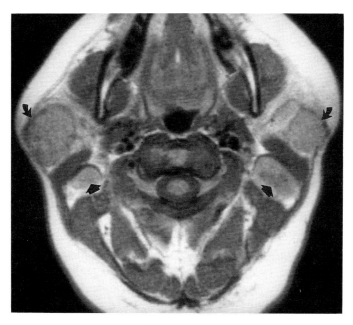

SE 700/20

*Figure 8-4.* Parotid gland sarcoidosis. Axial T1-weighted MR images show large, bilateral, isointense masses in the parotid glands. These masses cause diffuse enlargement of the superficial lobes bilaterally (curved arrows), with lesser involvement of the deep lobes. There are also multiple extraparotid nodes adjacent to the glands posteriorly, in the posterior cervical triangle and in the occipital regions bilaterally (straight arrows).

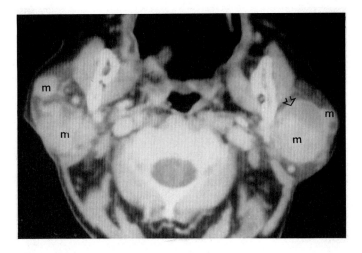

*Figure 8-5.* Bilateral Warthin's tumors. Postcontrast axial CT scan shows multiple bilateral parotid masses (m). The lesions are smoothly marginated, and cystic change is seen in the largest lesion on the left (arrow).

cystic lesions of widely varying size seen in the test patients are unlikely to represent sarcoidosis, which is usually characterized by fewer, larger, and often more uniformly sized solid lesions. In addition, the presence of enlarged adenoids in a male patient with no history of chest disease does not suggest sarcoidosis. The differential diagnosis of sarcoidosis includes other granulomatous diseases such as tuberculosis and atypical myco-bacterial infections.

Warthin's tumors (papillary cystadenoma lymphomatosum) (Option (C)) are the second most common benign tumors of the parotid gland (after pleomorphic adenomas [benign mixed tumors]). They represent 5 to 15% of all benign parotid tumors and are the most common parotid neoplasms to present bilaterally. Typically, they are found in men over the age of 50 years and they present as slow-growing tumors in the parotid gland tail. On both CT and MRI, these tumors are usually well marginated and, when small, are homogeneous in appearance. When they are large, they typically undergo cystic change and on imaging have a less homo-geneous appearance than the lesions in the test case (Figure 8-5). Cervical adenopathy and enlarged adenoids are not findings suggestive of Warthin's tumors.

Non-Hodgkin's lymphoma (Option (D)) may occasionally arise as a primary tumor in the parotid gland; however, most often the parotid gland is involved as part of a generalized lymphomatosis disease process.

Overall, involvement of the salivary glands by non-Hodgkin's lymphoma is rare, occurring in only 5% of cases. Non-Hodgkin's lymphoma of the parotid glands usually appears on CT or MRI as several smoothly marginated solid tumors, possibly in association with cervical adenopathy (Figure 8-6). The occasional presence of central tumor necrosis may cause some lesions to appear heterogeneous; however, frank cysts like those in the test images are rare.

Multiple abscesses in the parotid gland (Option (E)) are rare, and today they usually develop in immunocompromised or diabetic patients. Several decades ago, such abscesses used to occur as an expected postoperative complication secondary to dehydration and poor oral hygiene, which allowed infections in the mouth to ascend to the parotid glands. However, with today's better postoperative care, such postoperative abscesses rarely occur.

The typical parotid abscess develops following an indolent course of sialadenitis, typically untreated. Usually the abscess remains confined to the parotid gland because pain secondary to adjacent cellulitis causes the patient to seek medical attention promptly. Clinically, the abscess presents as a painful swelling of the parotid gland. Fever and trismus are typical, and cervical adenopathy is occasionally present. The clinical diagnosis of abscess is usually made because of a lack of a response to antibiotic therapy. Uncomplicated sialadenitis usually responds to such therapy.

CT or MRI documents the presence of parotid abscesses as discrete, fluid-filled cavities. An abscess typically has thickened, slightly irregular borders, which show intense enhancement after administration of contrast agent. Reactive changes in the overlying soft tissues are almost always present, reflecting an associated cellulitis (Figure 8-7). The test images do not show evidence of cellulitis, there are many smooth-walled cysts, and there was no history of pain; therefore, parotid abscess is an unlikely diagnosis.

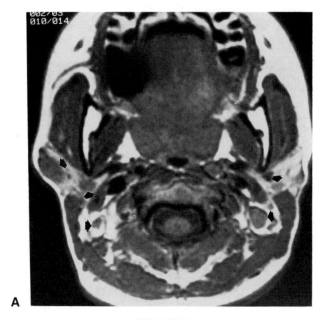

SE 600/20

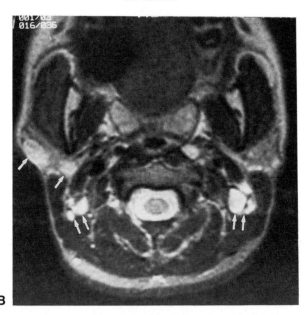

SE 2,800/70

*Figure 8-6.* Bilateral intra- and extraparotid non-Hodgkin's lymphoma. (A) Axial T1-weighted MR image shows that the normal palatine tonsils have isointense signal (compared to muscle), as do the multiple nodes in the parotid gland and in the posterior cervical triangles (arrows). (B) Axial T2-weighted MR image shows relatively increased signal intensity within the nodal masses bilaterally (arrows).

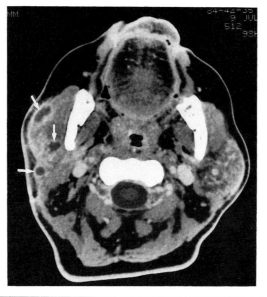

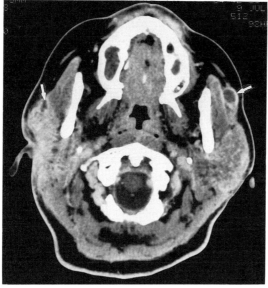

*Figure 8-7.* Multiple bilateral parotid abscesses. Postcontrast axial CT images show several cystic areas (arrows) with ringlike enhancement in both parotid glands, which are also noted to be enlarged. There is extensive soft tissue swelling and enhancement of the fascial planes overlying the parotid glands, consistent with associated cellulitis.

# Question 39

Concerning lymphoepithelial parotid cysts,

(A) patients are nearly always infected with human immunodeficiency virus
(B) enlarged adenoids are an associated finding
(C) they are often associated with diffuse reactive cervical lymphadenopathy
(D) they are a direct precursor of Kaposi's sarcoma

Since the initial descriptions of the acquired immunodeficiency syndrome (AIDS) and AIDS-related complex (ARC), an increasing understanding of the varied clinical manifestations of the disease spectrum has developed. The identification of HIV as the etiologic agent and the understanding of its mode of transmission have broadened investigations to include the study of asymptomatic individuals seropositive for HIV and patients at risk for HIV infection. Head and neck manifestations in patients with AIDS include various mucosal infections (particularly candidiasis), cervical adenopathy, Kaposi's sarcoma, and non-Hodgkin's lymphoma. Patients who do not have AIDS but who are HIV positive may demonstrate diffuse cervical adenopathy and parotid gland enlargement. The involvement of the parotid gland consists of benign lymphoepithelial infiltration and lymphoepithelial cysts, as in the test patients (Figures 8-1 and 8-2). Virtually all cases of multiple parotid cysts and diffuse cervical adenopathy occur in patients who are HIV positive and in some patients who have not yet become seropositive for HIV but are infected by the virus **(Option (A) is true).**

Surgical specimens from patients with HIV infection and parotid lymphoepithelial cysts demonstrate diffuse lymphoid infiltration. Microscopic evaluation reveals epithelial islands, partially encapsulated by fibrous tissue, within the lymphoid infiltration. Lymphoepithelial cysts are thought to result from entrapment of ducts by surrounding hyperplastic lymphoid tissue, leading to ductal dilatation and cyst formation. Alternatively, the cysts may develop from salivary ductal epithelium trapped within intraparotid lymph nodes. The cysts are lined with cuboidal epithelium and typically show dense surrounding lymphoid infiltration. Such cysts range from several millimeters to several centimeters in diameter, are often multiple, contain serous fluid, and may contain cholesterol crystals. Germinal centers are seen in the lymphoid tissue surrounding the cysts. The presence of HIV RNA particles in the inflammatory cells within the zones of lymphoid infiltration, but not within the salivary gland tissue itself, has been confirmed. Intraglandular lymph node enlargement has also been documented.

Progressive swelling of the parotid glands may be present in adult patients who do not meet the diagnostic criteria for AIDS, who may or may not have the generalized adenopathy associated with ARC, or who occasionally are HIV seronegative, but who have risk factors for HIV infection. The swelling may be unilateral or bilateral and is sometimes associated with a dull ache. Multiple discrete masses within the parotid gland are occasionally palpable clinically. In most patients who are ultimately shown to have benign lymphoepithelial infiltration or lymphoepithelial cysts, fever is absent and opportunistic infection is not present. Cervical adenopathy is almost always present, and enlarged adenoids are present in 30 to 50% of patients **(Options (B) and (C) are true).**

CT and MRI play an important role in the evaluation of HIV-positive patients with lymphoepithelial cysts. The CT scans typically reveal multiple homogeneous cystic intraparotid masses, which are frequently bilateral, even in patients whose clinical evaluation suggests unilateral disease. These cysts are thin walled and well circumscribed, with peripheral enhancement. There is a predominance of cysts in the superficial portion of the gland, and the central cyst attenuation values range from 10 to 25 HU. The remainder of the gland may show patchy areas of contrast enhancement; however, no changes are seen in the surrounding subcutaneous tissues. Almost all patients also demonstrate extensive cervical adenopathy, with lymph nodes measuring 0.5 to 2 cm in diameter within the submental, submandibular, internal jugular, and posterior triangle lymph node regions.

Evaluation by MRI reveals lesions that are isointense to the normal parotid gland on T1-weighted images and hyperintense on T2-weighted images. Following administration of gadolinium chelates, the remaining normal glandular tissue enhances but the cysts do not. In patients with associated cervical adenopathy, the nodes are homogeneous without central necrosis. MRI demonstrates benign enlargement of the adenoids and possibly of the palatine and lingual tonsils in addition to the cervical lymphadenopathy.

Treatment of patients with lymphoepithelial parotid cysts usually provides symptomatic relief, and a superficial parotidectomy is currently the treatment of choice. Pain may be reduced postoperatively, but cysts may recur in the deeper portions of the gland. An increased incidence of Kaposi's sarcoma, parotid adenoid cystic carcinoma, and non-Hodgkin's lymphoma has been reported in HIV-positive patients, and early diagnosis improves further treatment options. There is no evidence that these lymphoepithelial cysts will degenerate into Kaposi's sarcomas **(Option**

**(D) is false).** Recognition of benign lymphoepithelial cysts in patients who are at risk for HIV infection but are not HIV positive suggests the need for close follow-up. It has not yet been proven whether the development of lymphoepithelial cysts is a prognostic indicator regarding the future development of AIDS or ARC.

## Question 40

Concerning parotid tumors,

(A) they usually have low signal intensity on T1-weighted MR images
(B) most high-grade malignant ones have high signal intensity on T2-weighted MR images
(C) most benign ones lie deep to the facial nerve
(D) the Warthin's variety rarely enhances following intravenous administration of contrast agents

The parotid gland is composed of glandular parenchyma situated within the parotid fossa. The parotid fossa is bordered superiorly by the zygomatic arch; anteriorly by the back of the ramus of the mandible, the masseter muscle, and the pterygoid muscles; posteriorly by the mastoid process, the external auditory canal, the sternocleidomastoid muscle, and the posterior belly of the digastric muscle; and medially by the posterior belly of the digastric muscle, the styloid process and its musculature, the stylomandibular ligament, the internal carotid artery, and the internal jugular vein. The parotid gland has one capsule and no separate anatomic lobes; however, for descriptive purposes it is divided into superficial and deep lobes by the plane of the facial nerve. The tissue lying lateral to the facial nerve is considered superficial, and the tissue lying medial to this nerve is considered deep. The facial nerve exits the cranium via the stylomastoid foramen, where it passes through fatty tissue as it extends to the posterior belly of the digastric muscle. It then runs along this muscle until it pierces the posterior capsule of the parotid gland. The nerve then divides into its five main branches to supply the facial muscles. Within the parotid gland, the nerve courses lateral to the retromandibular vein and the external carotid artery.

Histologically, the parotid is a tuboacinar gland composed of a series of branching ducts terminating in acini; the acini within the parotid gland are almost entirely serous. The surrounding parenchyma is arranged in lobules, divided to an extent by delicate fibrous septa.

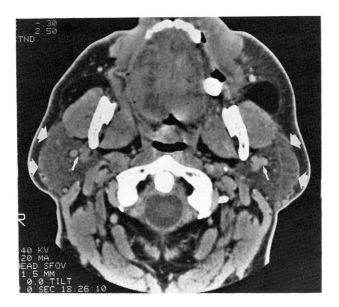

*Figure 8-8.* Normal parotid. Postcontrast axial CT scan clearly shows the normal appearance of an enhanced parotid gland (wide arrows). The density of the gland is lower than that of muscle but higher than that of the adjacent fat. Note the vascular bundles (external carotid artery laterally and retromandibular vein medially), which show enhancement (thin arrows). The facial nerve lies immediately lateral to the vascular bundle.

The anatomy of the normal parotid gland is well depicted by both CT and MRI. Imaging is done routinely in both the axial and coronal projections. Modified CT projections or sagittal images may be necessary to avoid dental artifacts produced either by metallic fillings or by dental prostheses. The normal parotid tissue has relatively low density on CT, ranging from just below that of the surrounding muscle to just above that of fat. Following infusion of contrast material, there is some glandular enhancement and improved definition of the intraparotid vessels (Figure 8-8).

The gland is well visualized on both T1-weighted and T2-weighted MR images. On T1-weighted images, the signal from the intermediate signal intensity separates the gland from its neighboring structures (muscle, fat, and bone) (Figure 8-9A). On T2-weighted images, the gland has a relatively high signal intensity compared with the low signal intensity of the surrounding muscles (Figure 8-9B). Following infusion of gadolinium chelates, normal glandular tissues enhance markedly (approximately 125%). Whenever a mass is palpated in the parotid gland, it is important to determine whether the lesion is actually an intraparotid

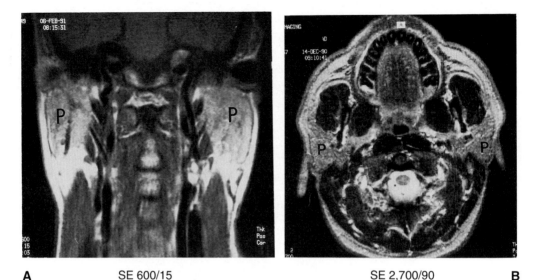

SE 600/15    SE 2,700/90

*Figure 8-9.* Normal parotid. (A) Coronal T1-weighted MR image of the parotid glands shows that the signal intensity of the glands is higher than that of muscle but lower than that of the surrounding fat. (B) Axial T2-weighted MR image shows that the parotid glands are of higher signal intensity than the adjacent muscles but of nearly equivalent signal intensity to the surrounding fat. P = parotid glands.

mass or whether it is of extraparotid origin. This information is essential for proper surgical planning. If a mass is medial to the gland in the parapharyngeal space, its site of origin is best identified in the axial plane by identifying the presence or absence of a fat plane between the deep lobe of the parotid and the posterolateral aspect of the mass. If there is an intact fat plane on all scans through the mass, the lesion has an extraparotid origin. Obliteration of the fat plane suggests an intraparotid lesion.

Tumors of the parotid gland account for 75 to 85% of all salivary gland tumors but for fewer than 3% of head and neck neoplasms. Parotid masses, at least histologically, can be divided into benign tumors, low-grade cancers, and high-grade cancers. Benign tumors are the most frequent, accounting for 80% of parotid neoplasms. The most common benign tumors in infants and young children are hemangioma and pleomorphic adenoma (Figure 8-10). The most common benign tumors in adults are pleomorphic adenoma and Warthin's tumor (papillary cystadenoma lymphomatosum). Pleomorphic adenomas (benign mixed tumors) account for 70 to 80% of the benign parotid neoplasms; they occur

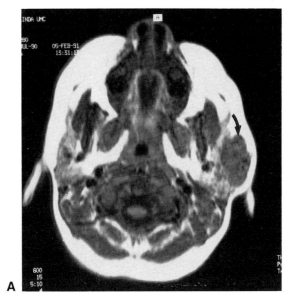

SE 600/15

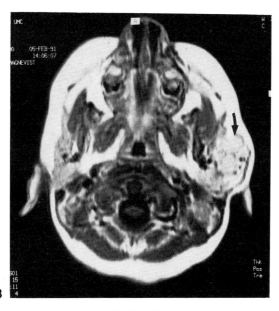

SE 600/15

*Figure 8-10.* Pleomorphic adenoma. (A) Noncontrast T1-weighted axial MR image shows a single, well-demarcated mass in the superficial lobe of the left parotid gland (arrow). The tumor is somewhat heterogeneous in appearance and has a lower signal intensity than the remainder of the parotid gland and the surrounding fat. (B) Postcontrast T1-weighted axial MR image shows dramatic enhancement of the tumor (arrow). Note also the enhancement of the parotid gland, which makes it difficult to separate the margins of the tumor from the gland.

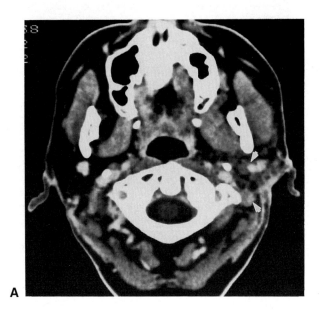

**A**

*Figure 8-11.* Recurrence of pleomorphic adenoma. (A and B) Postcontrast axial CT scans. This patient had resection of a left parotid pleomorphic adenoma and now has multiple palpable subcutaneous nodules. Note the presence of the subcutaneous nodules within the resected tumor bed (arrows in panel A) and in the regions of the carotid sheath and submandibular gland (arrows in panel B). (C) Sagittal T1-weighted MR scan clearly shows the multiple scattered subcutaneous nodules filling the left side of the neck (arrows).

most commonly in the superficial portion of the parotid gland. The majority of Warthin's tumors and other benign parotid tumors also occur most commonly in the superficial portion of the parotid gland **(Option (C) is false).** Histologically, pleomorphic adenomas are characterized by marked diversity with epithelial and myoepithelial components in varied patterns. Islands of cartilage, bone, or epithelium may be present. Pleomorphic adenomas present as solitary round or pedunculated lesions and usually occur in women over 50 years of age. Primary multicentric tumors are estimated to occur in only 0.5% of cases. However, multiple recurrent tumors following resection of a tumor whose capsule was violated are significantly more common (Figure 8-11).

CT evaluation of a pleomorphic adenoma reveals a solid mass that may contain focal calcifications. On MRI, the tumor appears as an area of low signal intensity on T1-weighted images and as an area of high signal intensity on T2-weighted images with relatively well-defined margins (Figure 8-12). Following administration of contrast agents, there

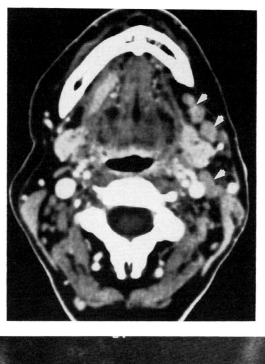

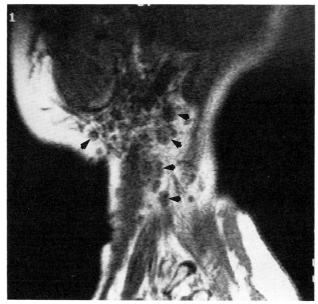

SE 600/20

may be heterogeneous enhancement as a result of areas of internal necrosis within the tumor.

Warthin's tumors represent 5 to 15% of parotid tumors and have both epithelial and lymphoid elements. These tumors are the only salivary

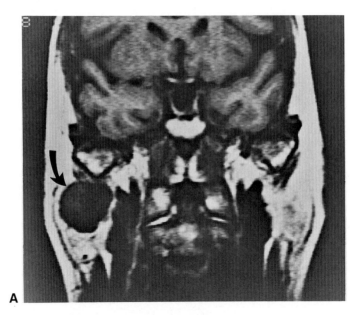

SE 500/20

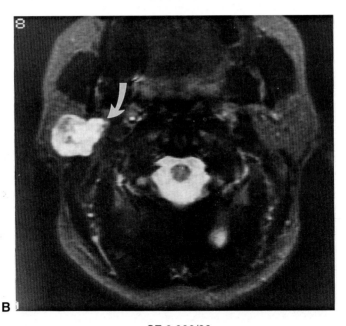

SE 2,000/80

*Figure 8-12.* Pleomorphic adenoma involving the superficial and deep lobes of the right parotid gland. (A) On the T1-weighted coronal MR image, the large tumor mass (arrow) appears hypointense relative to the signal in the parotid gland. (B) On the T2-weighted axial MR image, the tumor shows considerable T2 prolongation. A portion of the tumor extends through the stylomandibular tunnel into the deep lobe of the right parotid gland (arrow). (Reprinted with permission from Hasso AN. Malignant otitis externa. In: Siegel BA, Theros EG (eds), Magnetic resonance test and syllabus. Reston, VA: American College of Radiology; 1991:542–565.)

gland neoplasms that are more common in men than in women, and the lesions tend to occur in the caudal portions of the gland. They may be cystic or solid and may occur multiply either unilaterally or bilaterally. On CT, Warthin's tumors appear as well-marginated masses, often with areas of cyst formation. There is prominent contrast enhancement of the tumor in most cases **(Option (D) is false).** On MRI, Warthin's tumors are sharply defined lesions with a decreased signal intensity on T1-weighted images and an intermediate signal intensity on T2-weighted images. Areas of cyst formation have low and high signal intensity on T1- and T2-weighted images, respectively. Following infusion of gadolinium chelates, there is enhancement of the tumor. Pleomorphic adenomas and Warthin's tumors share benign features such as well-defined margins, a tendency to occur in the superficial portion of the parotid gland, and an increased signal intensity on T2-weighted images relative to the normal parotid gland. However, these imaging features are the same as those of the low-grade cancers, and biopsy is necessary for accurate histologic diagnosis.

The low-grade cancers of the parotid gland are most commonly low-grade mucoepidermoid carcinomas, some acinic cell carcinomas, and some adenoid cystic carcinomas. These tumors are sufficiently differentiated that they contain watery serous and mucoid contents and their MR signal intensities are essentially those of water, namely a low T1-weighted and a high T2-weighted signal intensity. This is the same imaging appearance as a benign neoplasm. The imaging evaluation of tumor margins may also be misleading since the pseudocapsule present around the low-grade cancers will appear as the true capsule of a benign lesion (Figure 8-13). Following gadolinium chelate administration, most of the benign and low-grade lesions exhibit tumor enhancement.

The most common aggressive or high-grade parotid cancers are high-grade mucoepidermoid carcinomas, undifferentiated carcinomas, adenocarcinomas, and squamous cell carcinomas. These tumors differ from the benign lesions and low-grade cancers in that they are highly cellular. They contain little serous or mucinous material. This alters their appearance, particularly on T2-weighted MR images, where they tend to have a low signal intensity compared with the normal parotid gland **(Option (B) is false).** However, the T1-weighted images show decreased signal intensity typical of nearly all parotid tumors **(Option (A) is true).** Malignant tumors tend to occur with a greater frequency in the deep portion of the gland (rather than in the superficial portion), and their margins are typically poorly defined or infiltrative, often involving the surrounding glandular tissue and occasionally extending into the adja-

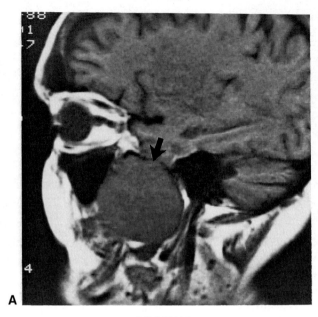

SE 800/15

*Figure 8-13.* Adenoid cystic carcinoma (low-grade parotid cancer). (A) A sagittal T1-weighted MR scan shows a large, solitary, homogeneous tumor between the mandible and maxillary sinus (arrow). (B) An axial proton-density MR image shows a well-outlined tumor with a pseudocapsule (arrows). The mass originates from the deep lobe of the parotid; it lies lateral to the parapharyngeal space and medial to the mandible.

cent extraparotid tissues. Enhancement with gadolinium chelates is usually quite prominent and helps define the tumor extent and any invasion of surrounding structures.

Assessment of contrast enhancement is quite helpful in differentiating recurrent parotid neoplasms from postoperative fibrosis. Fibrosis has low signal intensity on both T1- and T2-weighted MR images; however, there is little if any enhancement following gadolinium chelate administration.

*Anton N. Hasso, M.D.*
*Monika L. Kief-Garcia, M.D.*
*Paul S. Kim, M.D.*

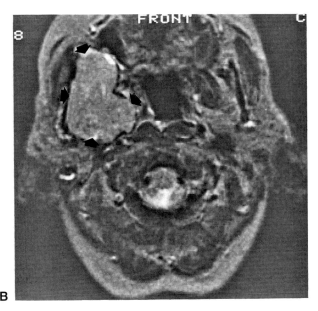

B

SE 2,000/30

## SUGGESTED READINGS

### BENIGN LYMPHOEPITHELIAL PAROTID CYSTS

1. Finfer MD, Schinella RA, Rothstein SG, Persky MS. Cystic parotid lesions in patients at risk for the acquired immunodeficiency syndrome. Arch Otolaryngol Head Neck Surg 1988; 114:1290–1294

2. Goddart D, Francois A, Ninane J, et al. Parotid gland abnormality found in children seropositive for the human immunodeficiency virus (HIV). Pediatr Radiol 1990; 20:355–357

3. Holliday RA, Cohen WA, Schinella RA, et al. Benign lymphoepithelial parotid cysts and hyperplastic cervical adenopathy in AIDS-risk patients: a new CT appearance. Radiology 1988; 168:439–441

4. Kirshenbaum KJ, Nadimpalli SR, Friedman M, Kirshenbaum GL, Cavallino RP. Benign lymphoepithelial parotid tumors in AIDS patients: CT and MR findings in nine cases. AJNR 1991; 12:271–274

5. Shugar JM, Som PM, Jacobson AL, Ryan JR, Bernard PJ, Dickman SH. Multicentric parotid cysts and cervical adenopathy in AIDS patients. A newly recognized entity: CT and MR manifestations. Laryngoscope 1988; 98:772–775

6. Soberman N, Leonidas JC, Berndon WE, et al. Parotid enlargement in children seropositive for human immunodeficiency virus: imaging findings. AJR 1991; 157:553–556

7. Tunkel DE, Loury MC, Fox CH, Goins MA III, Johns ME. Bilateral parotid enlargement in HIV-seropositive patients. Laryngoscope 1989; 99:590–595

## SARCOIDOSIS

8. Batsakis JG. Tumors of the head and neck, clinical and pathological considerations, 2nd ed. Baltimore: Williams & Wilkins; 1979:103
9. Iko BO, Chinwuba CE, Myers EM, Teal JS. Sarcoidosis of the parotid gland. Br J Radiol 1986; 59:547–552
10. Som PM, Shugar JM, Biller HF. Parotid gland sarcoidosis and the CT sialogram. J Comput Assist Tomogr 1981; 5:674–677

## PAROTID TUMORS

11. Finkelstein DM, Noyek AM, Chapnik JS. Multiple bilateral synchronous Warthin's tumors: a case report and review of the literature. J Otolaryngol 1989; 18:357–361
12. Richardson GS, Clairmont AA, Erickson ER. Cystic lesions of the parotid gland. Plast Reconstr Surg 1978; 61:364–370
13. Som PM, Biller HF. High-grade malignancies of the parotid gland: identification with MR imaging. Radiology 1989; 173:823–826
14. Som PM, Shugar JM, Sacher M, Stollman AL, Biller HF. Benign and malignant parotid pleomorphic adenomas: CT and MR studies. J Comput Assist Tomogr 1988; 12:65–69
15. Swartz JD, Rothman MI, Marlow FI, Berger AS. MR imaging of parotid mass lesions: attempts at histopathologic differentiation. J Comput Assist Tomogr 1989; 13:789–796
16. Turnbull AD, Frazell EL. Multiple tumors of the major salivary glands. Am J Surg 1969; 118:787–789

## NON-HODGKIN'S LYMPHOMA

17. Almac A, Undar L, Goze F. Small lymphocytic lymphoma presenting with simultaneous involvement of parotid and submandibular glands bilaterally, maxillary sinus, hard palate and optic nerve. J Laryngol Otol 1991; 105:584–587
18. Pollei SR, Harnsberger HR. The radiologic evaluation of the parotid space. Semin US CT MR 1990; 11:486–503

## ABSCESSES

19. Berman J, Myssiorek D, Reppucci A, Zito J. Sump catheter drainage of parotid abscess: an alternative to surgery. Ear Nose Throat J 1991; 70:393–395
20. Duff TB. Parotitis, parotid abscess and facial palsy. J Laryngol Otol 1972; 86:161–165
21. Magaram D, Gooding GA. Ultrasonic guided aspiration of parotid abscess. Arch Otolaryngol 1981; 107:549

*Notes*

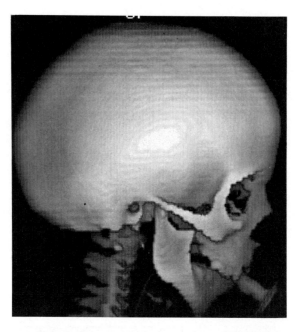

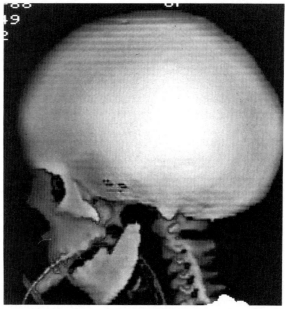

*Figure 9-1.* You are shown a series of three-dimensional CT images of the calvarium and face of a 6-year-old boy.

# Case 9: Hemifacial Microsomia

## Question 41

Which *one* of the following is the MOST likely diagnosis?

(A) Crouzon's disease
(B) Treacher Collins syndrome
(C) Pierre Robin syndrome
(D) Hemifacial microsomia
(E) Apert's syndrome

The test images (Figure 9-1) show that the calvarial and facial structures are normal on the right side but have distinct abnormalities on the left side, which are most consistent with hemifacial microsomia (see Figure 9-2) **(Option (D) is correct)**.

Hemifacial microsomia is characterized by multiple maxillofacial anomalies including hypoplasia of the zygoma (malar eminence), maxilla, and mandible. There are severe deformities of the ramus and condyle of the mandible and of the temporomandibular joint. The abnormalities involve the first and second branchial arches and are typically manifested unilaterally. Occasionally there are similar but far less severe findings on the contralateral side.

The principal radiographic feature of hemifacial microsomia is asymmetry of the mandible secondary to hypoplasia or agenesis of an affected condyle. With increasing severity, the condylar process and superior portions of the ramus become less recognizable and the gonial angle of the mandible becomes very obtuse. Hemiatrophy of the mandible becomes apparent as the affected side of the mandible loses its ability to grow in concert with the normal, contralateral side. The maxilla and zygomatic bones on the affected side of the face are also proportionately hypoplastic.

The test images document severe unilateral hypoplasia of the zygoma, maxilla, and mandible. The defects involve the posterior portion of the

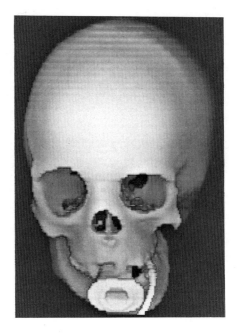

*Figure 9-1 (Continued)*

zygomatic arch, temporomandibular joint, and mandible, as well as atresia of the external auditory canal and hypoplasia of the mastoid process and mastoid air cells. These features are typical of hemifacial microsomia.

Crouzon's disease (craniofacial dysostosis) (Option (A)) includes multiple craniofacial abnormalities. The syndrome was originally described in 1912 by Crouzon. The inheritance pattern of this disease is autosomal dominant with variable penetrance. Approximately 25% of reported cases are sporadic and are presumed to represent new mutations.

Clinical features of Crouzon's disease include craniosynostosis with variable closure of the coronal, sagittal, and lambdoidal sutures and palpable ridging along these sutures. The head usually exhibits a short anteroposterior diameter with a high vertex and frontal bossing. The lateral dimension of the cranium may be widened, resulting in an acrocephalic appearance. There are increased digital markings relating to the craniosynostosis (Figure 9-3). Additional features of Crouzon's disease include intracranial anomalies such as hydrocephalus and agenesis of the corpus callosum.

Facial features of Crouzon's disease include maxillary hypoplasia, a "parrotlike" nose, prognathism, and a narrow nasopharynx. There may

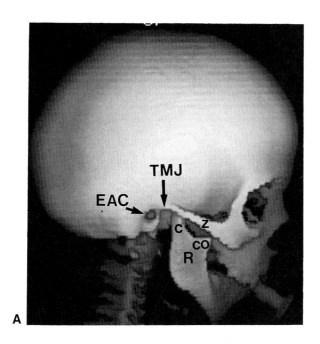

*Figure 9-2* (Same as Figure 9-1).   Hemifacial microsomia. 3-D CT of the skull and face performed under general endotracheal anesthesia. There is an airway device and a monitoring tube in the patient's mouth. (A) Right lateral view shows normal calvarial and facial structures on the right side. C = mandibular condyle; CO = coronoid process; EAC = external auditory canal; R = mandibular ramus; TMJ = temporomandibular joint; Z = zygomatic arch. (B) Left lateral view shows that the left side of the face is distinctly abnormal by comparison. There is partial absence of the zygomatic arch (Z) and mandibular ramus (R). There is agenesis of the coronoid process and mandibular condyle, and there is atresia of the external auditory canal. (C) In the anteroposterior view, the cleft in the left side of the face is apparent. Note also the hypoplasia of the left orbit when compared with the normal right orbit. The findings are diagnostic of left hemifacial microsomia. Note apparent holes (arrows) in the inferomedial walls of both orbits. These are examples of pseudo-foraminae, created because of the very thin lamina papyracea and volume-averaging error with the air-filled ethmoid sinuses.

be shallow orbits with hypertelorism. The palate has an inverted-V shape and may be cleft. Occasionally, there is atresia of the external auditory canal. The findings are typically bilateral, unlike the unilateral hypoplastic zygoma, mandible, maxilla, and external auditory canal seen in the test images. Craniosynostosis is a constant feature in Crouzon's disease but is not seen in the test images.

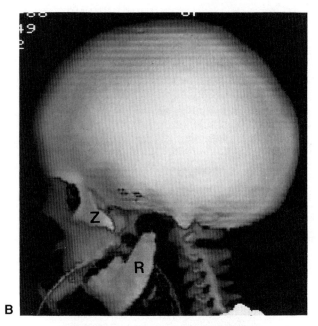

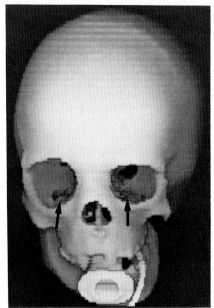

Treacher Collins syndrome (Option (B)) is a heterogeneous branchial arch anomaly that includes multiple craniofacial defects. The most constant feature is diffuse mandibular hypoplasia (Figure 9-4). This is typi-

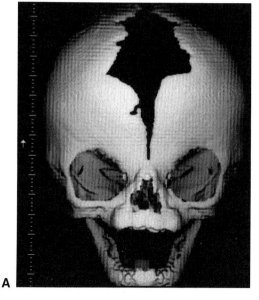

A

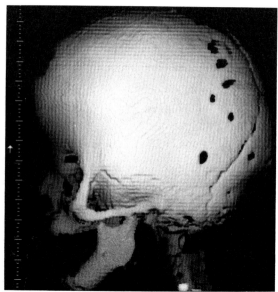

B

*Figure 9-3.* Crouzon's disease in a 3-month-old infant. 3-D CT images of the skull and face. (A) In the anteroposterior view, the metopic suture and anterior fontanelle are wide open but the coronal sutures have fused. Note the marked hypoplasia of the maxilla. There is associated hypertelorism. (B) In the left lateral view, the skull is brachycephalic and prominent convolutional markings are seen near the left lambdoidal suture, which remains patent. (C) In the posteroanterior view, the posterior fontanelle and lambdoidal sutures are patent. The extensive prominent convolutional markings are seen as scattered areas of bone thinning in both the midline occipital and lateral parietal bones. (D) Axial image from the CT data set used to obtain the 3-D images shows severe hypoplasia of the maxilla with small maxillary sinuses (white arrows). The petrous temporal bones are unremarkable. The convolutional markings in the occipital squamae are clearly visible (black arrows).

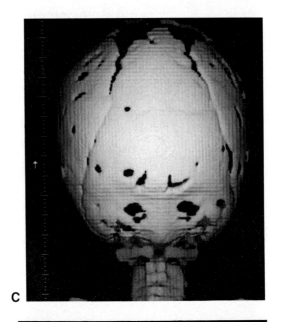

C

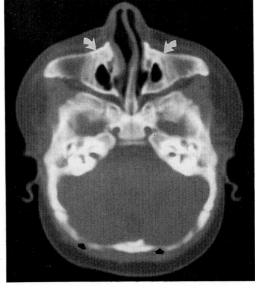

D

cally associated with bilateral hypoplasia of the malar eminences with or without clefts in the zygomatic bones. The petrous temporal bones are nearly always involved, with abnormalities of the outer, middle, and inner ears. There is complete lack of pneumatization of the mastoid air cells and there are small hypoplastic tympanic cavities, which appear

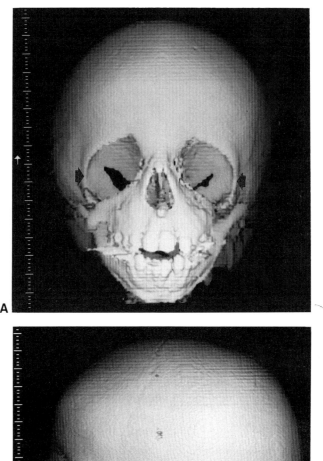

A

B

*Figure 9-4.* Treacher Collins syndrome. 3-D CT of the skull and face. (A) Anteroposterior view shows severe hypoplasia of the maxilla with flattening of the inferior orbital rims bilaterally. Note the severe hypoplasia of the zygomas with marked thinning of the lateral orbital rims (arrows). (B) Left lateral view shows hypoplasia of the body and ramus of the mandible. The coronoid process is prominent and extends superiorly into the region of the absent zygomatic arch. The condylar process is small and lies outside the temporomandibular joint (curved arrow). The gonial angle of the mandible is obtuse (straight arrow) and forms an antigonial notch. The findings are characteristic of Treacher Collins syndrome. Note the apparent holes in the medial wall of the orbit. These are examples of pseudoforaminae (see Figure 9-2).

"slit-like." The test images show a unilateral deformity of the external ear, zygoma, maxilla, and mandible, unlike the Treacher Collins syndrome, which is a bilateral phenomenon.

Pierre Robin syndrome (Option (C)) has no known genetic inheritance pattern and usually occurs in otherwise normal neonates. The Robin sequence is probably a better term for the disorder since its single initiating factor may be intrauterine hypoplasia of the mandible. This single defect can cause additional malformations such as posterior placement of the tongue, which inhibits closure of the palate. The resulting cleft palate is unusual and has a characteristic rounded shape. Glossoptosis and upper airway obstruction are invariably present. Neonates with the Robin sequence have an excellent prognosis if they survive beyond the initial period of respiratory distress.

The clinical features of Pierre Robin syndrome may be associated with other known genetic syndromes such as trisomy 18. There are no associated osseous deformities other than the mandibular hypoplasia in patients with Pierre Robin syndrome; the test images show other osseous abnormalities, making this diagnosis unlikely.

Apert's syndrome (or acrocephalosyndactyly) (Option (E)) was first reported in 1894. Additional cases were described by Apert in 1906. The syndrome demonstrates autosomal dominant transmission in offspring of affected individuals. Most cases appear to be sporadic and represent fresh mutations.

The clinical features of Apert's syndrome include irregular craniosynostosis, commonly with unilateral or bilateral involvement of the coronal and lambdoidal sutures (Figure 9-5A and B). The head classically has a short anteroposterior diameter with a high, broad, flat forehead and a flat occiput. The head shape is frequently classified as turribrachycephalic. Often, a horizontal supraorbital groove is present. The syndrome may be accompanied by a cloverleaf skull deformity, which occurs whenever the coronal, lambdoidal, and sagittal sutures are all prematurely fused.

Anomalies of the brain parenchyma are not a constant feature of this syndrome, but brain dysgenesis may be an associated finding. Convolutional atrophy has also been reported, as has agenesis of the corpus callosum, septum pellucidum, and other midline structures. This syndrome occurs with or without hydrocephalus.

Several other craniofacial features of Apert's syndrome are well known. Patients usually have a flat face with a full forehead and a flat occiput. The nose is small and has a depressed nasal bridge. The mandible is usually also hypoplastic. The palate is commonly narrow, high, and

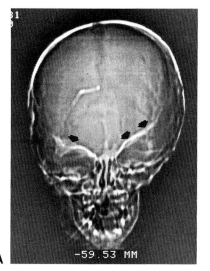
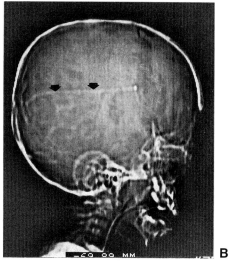

*Figure 9-5.* Apert's syndrome. (A and B) Anteroposterior and lateral views from the CT localizer images (scout views). Anteroposterior view shows the prominent bilateral convolutional markings with asymmetry of the calvarium. Note the bilateral harlequin eyes, more prominent on the left side (arrowheads). Lateral view shows extensive irregular convolutional markings, both anteriorly and posteriorly. The overall head shape is acrocephalic with a prominent forehead and flat occiput. Note the presence of a shunt tube, which was inserted for treatment of hydrocephalus (arrowheads). (C) Coronal CT image of the mid-face shows the high arched partially cleft hard palate (curved arrows). The bilateral harlequin eyes are again well demonstrated (straight arrows). (D) Axial CT image of the skull base shows severe plagiocephaly due to the craniosynostosis. The left middle and posterior cranial fossae are smaller than those on the right. (E) CT image of the right petrous temporal bone shows a congenital anomaly of the right inner ear. The right vestibule and semicircular canals form a single cavity (arrow). The visualized external and middle ears are normal bilaterally.

arched. A median groove or cleft palate may be present (Figure 9-5C). The orbits are typically shallow and hyperteloric. There may be hearing impairment, most frequently caused by congenital fixation of the stapes, although anomalies of the inner ear have been noted by many authors (Figure 9-5D and E). The syndrome includes other structural abnormalities such as syndactyly and a broad distal phalanx of the thumbs and big toes.

Conventional radiographs and three-dimensional computed tomography (3-D CT) frequently feature harlequin eyes, which are associated

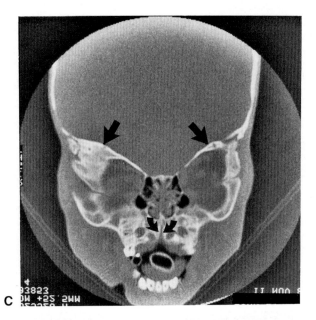

C

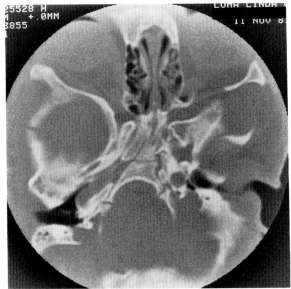

D

with coronal craniosynostosis. The head is brachycephalic with irregular convolutional markings, in contrast to the head in the test images, which is normal in shape. Irregular convolutional markings are a constant feature in Apert's syndrome and are not seen in the test images.

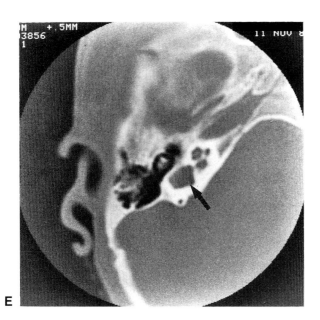

E

## Question 42

Features of the Treacher Collins syndrome include:

    (A)  antimongoloid slant of the palpebral fissures
    (B)  colobomas of the eyelids
    (C)  deformed auricles
    (D)  stenosis of the external auditory canals
    (E)  abnormal course of the facial nerve
    (F)  mandibular hypoplasia

    The Treacher Collins syndrome (mandibulofacial dysostosis) was first reported in 1846. To date, more than 250 cases of this anomaly have been reported. The inheritance pattern of the disorder is autosomal dominant, with more than 60% of cases representing fresh mutations. The variable expression of the syndrome in different patients is a well-documented phenomenon.

    The clinical manifestations of Treacher Collins syndrome typically involve the face and the base of the skull most severely. The head shape is usually normal, without evidence of craniosynostosis. Orbital and ocular findings may be extensive, including antimongoloid slant of the palpebral fissures, colobomas of the eyelids, and microphthalmia (**Op-**

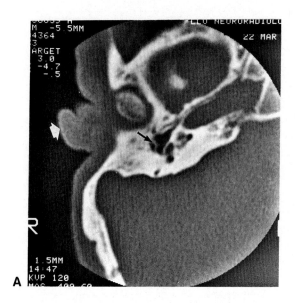

A

*Figure 9-6.* Treacher Collins syndrome. (A and B) In these axial CT scans through the right petrous temporal bone, the stigmata of a first branchial arch anomaly are clearly seen with atresia of the external auditory canal, maldevelopment of the middle ear, and an osseous atresia plate. The ossicles are fused to the thick atresia plate (black arrows). The middle ear cavity is reduced to a slitlike aperture, and the development of the mastoid air cells is poor. There is severe microtia with skin tags forming the outer ear (white arrows). The temporomandibular joint is abnormally positioned posteriorly. (C) Coronal CT scan shows that because of involvement of the second branchial arch, the facial nerve is unimpeded in its anterior migration and lies more anteriorly within the floor of the middle ear (arrows). This first and second branchial arch anomaly is consistent with the Treacher Collins syndrome.

**tions (A) and (B) are true).** Hypoplasia of the maxilla and malar eminence with or without a zygomatic cleft is almost always present (Figure 9-4). This may lead to underdevelopment of the paranasal sinuses. The palatine bones are usually hypoplastic or absent. Micrognathia is almost always present and is one of the most notable characteristics.

Additional manifestations of the Treacher Collins syndrome include extensive involvement of the ears. The external ears typically demonstrate auricular malformations with severe external auditory canal stenosis **(Options (C) and (D) are true).** Involvement of the middle ear frequently presents as conductive hearing loss secondary to absence or fusion of the ossicles (Figure 9-6A and B). The hypoplastic middle ear

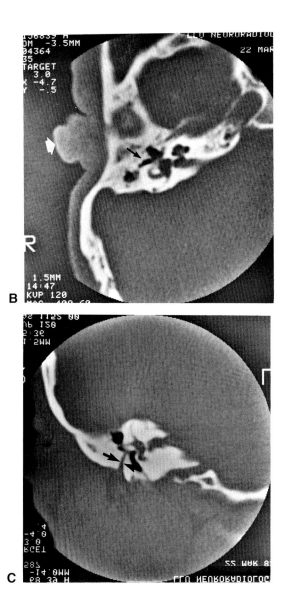

leads to an abnormal course of the facial nerve, which lies in the floor of the middle ear cleft **(Option (E) is true)** (Figure 9-6C). The inner ear may be deficient, with abnormalities of the cochlea and vestibular apparatus.

The mandible is usually hypoplastic and sometimes aplastic with an obtuse gonial angle **(Option (F) is true)** (Figure 9-4). The oropharynx may exhibit numerous developmental abnormalities including a cleft palate, incompetent soft palate, choanal atresia, or high arched palate. The nasopharynx and upper airway are commonly hypoplastic with a narrow anteroposterior dimension.


## Question 43

Concerning hemifacial microsomia,

(A) the external auditory canal is hypoplastic
(B) macrostomia is typically present
(C) the inner ear is usually involved
(D) the temporomandibular joint is typically involved
(E) the lateral orbital rim is hypoplastic

Hemifacial microsomia is occasionally referred to as the first and second branchial arch syndrome, since the first two branchial arches tend to be the most severely involved. The incidence of this anomaly is between 1 in 3,000 and 1 in 5,000 births, and boys are more likely to be affected than girls. The syndrome tends to be sporadic, although an autosomal dominant pattern has been suggested in some cases.

The clinical features are variable, but they tend to be asymmetric and are unilateral in up to 70% of cases. Head shape may be characterized by frontal bossing, an open anterior fontanelle, or a bony defect at the vertex. Associated intracranial dermoid cysts and occipital encephaloceles may occur. The orbits may be involved, yielding microphthalmia or macrophthalmia. The palate may be high arched or cleft. The lateral orbital rim is often hypoplastic **(Option (E) is true).** The maxilla and mandible are typically hypoplastic, with resultant microstomia **(Option (B) is false)** (Figures 9-1 and 9-2). A lateral facial cleft commonly occurs (Figure 9-7). Ear involvement is usually in the form of preauricular tags or pits. A narrow external ear canal (or microtia) may also be present **(Option (A) is true).** The middle ear is severely deformed, with absence or fusion of the ossicles. Although there is severe hypoplasia of the petrous temporal bone, the inner ear structures are usually uninvolved **(Option (C) is false)** (Figure 9-7). The mandible is frequently hypoplastic; therefore the temporomandibular joint is affected and may be anteriorly located or absent **(Option (D) is true)** (Figures 9-1 and 9-2).

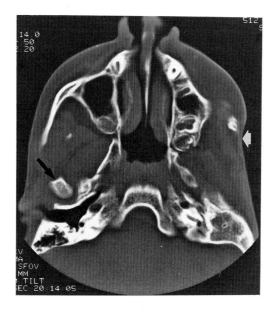

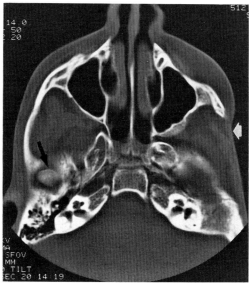

*Figure 9-7.* Same patient as in Figure 9-1. Hemifacial microsomia. Axial CT images through the mid-face and petrous temporal bones show the left facial cleft due to the partial agenesis of the left zygomatic arch (arrowheads). The right temporomandibular joint is normal (arrows). The left temporomandibular joint is atretic. There is similar atresia of the left external auditory canal, middle ear, and mastoid air cells. The inner ears are normal and symmetric bilaterally. The findings confirm the diagnosis of left hemifacial microsomia with marked agenesis of structures originating from the left first and second branchial arches.

# Question 44

Concerning craniosynostosis of the skull,

  (A) head dimensions perpendicular to the affected suture are increased
  (B) involvement of the sagittal suture results in brachycephaly
  (C) involvement of the coronal sutures results in scaphocephaly
  (D) it is usually associated with one of the craniofacial syndromes
  (E) most patients have a symmetric cranial deformity

Craniosynostosis refers to the premature closure or the cessation of growth of one or more cranial sutures. The pathogenesis of this disease is poorly understood and probably has numerous etiologies. Primary craniosynostosis is most often an isolated abnormality. Fewer than 10% of cases are associated with various congenital craniofacial syndromes **(Option (D) is false).** Secondary craniosynostosis results from diverse insults including trauma, atrophy, surgically arrested hydrocephalus, rickets, and hypophosphatasia (Figure 9-8).

Craniosynostosis produces abnormal head growth. In general, head dimensions perpendicular to the affected suture are decreased **(Option (A) is false).** Head growth in the opposite direction usually increases to compensate. The resultant aberrant head shape may be quite striking.

Several terms are used in describing the abnormal head shape in craniosynostosis. Sagittal craniosynostosis typically produces a narrow and elongated cranium, which is called dolichocephaly or scaphocephaly **(Option (B) is false).** Brachycephaly or acrocephaly refers to a short, wide cranium which may be produced by premature closure of both coronal sutures or both lambdoidal sutures **(Option (C) is false).** Premature closure of the sagittal and coronal sutures together results in a tall cranium with a narrow transverse diameter. This configuration is called turricephaly or oxycephaly. Other combinations of complete or partial premature suture closure are possible. The resultant asymmetric calvarium is referred to as plagiocephaly and is present in nearly all cases **(Option (E) is false).** A severe form of craniosynostosis is a trilobed skull deformity, which is characterized by fusion of the sagittal, coronal, and lambdoidal sutures. This skull deformity is described as "cloverleaf" or as the kleeblattschädel anomaly.

The major clinical feature of craniosynostosis is the cosmetic problem. Mental retardation occurs in approximately 5% of cases. Hydrocephalus may also be present. Less frequently, there may be seizures, visual disturbances, or other complications of cranial compression.

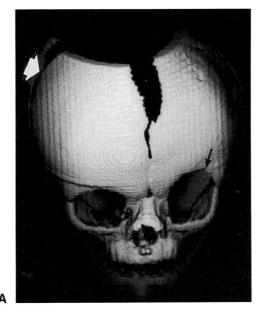

A

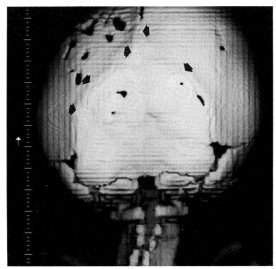

B

*Figure 9-8.* Craniosynostosis. CT scans of the skull and face (the very top of the calvarium is not scanned and is cut off from the images). (A) In the 3-D anteroposterior view, the metopic suture and anterior fontanelle are widely patent, as is the right coronal suture (white arrow). The left coronal suture is fused. Note the unilateral left harlequin eye (black arrow). (B) In the 3-D posteroanterior view, there is craniosynostosis of the posterior portion of the superior sagittal suture and both lambdoidal sutures (arrows). Note the irregular convolutional markings, most prominent in the left parietal bone. (C) In the axial CT image of the brain, the left hemisphere is smaller with an expansion of the body of the left lateral ventricle. This confirms the diagnosis of left hemicerebral atrophy with secondary craniosynostosis.

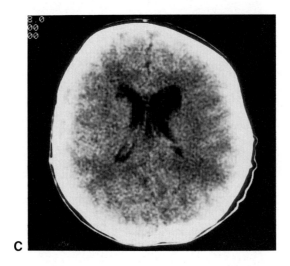

c

Early detection and cosmetic reconstructive surgery are imperative to avoid delayed complications. Before the advent of CT, radiography was the diagnostic modality of choice. The findings on radiographs include skull asymmetry, parasutural sclerosis, and increased inner table convolutional markings. Conventional CT yields better resolution than radiography and has been used to demonstrate more accurately the presence and extent of craniosynostosis. The advent of 3-D CT has dramatically aided the early detection of craniosynostosis and improved surgical planning. Sites of suture closure can be precisely localized presurgically on the patient's skin. The full extent of suture fusions can be visualized. The craniectomy sites can be chosen and mapped out on the basis of the 3-D CT landmarks. Simulation of the cosmetic surgery is possible with 3-D CT. Such presurgical planning may save the patient up to 30 minutes of operative time. Postoperatively, 3-D CT is used for evaluation of the cosmetic results and for comparison with the presurgical images.

# Discussion

*Technical Considerations of 3-D CT. (i) Hardware versus software.* Two components are necessary to implement the 3-D computing algorithms: hardware and software. Hardware refers to the actual computer circuitry or components of the computer. These are tangible elements of the system. Software consists of the programming packages or sets of instructions for the hardware to perform. All systems use a mixture of hardware and software to accomplish specific tasks. The types of hardware and software will directly affect the speed, flexibility, utility, and cost of a given system.

Dedicated hardware refers to circuitry that has been specifically designed on a circuit board or computer chip to perform a specific task. The main advantage of such a system for 3-D imaging is computing speed. Dedicated hardware systems tend to be much faster than systems that use predominantly software. This advantage is steadily decreasing in significance as general-purpose computers increase in speed.

Another technological aspect of hardware to consider is the choice of single versus parallel processing. Traditionally, computers have used one microprocessor to perform all the computational tasks. Because of this, computational time may become prohibitively long for complicated tasks. The graphics and spatial relationships involved in 3-D imaging require innumerable computing steps. Thus, high-speed hardware is necessary. One way to gain speed without using dedicated hardware is to use parallel processing. Parallel processing takes advantage of the fact that most computational tasks can be subdivided into smaller tasks. In this procedure, several different microprocessors can be used simultaneously to perform computations, thus decreasing the overall computational time. This concept is similar to that of an office manager dividing a large task into several smaller tasks to be split among several employees. The job can be completed sooner and more efficiently. The various subtasks can be controlled and reassembled by one microprocessor (or, in the example, by the boss). The tradeoff for an increase in speed is usually an increase in the initial cost of the system.

The main disadvantage of predominantly software-based systems is decreased speed. As general-purpose computing speeds increase, there will be less overall computing time. The advantages of software-based systems are lower expense and easy maintenance since new and more rapid algorithms can easily and quickly be used by planned upgrading of the software. Another advantage is that software computing flaws can be corrected more quickly and easily than hardware flaws.

Several disadvantages of dedicated hardware systems exist. First, as mentioned above, more sophisticated hardware generally costs more to purchase and maintain. Second, rapid advancement in computer technology may cause the hardware to become obsolete quickly. Third, algorithm flaws in the dedicated hardware may be difficult to fix without replacing some hardware components. As the size of the circuitry decreases and the complexity increases, the possibility of a flaw in the circuitry is significant. Finally, new and more rapid algorithms are constantly being developed. An algorithm change cannot be implemented as quickly in dedicated hardware as it can with software.

*(ii) Interactive versus static.* Two different programming modes are available to view the generated 3-D images: interactive and static. In static programs, the images are presented in a predetermined sequence of set orientations. The user has minimal ability to manipulate the presentation of the images. In the interactive mode, the user is able to manipulate the data presentation. The image may then be presented in unique orientations, e.g., rotated or tilted, for optimal evaluation of spatial relationships. Surgical procedures can be planned with simulated osteotomies that remove a specific portion of a bone. Thus, the image presentation can be modified in the interactive mode to best suit the needs of the clinician. On the other hand, interactive programs tend to be more expensive and demand more user time than static programs.

*(iii) Volume- versus surface-based imaging.* The rendering technique, which refers to the type of algorithm used to convert conventional 2-D CT images to a 3-D format, is an important factor in 3-D imaging. The two major classes of rendering techniques are volume-based and surface-based algorithms.

Image acquisition in both algorithms is the same as in conventional 2-D imaging. No additional imaging information is gleaned from the 3-D system that is not present on the 2-D images. In both algorithms, the acquired data must then be stored in a geographic matrix with each geographic point assigned an appropriate density. Each geographic point, from a practical computational standpoint, must have a finite volume. This volume is called a voxel. The use of very small volumes requires a tremendous amount of memory. To conserve memory without sacrificing resolution, an optimal voxel size must be used. The optimal voxel size is highly dependent on the speed and memory capabilities of a given system. The average density of the voxel is determined and stored in the geographic matrix. Obviously, a system that uses smaller voxels will have better resolution. However, such a system is more expensive and requires more money and computing time than a system that uses large voxels.

The difference in the two rendering techniques is at the level of density classification within the geographic matrix. Surface-based algorithms require the user to specify the objects of interest. Usually the user specifies a threshold density in Hounsfield units. The result is a binary system with densities below the threshold represented by 0 and those above the threshold represented by 1. This scheme reduces the amount of data stored in the geometric matrix, thus conserving memory space and reducing the data manipulation required for 3-D representation.

Volume-based algorithms attempt to conserve density data. One method of volume imaging is to divide each voxel into tissue types, e.g., air, fat, soft tissue, or bone. Each tissue type is assigned upper and lower threshold limits. Each voxel is then classified by identifying its average density with the appropriate tissue type. More complicated volume-based systems may classify density into more user-specific schemes. For example, soft tissue may be subdivided into thresholds to differentiate a soft tissue tumor from surrounding soft tissue of slightly different density. The densities are coded as different shades of gray in the geographic matrix. Volume-based systems require more memory and more data manipulation than surface-based systems do.

*(iv) Slice thickness.* Slice thickness directly affects the resolution of the 3-D images. Thinner slices increase resolution. The price for increased resolution includes longer scan times, larger memory requirements, and increased patient exposure to ionizing radiation. Furthermore, the thinner slices require more time to cover the area of interest. During the time when the scans are obtained, the patient must remain motionless for optimal 3-D reconstruction of the slices.

*Applications of 3-D CT.* 3-D CT offers a number of distinct advantages over conventional 2-D CT. Spatial relationships can be shown in familiar anatomic formats. In addition, spatial relationships between multiplanar objects can be determined more precisely, and life-size images may be produced to aid in the manufacture of prostheses or other surgical devices. With 3-D CT, computer-assisted disarticulations may be performed, which will help in designing a prosthetic device. Direct pre- and postoperative comparisons of surgical results can be made with great precision. In cases of trauma, there is a clear perception of the extent of major fractures and the direction of displacement (Figure 9-9). This improved detail of fractures has been shown to alter management in 20 to 30% of patients when compared with conventional 2-D CT.

The ability to disarticulate structures and to view fractures from a surgeon's perspective is particularly helpful in preoperative planning for trauma patients. This saves considerable time relative to the tedious task of comparing multiple 2-D CT slices. 3-D CT is now frequently used in the evaluation of mandibular fractures and complex malar fractures including LeFort fractures (Figure 9-10). 3-D CT may also be used in the evaluation of complex orbital fractures. Unfortunately, fractures of the medial and inferior orbital walls are difficult to detect reliably on 3-D CT. Artifacts known as pseudoforamina may be produced in these regions by volume-averaging errors. These artifacts are particularly common in regions where the orbital wall is thin and is surrounded by the paranasal

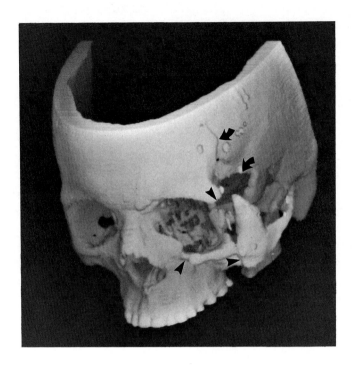

*Figure 9-9.* Disarticulated 3-D CT of the anterior portion of the calvarium and face; oblique view. There is a complex fracture of the left squamous temporal bone (arrows) and a markedly displaced fracture of the left zygoma (arrowheads). Multiple bony fragments are noted within the left orbit. Note the clear depiction of the direction and extent of displacement of the major and minor fractures.

sinuses. Volume-averaging errors can be minimized in these regions by using thin sections and overlapping slices. Because of these limitations, 3-D CT is best used in conjunction with 2-D CT and radiographs.

3-D CT has proven to be an essential tool for early diagnosis and for surgical planning in patients with craniofacial deformities. Prosthetic devices can be tailored to the individual patient's needs before surgery actually occurs. In patients with neoplasms, the tumors are more accurately staged by using 3-D CT since the size, shape, margins, and relationships to adjacent structures may be optimally visualized. In addition, radiation therapy is enhanced by 3-D CT, which maximizes the ability to target the tumor and spare the surrounding normal tissues.

The future of 3-D CT applications may already be emerging as work proceeds on merged multimodality imaging. The premise of such technology is that multiple imaging modalities can be referenced to common

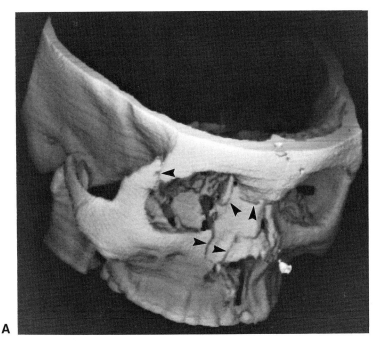

A

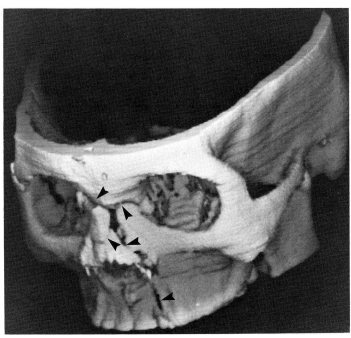

B

*Figure 9-10.*   Disarticulated 3-D CT of the face and orbits. (A) Oblique right lateral view. (B) Oblique left lateral view. Note the complex multiple bilateral facial fractures (arrowheads). On the right side, there is a non-displaced tripod fracture of the right zygoma. Fractures are noted within the right orbit and extending across the anterior maxilla into the central portion of the premaxilla. Because of the involvement of the posterior portion and lateral wall of the right orbit, this is consistent with a LeFort type III fracture. A similar fracture is present on the left side without disruption of the left zygoma. This is consistent with a LeFort type II fracture. Note also the extensive fracturing involving the nasal bones.

anatomic landmarks. Thus, the diverse information obtained from two or more imaging modalities is merged with computer reconstruction. Such merged images would provide better characterization of the structures under study. Additional technological advances will produce better resolution, increased signal-to-noise ratios, more rapid reconstruction times, and decreased acquisition times. With more widespread availability of 3-D CT, applications will no doubt affect an increasingly diverse patient population.

*Anton N. Hasso, M.D.*
*Thomas E. Wiley, M.D.*
*Alix Vincent, M.D.*

*SUGGESTED READINGS*

CRANIOFACIAL SYNDROMES

1. Hasso AN, Broadwell RA. Congenital abnormalities. In: Som PM, Bergeron RT (eds), Head and neck imaging. Chicago: Mosby-Year Book; 1991:960–992
2. Naidich TP, Osborn RE, Bauer BS, McLone DG, Kernahan DA, Zaparackas ZG. Embryology and congenital lesions of the midface. In: Som PM, Bergeron RT (eds), Head and neck imaging, 2nd ed. St. Louis: Mosby-Year Book; 1991:1–50

CRANIOSYNOSTOSIS

3. Hardesty RA, Marsh JL, Vannier MW. Unicoronal synostosis. A surgical intervention. Neurosurg Clin North Am 1991; 6:641–653
4. Parisi M, Mehdizadeh HM, Hunter JC, Finch IJ. Evaluation of craniosynostosis with three-dimensional CT imaging. J Comput Assist Tomogr 1989; 13:1006–1012
5. Pilgram TK, Vannier MW, Hildebolt CF, et al. Craniosynostosis: image quality, confidence, and correctness in diagnosis. Radiology 1989; 173:675–679
6. Vannier MW, Hildebolt CF, Marsh JL, et al. Craniosynostosis: diagnostic value of three-dimensional CT reconstruction. Radiology 1989; 173:669–673

THREE-DIMENSIONAL CT

7. DeMarino DP, Steiner E, Poster RB, et al. Three-dimensional computed tomography in maxillofacial trauma. Arch Otolaryngol Head Neck Surg 1986; 112:146–150

8. Fishman EK, Magid D, Ney DR, et al. Three-dimensional imaging. Radiology 1991; 181:321–337

9. Howard JD, Elster AD, May JS. Temporal bone: three-dimensional CT. Part I. Normal anatomy, techniques, and limitations. Radiology 1990; 177:421–425

10. Howard JD, Elster AD, May JS. Temporal bone: three-dimensional CT. Part II. Pathologic alterations. Radiology 1990; 177:427–430

11. Schellhas KP, el Deeb M, Wilkes CH, et al. Three-dimensional computed tomography in maxillofacial surgical planning. Arch Otolaryngol Head Neck Surg 1988; 114:438–442

12. Zonneveld FW, Lobregt S, van der Meulen JC, Vaandrager JM. Three-dimensional imaging in craniofacial surgery. World J Surg 1989; 13:328–342

SE 2,200/20

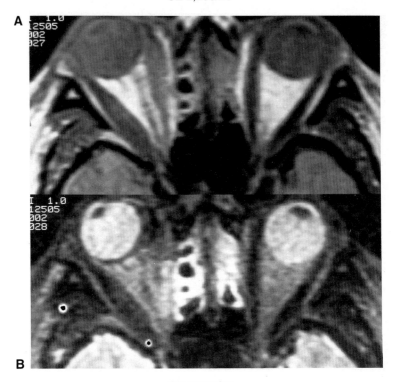

SE 2,200/80

*Figure 10-1.*   This 42-year-old woman has painful proptosis of the right eye. You are shown proton-density (A), T2-weighted (B), fat-suppressed STIR (C), and postcontrast T1-weighted (D) MR scans.

# Case 10: Myositic Orbital Pseudotumor

## Question 45

Which *one* of the following is the MOST likely diagnosis?

(A) Dysthyroid orbitopathy
(B) Myositic orbital pseudotumor
(C) Lymphoma
(D) Metastasis
(E) Rhabdomyosarcoma

The proton-density and T2-weighted MR scans (Figure 10-1A and B) show enlargement of the right medial and lateral rectus muscles (see Figure 10-2A and B). The right medial rectus muscle has a ragged, fluffy border and appears slightly hyperintense to normal muscle on the proton-density MR image and hyperintense to other muscles on the T2-weighted MR image. This is due to associated diffuse edema of the right medial rectus muscle. The short-inversion-time inversion-recovery (STIR) MR scan (Figure 10-1C) shows enlargement of the right medial and lateral rectus muscles. There is marked edema of the right medial rectus muscle, evidenced by the increased signal intensity of this muscle (arrow, Figure 10-2C). The T1-weighted MR scan obtained after administration of gadolinium DTPA (Figure 10-1D) shows enlargement of the right lateral and medial rectus muscles. There is some enhancement of the involved rectus muscles. The swelling of these muscles extends to involve their tendons (arrows, Figure 10-2D).

The clinical presentation of proptosis and pain and the MR findings of enlargement of the extraocular muscles, including swelling of the right medial and lateral rectus tendons and marked edema of the right medial rectus muscle, are characteristic of idiopathic orbital inflammation of a myositic type. Myositic orbital pseudotumor is therefore the most likely diagnosis **(Option (B) is correct).**

In patients with dysthyroid orbitopathy (Option (A)), the muscle involvement is usually bilateral and symmetric. CT or MR scanning of

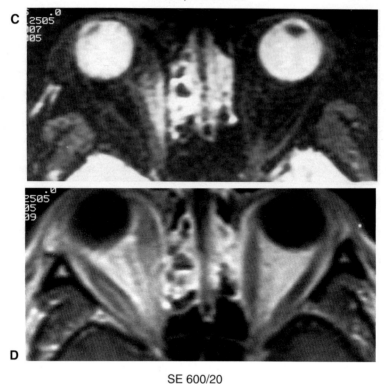

SE 600/20

*Figure 10-1 (Continued)*

patients with dysthyroid orbitopathy almost always shows that the swelling of the muscle belly spares the tendons.

Orbital lymphoid tumors (Option (C)) tend to have an insidious and clinically quiet onset, without the pain and inflammatory signs of the orbital pseudotumor. Orbital lymphomas can involve any area of the orbit but are commonly situated in the superior and anterior orbit, involving the lacrimal gland, conjunctiva, or lids.

The clinical presentation of orbital metastasis (Option (D)) is often sudden, with proptosis, lid swelling, visual loss, and pain. It is not uncommon for orbital metastasis to present clinically before the primary tumor is discovered. Metastatic tumor may involve the bony orbit, the extraconal space (including the lacrimal glands), the extraocular muscles (conal space), optic nerves and other parts of the intraconal space, as well as the globe. Metastasis to extraocular muscles often results in irregular or segmental muscular enlargement. In addition, the margin of the involved muscle is often irregular.

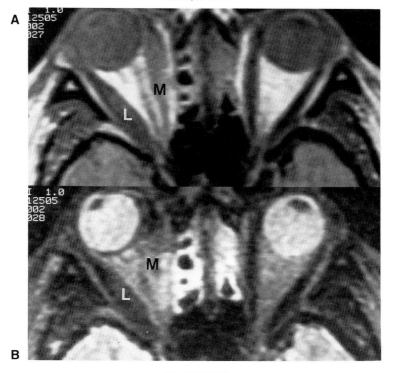

*Figure 10-2* (Same as Figure 10-1). (A and B) Proton-density and T2-weighted images show enlargement of the right medial (M) and lateral (L) rectus muscles. The medial rectus muscle has ill-defined borders and shows a more markedly increased signal intensity on the T2-weighted image. (C) Fat-suppressed STIR image shows marked edema of the right medial rectus muscle. Note the high signal intensity of the muscle (arrow). (D) Postcontrast T1-weighted image demonstrates enlargement and some enhancement of the right lateral and medial rectus muscles. The swelling of the involved muscles extends to involve their tendons (arrows).

Orbital rhabdomyosarcoma (Option (E)) is primarily a disease of childhood. Rapidly progressing unilateral proptosis is the hallmark of this lesion. Primary orbital rhabdomyosarcoma commonly fills the adjacent paranasal sinuses and nasal cavity. Rhabdomyosarcomas are aggressive and are capable of bone destruction and extraorbital extension.

The test patient has one of the several different types of inflammatory disease that may affect the orbit. Based on clinical presentation and the overall CT and MR appearance, the different types of infectious and

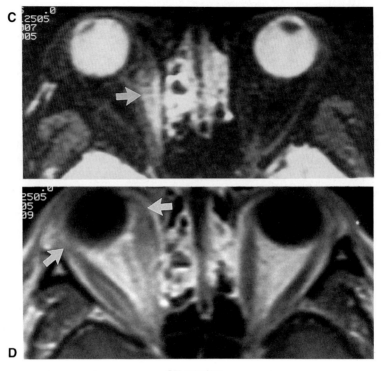

SE 600/20

noninfectious orbital inflammations are often difficult to differentiate. The following discussion addresses the key features of the infectious orbital inflammations and the noninfectious orbital inflammations or pseudotumors.

*Orbital infections.* Orbital infections account for about 60% of primary orbital disease processes. The orbital process may be acute, subacute, or chronic. Most acute orbital inflammatory disorders are secondary to infections of the paranasal sinuses (Figures 10-3 and 10-4). However, they may develop from an infectious process of the face or pharynx, from trauma, or from foreign bodies, or they may be secondary to septicemia. The bacteria most commonly involved are *Staphylococcus*, *Streptococcus* (including *S. pneumoniae), Pseudomonas, Haemophilus*, and *Mycobacterium* species and members of the family *Neisseriaceae*. Herpes simplex and herpes zoster viruses are the major causes of viral infections of the orbit. In immunosuppressed patients and patients with poorly controlled diabetes, opportunistic infections such as those caused by fungal and parasitic pathogens may be responsible for severe sinonaso-orbital infections. Acute inflammation is characterized by rapid development of

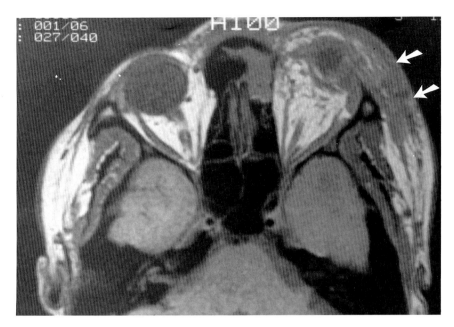

SE 2,000/20

*Figure 10-3.* Sinogenic orbital cellulitis. Axial proton-density MR scan shows marked edema of the left eyelid. Note the involvement of fascial planes with edema extending into the temporal region (arrows), characteristic of an inflammatory process. Also note the reticular infiltrations of the retrobulbar space.

tissue swelling, infiltration, loss of normal tissue planes, destruction, and abscess formation. The location of the process is important. The orbital septum is a fibrouslike sheet that extends from the superior bony orbital rim down to the superior tarsal plate and from the inferior bony rim up to the inferior tarsal plate. When the eyelids are closed there is thus a functional plane (the orbital septum) that separates the preseptal region from the retroseptal area (orbit). A preseptal infection rarely affects orbital functions. On the other hand, a retroseptal infection (Figure 10-4) may have a profound and sudden effect on optic nerve function and ocular motility. Pathologically, in acute bacterial inflammation, polymorphonuclear leukocytes are usually the dominant cells, and the process is often rapidly progressive with necrosis and destruction of tissue planes.

*Subperiosteal phlegmon and abscess.* As the reaction of the orbital infection begins and gradually advances, the edema of the eyelids and conjunctivae becomes more generalized and the eye begins to protrude. Inflammatory tissue and edema collect beneath the periosteum (Figure

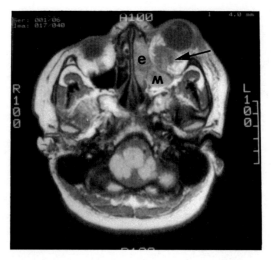

SE 2,000/20

*Figure 10-4.* Sinusitis and orbital cellulitis. Axial proton-density MR scan shows left ethmoid (e) and maxillary (m) sinusitis with marked retrobular cellulitis (arrow).

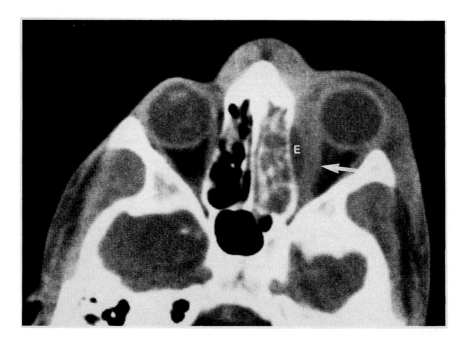

*Figure 10-5.* Ethmoid sinusitis and subperiosteal tissue reaction and edema. Axial CT scan shows left ethmoid sinusitis associated with fluid (edema) (E) and inflammatory reactions in the subperiosteal space, displacing the medial rectus muscle laterally (arrow).

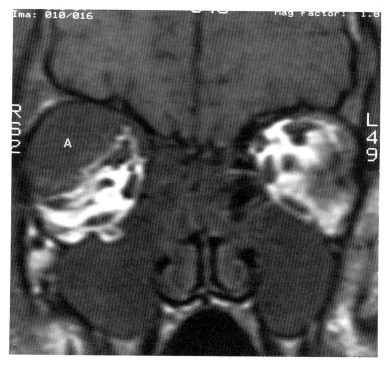

SE 800/20

*Figure 10-6.* Subperiosteal phlegmon. Coronal T1-weighted MR scan shows maxillary and ethmoid sinusitis. There is a large subperiosteal phlegmon/abscess (A) in the superior extraconal space.

10-5) to form a subperiosteal phlegmon (Figure 10-6). Subsequently, pus may form, causing a subperiosteal abscess (Figure 10-7). As the disease progresses, the inflammatory process may infiltrate the periorbital and retro-orbital fat to give rise to a true orbital cellulitis (Figure 10-4). The subperiosteal abscess and orbital cellulitis frequently coexist. At this stage, extraocular muscle motility is progressively impaired. With severe involvement, visual disturbances can result from optic neuritis or ischemia. Progression of intraorbital cellulitis or spread from the subperiosteal space leads to intraconal or extraconal loculation and abscess formation.

Ophthalmic vein thrombosis and cavernous sinus thrombosis are very serious complications of orbital and sinonasal infections. Cavernous sinus thrombosis is heralded by profound central nervous system deficit and orbital functional impairment.

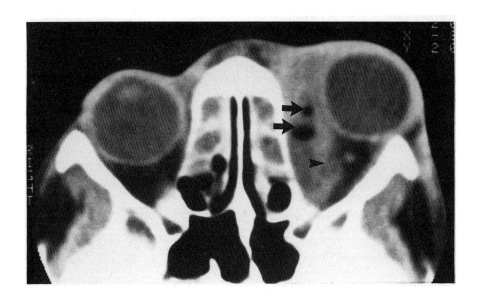

*Figure 10-7.* Subperiosteal abscess. Axial CT scan shows bilateral ethmoid sinusitis associated with a subperiosteal abscess (arrows). The medial rectus muscle is displaced (arrowhead).

*Acute, subacute, and chronic idiopathic orbital pseudotumors.* Idiopathic inflammatory syndromes are usually referred to as orbital pseudotumors, a clinically and histologically confusing category of lesions. Orbital pseudotumor is defined as a nonspecific, idiopathic inflammatory condition for which no local identifiable cause or systemic disease can be found. By definition, this excludes orbital inflammatory disease caused by entities such as Wegener's granulomatosis, retained foreign bodies, known granulomatous diseases (such as sarcoidosis or tuberculosis), sclerosing hemangioma, trauma, and sinusitis. Pseudotumors must be distinguished from both Graves' disease and lymphoma of the orbit.

Orbital pseudotumor was first described in 1905 by Birch-Hirschfield and has remained something of an enigma in the ophthalmology, radiology, and pathology literature. In addition to the variety of classification systems and diagnostic criteria that have been offered over the years, this disease can include a wide range of clinical presentations, and many of the symptoms are nonspecific. Both children and adults may be affected by pseudotumors. In children there may be evidence of papillitis or iritis, and bilaterality is quite common, occurring in about 40% of cases. In adults bilaterality is less common and is strongly suggestive of a systemic disease, such as lymphoma or Wegener's granulomatosis. Orbital involvement is one of the most common ophthalmic manifestations of Wegener's granulomatosis. The diagnosis of orbital Wegener's granulomatosis is often not straightforward because of confusion with orbital pseudotumors, lymphoma, and other entities that may present with similar features. Serum immunoglobulin G (IgG) antibodies against cytoplasmic components of neutrophils and monocytes, the so-called antineutrophil cytoplasmic antibody, have been a useful diagnostic adjunct for Wegener's granulomatosis. The classic triad of histopathologic findings in Wegener's disease comprises vasculitis, granulomatous inflammation, and tissue necrosis.

The histopathology of orbital pseudotumors can vary greatly from polymorphous inflammatory cells and fibrosis to a predominantly lymphocytic form, which may be related to lymphoma. The presence of germinal follicles and increased vascularity suggests a reactive lesion and is associated with a favorable prognosis and responsiveness to steroids. An association has been noted between diffusely distributed lymphoblasts, unresponsiveness to steroids, and a probable neoplastic lymphoid lesion. However, not all steroid-resistant pseudotumors are destined to become lymphomatous. The peculiar behavior of pseudotumors has led some authors to speculate that some forms of pseudotumor are the result of an autoimmune process. As the disease progresses, there is fibrous replacement of the extraocular muscles, orbital fat, and lacrimal gland. If follicular or diffuse lymphoid hyperplasia is marked, differentiation from orbital lymphoid tumors becomes more difficult. In pseudotumor, T lymphocytes predominate (about 70%) in the lesions, whereas in lymphomatoid tumor one may find a monoclonal predominance of B lymphocytes.

Pseudotumors may be classified as (1) acute and subacute idiopathic anterior orbital inflammation, (2) acute and subacute idiopathic diffuse orbital inflammation, (3) acute and subacute idiopathic myositic orbital inflammation, (4) acute and subacute idiopathic apical orbital inflammation, (5) idiopathic dacryoadenitis, and (6) perineuritis.

*Anterior orbital pseudotumor.* In the anterior orbital pseudotumor group, the main focus of inflammation involves the anterior orbit and the globe. The major presenting features are pain, proptosis, lid swelling, and decreased vision. Other findings may be ocular and include uveitis, sclerotenonitis (i.e., inflammation of Tenon's capsule), papillitis, and exudative retinal detachment. The extraocular muscle motility is usually unaffected. CT and MRI show thickening of the "uveal-scleral" rim with obscuration of the optic nerve junction, which enhances with contrast medium infusion (Figure 10-8). These findings are due to leakage of

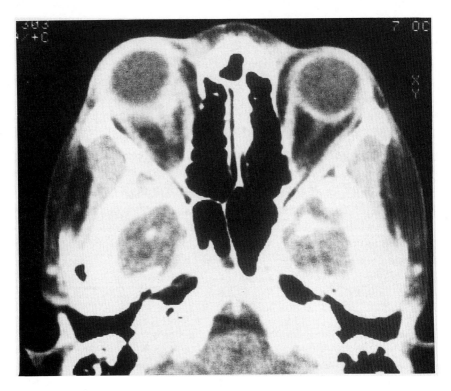

*Figure 10-8.* Orbital pseudotumor. Axial CT scan shows marked thickening of the right globe associated with increased enhancement around the globe and proximal right optic nerve. These changes are related to scleritis, as well as fluid and cellular infiltration in Tenon's space.

proteinaceous edema fluid into the interstitium of the uvea, sclera, Tenon's capsule, and Tenon's space secondary to inflammatory reaction. Fluid in Tenon's capsule has been well documented by ultrasonography (the T sign). Patients with posterior scleritis can develop retinal detachment and fundal masses, which simulate intraocular tumors (Figure 10-9). The clinical differential diagnosis of anterior orbital pseudotumor includes orbital cellulitis, ruptured dermoid cyst, hemorrhage within a vascular lesion (hemangioma, lymphangioma), collagen vascular disease, rhabdomyosarcoma, and leukemic infiltration.

*Diffuse orbital pseudotumor.* Diffuse orbital pseudotumor is similar in many respects to acute and subacute anterior inflammation, but the signs and symptoms are more severe. The diffuse (also called tumefactive or infiltrative) type of pseudotumor may fill the entire retrobulbar space and mold itself around the globe while respecting its natural shape (Figure 10-10). Even the largest of masses usually do not invade or distort

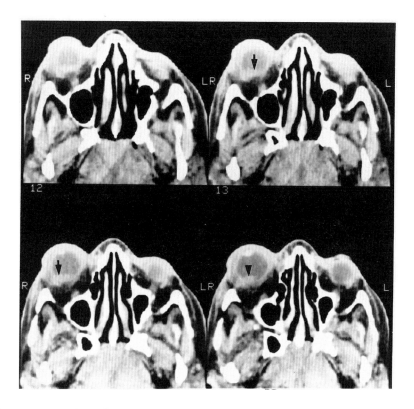

*Figure 10-9.* Pseudotumor. Axial CT scans in this patient with scleritis and retinal detachment show marked thickening of the wall of the right globe. There is dependent fluid in the subretinal space (arrow) and a mass (pseudotumor) in the posterior pole of the right globe (arrowhead). Although the fluid and the mass appear similar on CT, they can be distinguished clinically.

the shape of the globe or erode bone. This type (Figures 10-11 and 10-12) can be very difficult to differentiate from lymphoma. These large, bulky masses can be intraconal or extraconal or can be situated in both spaces, and they must be differentiated from true tumors of the orbit, e.g., cavernous hemangioma, hemangiopericytoma, optic nerve sheath meningioma, optic nerve glioma, orbital schwannoma, and metastasis. Sarcoidosis may have a CT and MR appearance identical to that of pseudotumors (Figure 10-13). True tumors do not respect the boundaries of the globe; they push or indent its surface. Also, bone erosion and extraorbital extension are more typical of true tumors than of pseudotumors. One of the important features of a pseudotumor is that it appears rather hypointense on T2-weighted MR scans (Figures 10-11B and 10-12)

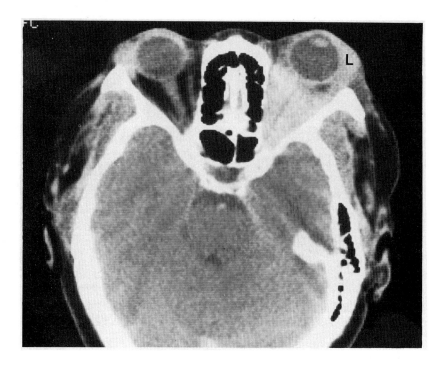

*Figure 10-10.* Pseudotumor. Axial CT scan shows diffuse infiltration of the left retrobulbar space. There is proptosis and slight enlargement of the left lacrimal gland (L). The lesion molds itself around the globe while respecting its natural shape. This is characteristic of pseudotumor as well as orbital lymphoma.

whereas true tumors, including some orbital lymphomas, appear hyperintense. Enhancement of pseudotumors can be best demonstrated on postcontrast fat-suppressed T1-weighted MR scans (Figure 10-14). In rare cases there is the picture of a sclerosing pseudotumor, with an excessive deposition of fibrosis leading to the wall-to-wall congealing of all of the orbital contents by the fibrosis, creating a "frozen orbit." Rarely, metastatic scirrhous carcinoma (of the breast) creates a similar picture (Figure 10-15).

*Orbital myositis.* Idiopathic orbital myositis is a condition in which one or more of the extraocular muscles are infiltrated primarily by an inflammatory process (Figure 10-16). Myositis can be acute, subacute, or recurrent. The patient usually presents with painful ocular movements, diplopia, proptosis, swelling of the lid, conjunctival chemosis, and inflammation over the involved muscle. This disorder may be bilateral. The most frequently affected muscles are the superior complex and the medial rectus (Figure 10-16). The major differential diagnosis is Graves' disease.

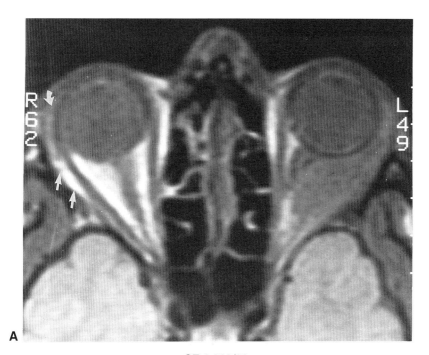

SE 2,000/20

*Figure 10-11.* Pseudotumor. (A) Axial proton-density MR scan shows an infiltrative process in the left retrobulbar space with involvement of the left lateral rectus, the extraconal fat lateral to the lateral rectus muscle, and the left lacrimal gland. The right extraconal fat (straight arrows) and right lacrimal gland (curved arrow) are normal. The lesion molds itself around the globe without invading it. (B) Axial T2-weighted MR scan. The pseudotumor appears mostly hypointense. (C) Axial STIR MR scan. The pseudotumor appears hyperintense in relation to normal fat. (D) Axial postcontrast T1-weighted MR scan. There is moderate enhancement of the left lacrimal gland and pseudotumor in the retrobulbar space.

However, dysthyroid orbitopathy is usually painless in onset, slowly progressive, and often associated with systemic manifestations of hyperthyroidism.

Trokel and Hilal state that the typical CT finding in orbital myositis is enlargement of the extraocular muscles, which extends anteriorly to involve the inserting tendon (Figure 10-16). Other helpful indicators of idiopathic inflammatory orbital myositis include a ragged, fluffy border of the involved muscle with infiltration and obliteration of the fat in the peripheral orbital space between the periosteum of the orbital wall and the muscle cone (Figure 10-14). There is also an inward bowing of the

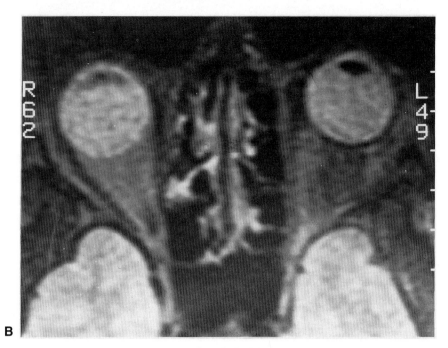

SE 2,000/80

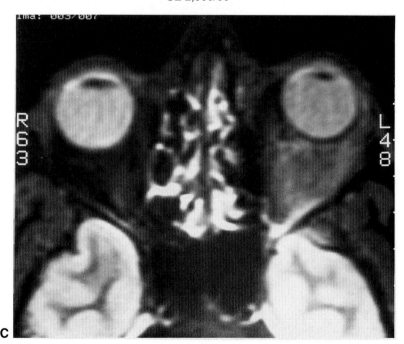

STIR 2,000/40/160

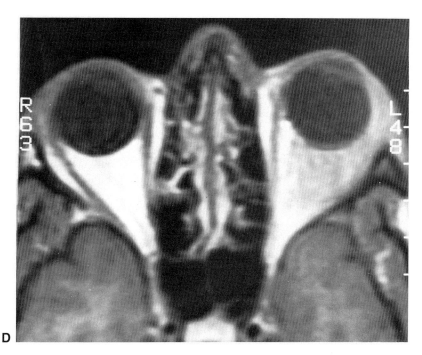

SE 600/20

medial contour of the muscle belly, forming a shoulder as it passes behind the globe (Figures 10-1 and 10-16). Another important finding is localized inflammation around the arc of contact of muscle with the globe as a result of tendinitis and local tenon fasciitis (Figure 10-14). All these findings can be attributed to local tendinitis, fasciitis, and myositis of the involved muscle. In contrast, the fusiform appearance of an enlarged muscle in dysthyroid myopathy is produced by myositis along the belly of the muscle only (see Figure 10-23). The muscle borders are sharply defined, the fat in the peripheral orbital space is preserved, and there is no tendinous infiltration. Less common causes of extraocular muscle enlargement include arteriovenous fistula (e.g., carotid-cavernous fistula) and primary or metastatic neoplasm (Figure 10-17).

*Acute and subacute idiopathic apical orbital inflammation.* Pseudotumor may present with infiltration of the orbital apex (Figure 10-18). Patients present with a typical apical orbital syndrome of pain, minimal proptosis, visual loss, diplopia, and restricted movement of extraocular muscles. The CT and MR findings include an irregular infiltrative process of the apex of the orbit with extension along the posterior portion of the extraocular muscles or the optic nerve (Figure 10-18). A specific localiza-

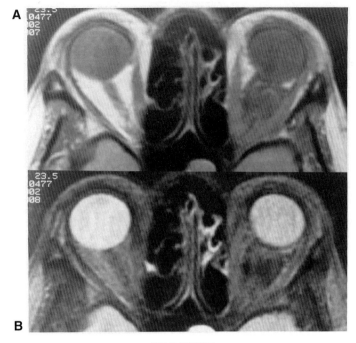

SE 2,000/80

*Figure 10-12.* Pseudotumor. Axial proton-density (A) and T2-weighted (B) MR scans show a large left retrobulbar mass, associated with enlargement of the lateral and medial rectus muscles. The lesion is hypointense in the T2-weighted scan. In this case, the clinical diagnosis was pseudotumor versus lymphoma. The differential diagnosis should include orbital meningioma and metastasis.

tion is seen in Tolosa-Hunt syndrome (one of the causes of superior orbital fissure syndrome), in which there is inflammation of the periosteum of the orbit along the superior orbital fissure, leading to partial or complete painful external ophthalmoplegia, sometimes with papillary signs (papilledema). This inflammatory infiltration may extend to involve the dura in the middle cranial fossa and may encroach on the cavernous sinus, resulting in constriction of the intracavernous portions of the carotid artery. The inflammation often has an explosive onset, and the disease is exquisitely sensitive to systemic corticosteroids. Any infiltrative process in the superior orbital fissure can cause symptoms and signs simulating Tolosa-Hunt syndrome. These diseases include tuberculosis (Figure 10-19), sarcoidosis (Figure 10-13), fungal infections, other granulomatous processes, lymphoma, en plaque meningioma, orbital extension

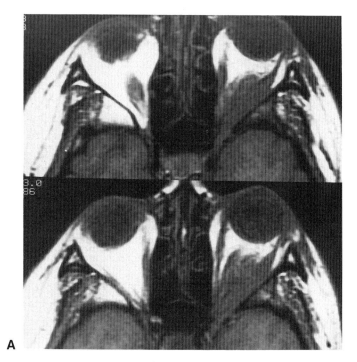

SE 400/25

*Figure 10-13.* Sarcoidosis presenting as pseudotumor. (A) Axial T1-weighted MR scans show an infiltrative mass in the left orbital apex associated with enlargement of the lateral rectus muscle. (B) Postcontrast axial T1-weighted MR scans show moderate enhancement of the orbital apical infiltrate. Enhancement along the border of the middle cranial fossa (arrow) is due to infiltration of the meninges. The enhancement of the normal extraocular muscles is better seen in panel C. (C) Postcontrast fat-suppressed axial T1-weighted MR scans show enhancement of the left apical infiltrate. The enhancement of the extraocular muscles is normal and is presumed to be related to their high vascularity; it should not be mistaken for a sign of abnormalities.

of paranasal sinus tumors, and metastatic diseases. In idiopathic Tolosa-Hunt syndrome, lymphocytes, histiocytes, and multinucleated cells have been found in histopathologic specimens.

*Lacrimal adenitis.* Acute idiopathic lacrimal adenitis presents with tenderness in the upper outer quadrant of the orbit in the region of the lacrimal gland. Viral dacryoadenitis (e.g., due to mumps, mononucleosis, or herpes zoster) may present in a similar manner. Adenopathy and lymphocytosis may be present. The differential diagnosis of nonspecific lacrimal adenitis and pseudotumors (Figures 10-20 and 10-21) includes

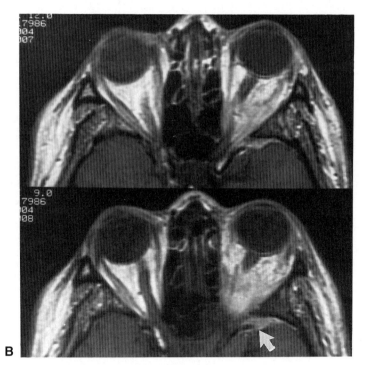

SE 400/25

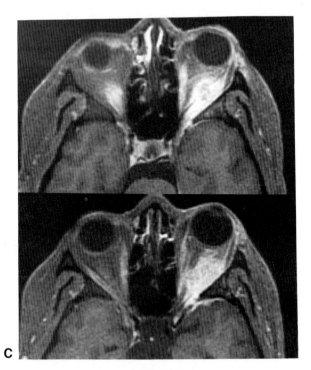

SE 600/25

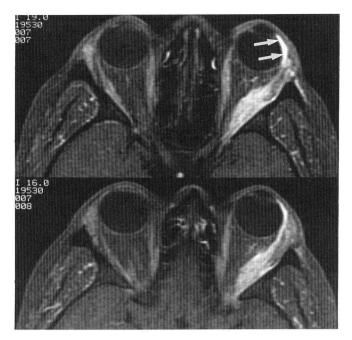

SE 800/15

*Figure 10-14.* Pseudotumor. These postcontrast fat-suppressed axial T1-weighted MR scans show enhancement of the left lateral rectus muscle and adjacent orbital infiltrate. Enhancement along the arc of contact of the left lateral rectus tendon with the left globe (arrows) is due to tendinitis and localized tenon fascitis.

viral and bacterial dacryoadenitis, rupture of a dermoid cyst in the lacrimal gland region, specific lacrimal gland inflammations such as sarcoidosis (Figure 10-22) and Sjögren's syndrome, lymphoproliferative or myeloproliferative disorders, cysts, and neoplasia in this region. Because of the wide variety of tumefactions of the lacrimal gland, biopsy of this accessible site is necessary to make the correct diagnosis.

*Perineuritis.* Idiopathic perineuritis (perineuritic pseudotumor) and orbital lymphoma can simulate optic neuritis by presenting with orbital pain, pain with ocular motility, decreased visual acuity, and disk edema. In contrast to optic neuritis, pain is exacerbated, with retrodisplacement of the globe, and there is mild proptosis. CT and MRI show a ragged, edematous enlargement of the optic nerve (see Figure 10-28).

Of the various CT and MR characteristics associated with different features of pseudotumors, the most common findings include moderate enhancement with intravenous contrast medium (95%), infiltration of the

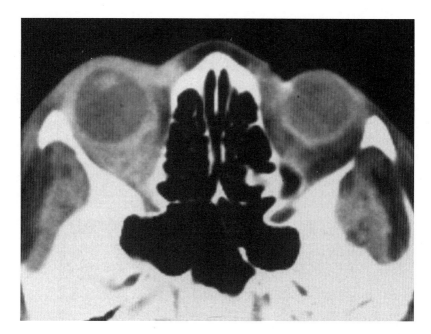

*Figure 10-15.* Metastatic scirrhous carcinoma of the breast simulating sclerosing pseudotumor. Axial CT scan shows diffuse right retrobulbar infiltrate without proptosis.

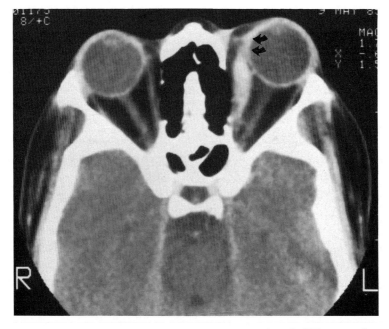

*Figure 10-16.* Pseudotumor (myositic type). Axial CT scan shows enhancement of the enlarged left medial rectus muscle. Note the involvement of its tendon (arrows) characteristically seen in orbital myositis.

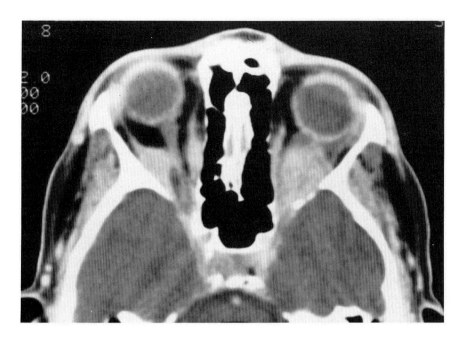

*Figure 10-17.* Metastatic deposits from breast carcinoma. Axial CT scan shows enlargement of the right lateral and medial rectus muscles, as well as a large left retrobulbar mass.

retrobulbar fat (76%), proptosis (71%), extraocular muscle enlargement (57%), apical fat infiltration and edema (48%), muscle tendon/sheath enlargement (43%), and optic nerve thickening (38%). On MRI, the enhancement of pseudotumors with gadolinium DTPA is best demonstrated on fat-suppressed images (Figures 10-14 and 10-18D). A key finding with pseudotumors is the virtual absence of bone erosion or distortion of the orbital contents. In contrast, distortion of the orbital contents is commonly present with both benign and malignant tumors.

There are no specific imaging characteristics or clinical signs to establish the diagnosis of pseudotumor with absolute certainty. Classically, the rapid development of unilateral, painful ophthalmoplegia, proptosis, and chemosis with a rapid and lasting response to steroid therapy in an otherwise healthy patient is highly suggestive of pseudotumor. Most pseudotumors encountered in practice are of the diffuse and myositic varieties. These forms must be differentiated primarily from a true orbital neoplasm and dysthyroid myopathy, respectively. A well-defined tumefactive pseudotumor with sharp borders cannot be reliably and absolutely distinguished from tumor by CT and MR criteria alone.

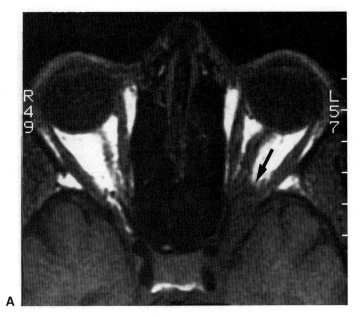

SE 400/20

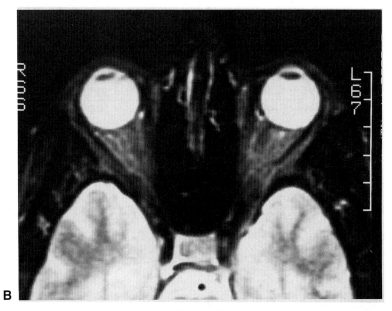

SE 2,200/80

*Figure 10-18.* Apical orbital pseudotumor. (A) Axial T1-weighted MR scan shows a left apical orbital infiltrate (arrow). (B) Axial T2-weighted MR scan. The left orbital infiltrate appears isointense to normal retrobulbar fat. (C) Axial postcontrast T1-weighted MR scan shows enhancement of the apical infiltrate (arrow). (D) Axial postcontrast fat-suppressed T1-weighted MR scan shows apparently marked enhancement of the apical infiltrate. In this pulse sequence the normal extraocular muscles also appear hyperintense.

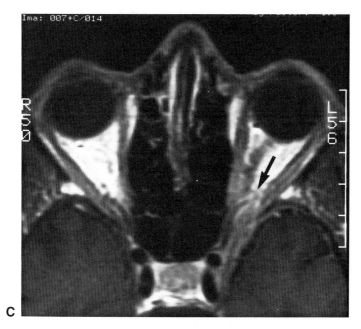

C

SE 400/20

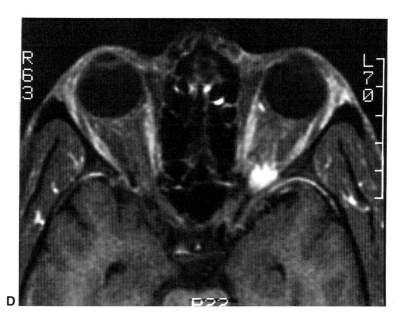

D

SE 400/15

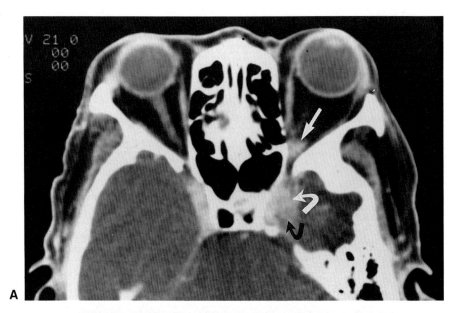

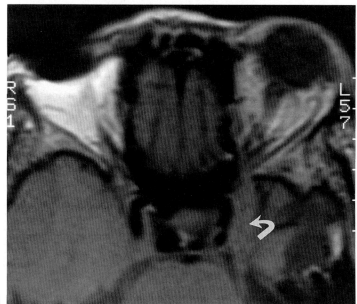

SE 2,000/20

*Figure 10-19.* Tuberculosis mimicking Tolosa-Hunt syndrome. (A) Axial
CT scan shows increased soft tissue with enhancement in the left orbital
apex (straight arrow). The left cavernous sinus is enlarged (curved arrows). (B) Proton-density axial MR scan shows infiltration within the left
cavernous sinus (arrow).

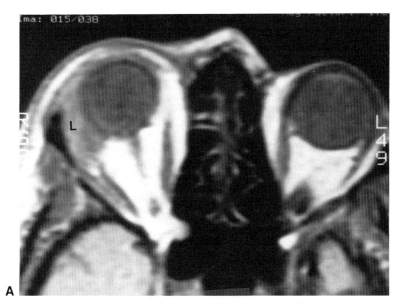

SE 2,200/25

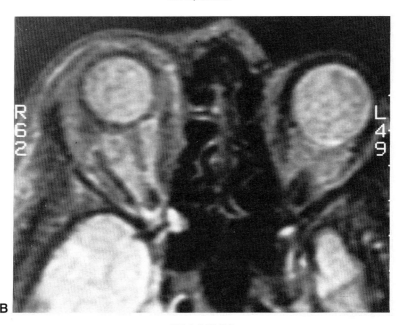

SE 2,200/80

*Figure 10-20.* Pseudotumor with predominant involvement of the lacrimal gland. (A) Axial proton-density MR scan shows enlargement of the right lacrimal gland (L). (B) Axial T2-weighted MR scan. The pseudotumor appears isointense or slightly hypointense to retrobulbar fat. (C) Axial STIR MR scan. The lacrimal gland pseudotumor appears hyperintense (arrows). (D) Axial postcontrast T1-weighted MR scan shows moderate enhancement of the right lacrimal gland pseudotumor (arrows).

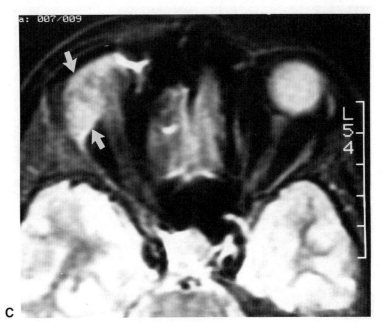

STIR 2,500/40/170

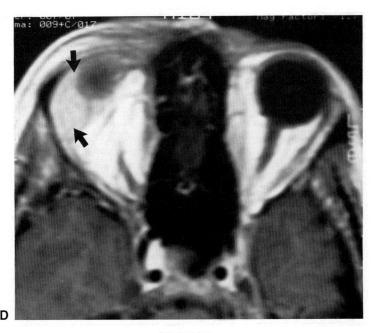

SE 600/20

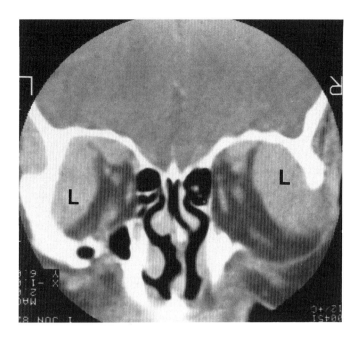

*Figure 10-21.* Lacrimal gland pseudotumors. This 80-year-old patient had swelling of both eyes. Coronal CT scan shows bilateral lobular enlargement of lacrimal glands (L). There is slight enlargement of the superior rectus muscles. A biopsy specimen showed a nonspecific granulomatous infiltrate of lacrimal gland.

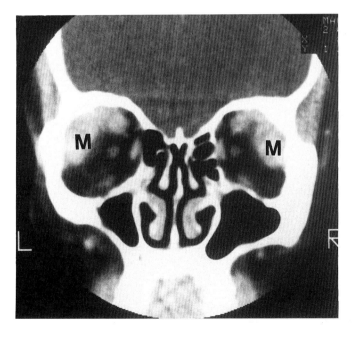

*Figure 10-22.* Sarcoidosis of the lacrimal glands. Coronal CT scan shows a mass (M) involving both lacrimal glands. This is due to diffuse infiltration of the glands by a granulomatous process.

Orbital manifestations of a systemic process, namely dysthyroid disease, lymphoma, leukemia, or metastases, are often diagnosed by exclusion. In the absence of a characteristic clinical presentation of pseudotumor or when there is a poor response to steroids, a biopsy is necessary. Myositic pseudotumor has the most reliable predictive CT and MRI characteristics as a result of its unilateral and usually single muscle enlargement that extends into the tendinous insertion (Figures 10-14 and 10-16).

## Question 46

Concerning dysthyroid orbitopathy,

(A) it is an autoimmune disorder
(B) pain is a common clinical presentation
(C) the lateral rectus muscles are most commonly involved
(D) enlargement of the muscle is usually limited to its belly
(E) bilateral enlargement of the extraocular muscles is less common than in pseudotumor

Ophthalmopathy is one of the characteristic features of Graves' disease. Although most commonly associated with hyperthyroidism, Graves' ophthalmopathy may also occur in patients with primary hypothyroidism or Hashimoto's thyroiditis and is sometimes found in the absence of identifiable thyroid disease. Graves' disease is presently believed to have an autoimmune etiology; a derangement in the B lymphocytes is thought to be responsible, although both T and B lymphocytes have been identified in affected orbital tissues **(Option (A) is true).** An antithyroid immunoglobulin called thyroid-stimulating immunoglobulin (TSI) (previously called long-acting thyroid stimulator) is thought to be responsible for hyperfunction of the thyroid gland. This immunoglobulin interacts with the thyroid-stimulating hormone receptors on the thyroid follicular cells. The thyroid gland thereby is stimulated to increase the rate of thyroid hormone synthesis and to release increased amounts of thyroid hormone into the peripheral blood. Levels of TSIs that are believed to cause thyrotoxicosis do not correlate with the presence, absence, or progression of ophthalmopathy. Approximately 50% of patients with Graves' disease may show ophthalmic signs and symptoms, which are frequently mild and benign. Fewer than 10% develop evidence of infiltrative myopathy, resulting in swelling of extraocular muscles and so

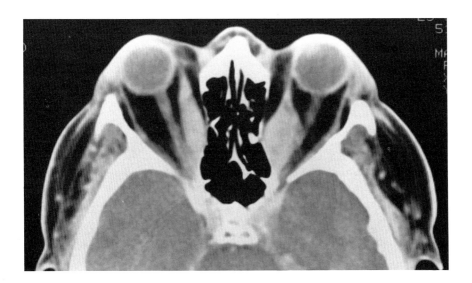

*Figure 10-23.* Dysthyroid orbitopathy. Axial CT scan shows marked enlargement of the belly of the medial rectus muscles. Their tendons are spared.

leading to proptosis, diplopia, extraocular muscle motility imbalance, and compressive optic neuropathy.

The principal pathologic feature of Graves' ophthalmopathy is inflammation of the orbital soft tissues and muscles. Histologically, the muscles show lymphocytic and plasmacytic infiltration, fibrosis of the muscle fibers, and increased levels of mucopolysaccharides. The earliest change in the extraocular muscles appears to be inflammation of the endomysial connective tissues, which seems to stimulate endomysial fibroblasts to produce first hyaluronic acid and then collagen. There is a conspicuous absence of inflammation in the surrounding orbital fat, which is a useful finding on CT and MR scanning (Figures 10-23 through 10-26), as well as pathologically, to distinguish orbital Graves' disease from idiopathic pseudotumors (Figure 10-27).

Dysthyroid orbitopathy occurs most commonly in middle-aged women. It is ophthalmologically characterized by exophthalmos and, in some patients, by the gradual onset of diplopia, usually the vertical type. Unlike the situation with orbital pseudotumor, pain is not a feature of dysthyroid orbitopathy **(Option (B) is false).** Initially, in the acute congestive phase, the retrobulbar orbital contents are markedly swollen and congested. A more chronic, noncongestive phase follows; in this phase a restrictive type of limited eye movement often develops, secondary to infiltration of the extraocular muscles and to subsequent loss of elasticity.

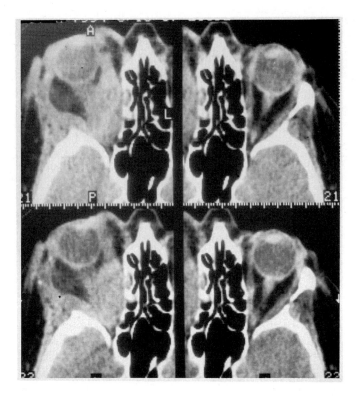

*Figure 10-24.* Unilateral dysthyroid orbitopathy. Axial CT scans show marked enlargement of the right medial and lateral rectus muscles. Their tendons also appear somewhat thickened. This thickening of the tendon is infrequent in dysthyroid orbitopathy. In myositic pseudotumor, thickening of the tendon is a frequent finding. Notice the post-decompression surgical changes (lateral orbitotomy) of the right lateral orbit.

The involvement can be unilateral (Figure 10-24) or bilateral (Figure 10-25); when it is bilateral it is often fairly symmetric (Figures 10-25 and 10-26). Bilateral involvement of the extraocular muscles is more common in dysthyroid orbitopathy than in pseudotumors **(Option (E) is false).** The inferior rectus muscle is most commonly involved, leading to a limitation of elevation of the involved eye **(Option (C) is false).** The medial rectus muscle and superior rectus elevator complex are also frequently involved, and the lateral rectus and superior oblique muscles are least commonly affected. The forced duction test result is almost always abnormal. Limitation of elevation is the most common disturbance of ocular motility in patients with Graves' disease. The myopathy may occur at any time in the course of Graves' disease; laboratory

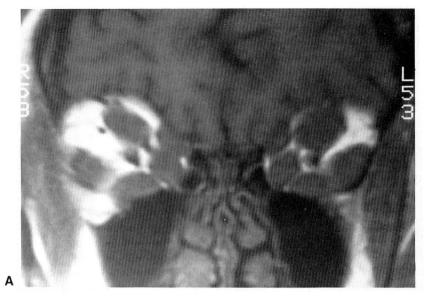

SE 500/20

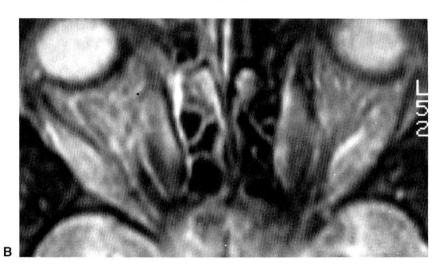

SE 2,000/80

*Figure 10-25.* Dysthyroid orbitopathy. (A) Coronal T1-weighted MR scan shows marked enlargement of all recti as well as superior oblique muscles of both eyes. (B) Axial T2-weighted MR scan shows the enlarged horizontal recti, which appear isointense to the brain.

evaluation may reveal hyperthyroidism, hypothyroidism, or euthyroidism. In fact, the disease is occasionally seen in patients who have been successfully treated for hyperthyroidism and who are euthyroid

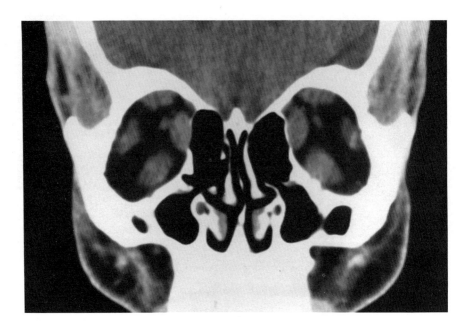

*Figure 10-26.* Dysthyroid orbitopathy. Coronal CT scan shows enlarged horizontal and vertical recti of both eyes. Notice the lack of infiltrate between the muscles. There is no infiltrative process involving the orbital fat lateral to the muscle. Compare this with Figure 10-27, which shows a case of pseudotumor.

when first seen. In a recent study by Rosen et al., orbital muscle, adipose tissues, and peripheral muscle from patients with Graves' ophthalmopathy were studied in *in situ* assays with monoclonal antibodies for immunoglobulin A1 (IgA1), IgA2, IgM, and IgG. Only connective tissue associated with extraorbital muscles and periorbital muscles (levator, Mueller's, and orbicular muscles) showed any reactivity. All positive reactions seen were localized to the endomysium and perimysium with no staining of the muscle fibers themselves. None of the antibodies reacted with sections of adipose tissue. Distinct IgA1 positivity was found in orbital muscle of patients with Graves' disease.

Extraocular muscle enlargement in patients with Graves' disease and associated compressive neuropathy, if any, can be visualized by CT and MR scanning (Figures 10-23 through 10-26). About 90% of patients with dysthyroid orbitopathy will have bilateral CT or MR abnormalities, even if the clinical involvement is unilateral. Typically, enlargement involves the muscle belly and spares its tendinous portion **(Option (D) is true).** Some patients do show thickening of the tendinous portion, but this is

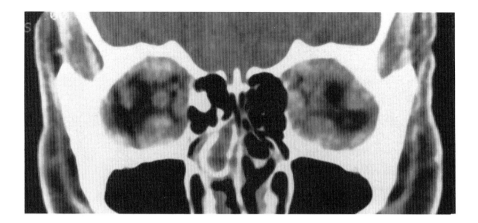

*Figure 10-27.* Reactive lymphoid hypertrophy (pseudotumor). Coronal CT scan shows enlargement of the horizontal and vertical recti of both eyes. Notice the soft tissue infiltrate between and lateral to the muscles, involving the orbital fat. This is characteristic of pseudotumor. Compare this with Figure 10-26.

rare. Another helpful finding is the presence of low-density areas within the muscle bellies of patients with dysthyroid orbitopathy. These are probably the result of focal accumulation of lymphocytes and mucopolysaccharide deposition. Other CT and MR findings are increased orbital fat, enlargement (engorgement) of the lacrimal glands, edema (fullness) of the eyelids, proptosis, and stretching of the optic nerve with or without associated "tenting" of the posterior globe. An important CT and MR finding is absence of inflammatory infiltration in the surrounding orbital fat (Figure 10-26), as opposed to the findings in patients with pseudotumors (Figure 10-27), lymphoma (Figure 10-28), and other types of myositis.

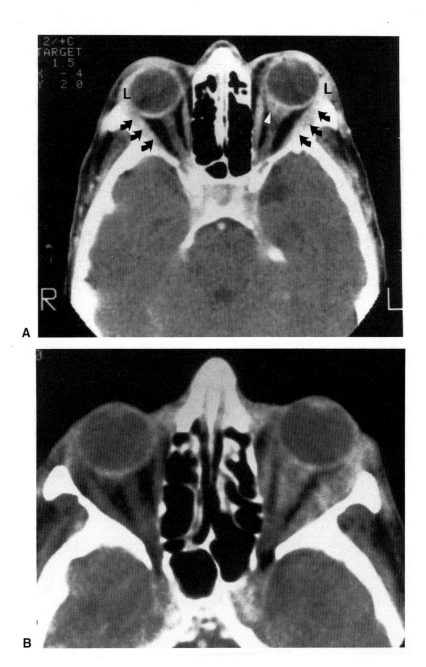

*Figure 10-28.* Orbital lymphoma. (A) Axial CT scan shows slight enlargement of lacrimal glands (L), soft tissue infiltration lateral to the
lateral rectus muscles (arrows), and increased soft tissue density adjacent
to the left optic nerve (arrowhead). (B) Axial CT scan obtained 10 months
later and after an initial response to a course of steroid therapy. The scan
shows progression of left orbital infiltration and slight resolution of right
orbital disease. A biopsy proved that lymphoma was present.

# Question 47

Concerning orbital lymphoma,

   (A) it accounts for 10 to 15% of orbital masses

   (B) it commonly occurs in the anterior portions of the orbit

   (C) when limited to extraocular muscles, it generally cannot be differentiated from myositic pseudotumor by CT or MRI

   (D) it demonstrates intense contrast enhancement on MRI

Lymphomas are solid tumors of the immune system. Most are composed of monoclonal B cells. The extranodal presentation of non-Hodgkin's lymphomas is common, occurring in from 21 to 64% of cases. Roughly 10% of non-Hodgkin's lymphomas present in the head and neck region. Lymphoid tumors account for 10 to 15% of orbital masses **(Option (A) is true).**

Lymphoid disorders of the orbit span a broad spectrum ranging from the malignant lymphomas to the benign pseudolymphomas or pseudotumors to the reactive and atypical lymphoid hyperplasias. There are no absolute imaging, clinical, or even laboratory tests that delineate all types of benign orbital lymphoid lesions from orbital lymphomas or lesions that can simulate them. A pleomorphic cellular infiltrate is correlated with more benign biologic activity. The more uniform the cellular appearance, the greater the likelihood that a malignant neoplasm is present. Of all patients with orbital lymphoma, 75% have or will have systemic lymphoma. There is extensive overlap histologically from one type to another, and some of the benign processes can transform over time into a more aggressive lymphoma. True lymphoid tissue in the eye is found in the subconjunctiva and lacrimal gland. This explains why most orbital tumors are commonly seen in anterior portions of the orbit **(Option (B) is true).** Most of the lymphoreticuloses develop at these sites. The most common cytologic forms of malignant lymphoma involving the orbit are large cell and lymphocytic in various degrees of differentiation.

*Diagnostic imaging.* Ultrasonography, CT, and MRI can be used to evaluate orbital lymphomas. CT and MRI have made possible a strong presumptive diagnosis of orbital lymphoma, especially when CT and MR features are examined in conjunction with the clinical characteristics. The CT and MR findings are usually nonspecific and at times are impossible to differentiate from those of orbital pseudotumors (Figures 10-28 and 10-29), lacrimal gland tumors, optic nerve tumors (Figure

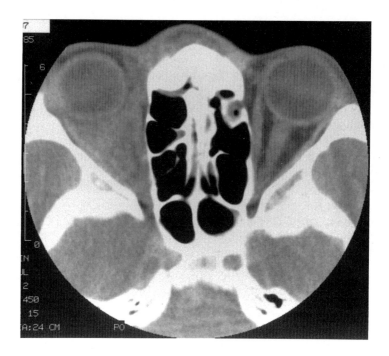

*Figure 10-29.* Lymphomatoid granulomatosis (T-cell lymphoma precursor). Axial CT scan shows diffuse infiltration of the intraconal space of the right orbit with puttylike molding of the disease process around the posterior globe. This CT appearance is virtually identical to those of pseudotumor, B-cell lymphoma, lupoid infiltration, and metastatic scirrhous carcinomas (of the breast and stomach) (see Figures 10-10 and 10-15).

10-30), Graves' orbitopathy, primary orbital tumors, orbital myositis, and orbital cellulitis. Differentiation of lymphoma from myositic tumor is not possible if only the extraocular muscles are involved **(Option (C) is true).** Involvement of multiple orbital structures is more characteristic of lymphoma (Figure 10-31). Orbital lymphomas are homogeneous masses of relatively high CT density and sharp margins; they are more common in the anterior portion of the orbit, retrobulbar areas (Figure 10-32), or the superior orbital compartment. There usually is mild to moderate contrast enhancement of the tumor.

The shared feature of all orbital lymphoid tumors is their tendency to mold themselves around the orbital structures without evidence of bone erosion (Figure 10-32). In particular, a bulky lesion in the region of the lacrimal fossa that does not produce any bone erosion is most likely to

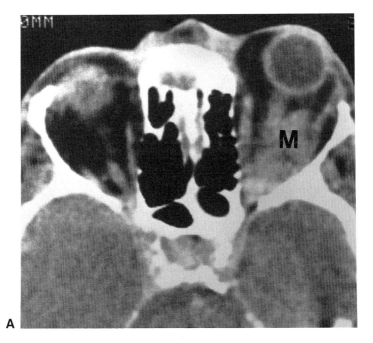

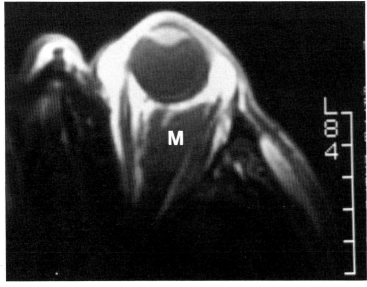

SE 600/20

*Figure 10-30.* Orbital lymphoma. (A) Axial CT scan shows an intraconal mass (M) in contact with the optic nerve. (B) T1-weighted axial MR scan shows the mass (M) to be hypointense to fat and almost isointense to muscle.

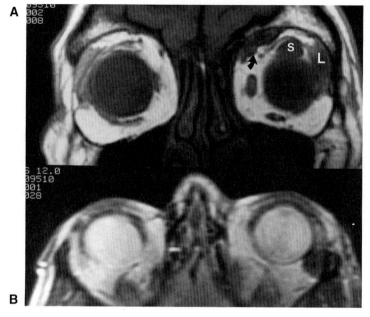

SE 2,000/80

*Figure 10-31.* Small cell lymphoma. Coronal T1-weighted (A) and axial T2-weighted (B) scans show abnormal soft tissue infiltration involving the left lacrimal gland (L) and the left superior rectus muscle (S), as well as infiltration in the subperiosteal space (arrow). Involvement of multiple orbital compartments should suggest lymphoma and pseudotumor.

be inflammatory or lymphoid (Figure 10-33). However, the aggressive malignant lymphomas can produce frank destruction of bone.

Lacrimal gland lymphoma displaces the globe medially and forward and appears on CT scans as a moderately enhancing mass in the lacrimal gland (Figure 10-32). Lacrimal gland lymphoma must be differentiated from other benign and malignant tumors of the lacrimal gland.

MRI has proved to be as sensitive as CT for the diagnosis of orbital lymphomas and pseudotumors. Both pseudotumors and lymphomas may have an intermediate or hypointense signal in T1-weighted (Figure 10-18A) and proton-density (Figures 10-11A and 10-12A) MR images and appear isointense to fat in T2-weighted MR images (Figures 10-11B, 10-12B, and 10-18B). Lymphomas may be hypointense to pseudotumors in T1-weighted images (Figures 10-30B and 10-31), and they may be hyperintense in T2-weighted images. Leukemic infiltration has a similar MR appearance to that of lymphomatous lesions (Figure 10-34). All

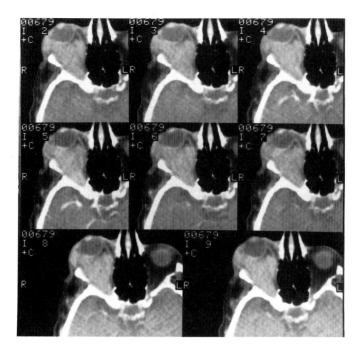

*Figure 10-32.* Orbital lymphoma. Serial dynamic axial CT scans, obtained after a rapid bolus injection of contrast agent in this patient with orbital lymphoma, show slight to moderate contrast enhancement of the retrobulbar mass. Lymphomas involving the orbit often do not show marked enhancement after intravenous injection of contrast medium.

criteria used for CT in the diagnosis of orbital pseudotumors and lymphomas in terms of morphology, location, homogeneity, and contouring may also be used in the diagnosis of these conditions by MRI. Both pseudotumors and lymphomas demonstrate mild to moderate contrast enhancement on CT and MRI **(Option (D) is false).** Enhancement on T1-weighted postcontrast MR scans is moderate (Figure 10-18C); however, enhancement on postcontrast fat-suppressed T1-weighted MR scans is more marked (Figure 10-18D). This is due to increased dynamic range with the fat-suppressed (Chemsat) technique. In general, the lesion appears less hypointense in precontrast fat-suppressed T1-weighted MR scans. It is therefore believed that the greater hyperintensity in fat-suppressed T1-weighted images is due partly to technique.

*Lymphoplasmacytic tumors (plasma cell tumors).* Tumors composed of pure plasma cells (plasmacytomas) and those composed of B lymphocytes and plasma cells (lymphoplasmacytoid tumors) are closely related to the

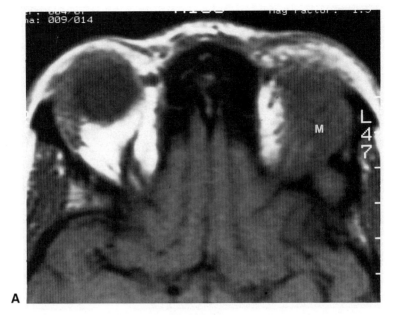

SE 450/25

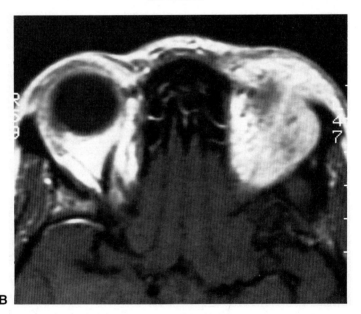

SE 450/25

*Figure 10-33.* Tumefactive pseudotumor simulating lacrimal gland tumor and true orbital lymphoma. (A) Axial T1-weighted MR scan shows an irregular large infiltrative mass (M) in the superior temporal portion of the left orbit. (B) Postcontrast axial T1-weighted MR scan shows moderate enhancement of the mass. The enhancement is slightly higher than that of normal right lacrimal gland. A biopsy revealed nonspecific inflammation.

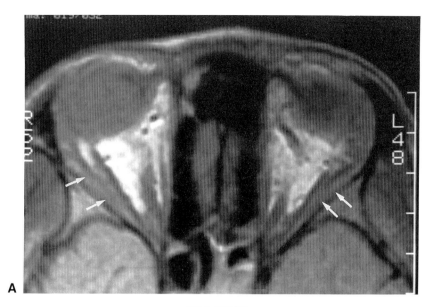

SE 2,000/20

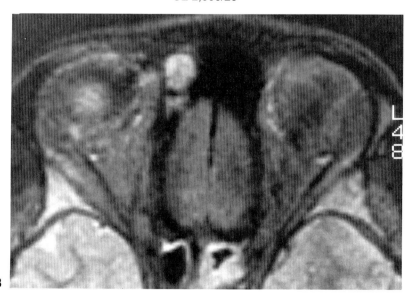

SE 2,000/80

*Figure 10-34.* Orbital leukemic infiltrate. (A) Axial proton-density MR scan shows soft tissue infiltration of the extraconal orbital fat (arrows), which is isointense to brain. (B) Axial T2-weighted MR scan shows that the process appears hypointense to the brain.

various lymphomas. The plasma cell is actually a B lymphocyte that has become modified to produce large quantities of immunoglobulin. The so-called plasmacytoid lymphomas may secrete IgM paraprotein in sufficient quantities to cause a monoclonal peak on serum electrophoresis; this is classically seen in Waldenström's macroglobulinemia. An important tumor of plasma cells is multiple myeloma. There are solitary forms of extramedullary plasmacytomas, which are not associated with systemic multiple myeloma. Plasma cell tumors, particularly as they affect the orbit and ocular structures, display the same spectrum of clinical involvement seen in the lymphoproliferative disorders. Isolated plasmacytoma and Waldenström's macroglobulinemia produce a mass that can be visualized by both CT and MRI. The mass may be lobulated, densely enhancing, and well-defined with or without bone erosion. In patients with systemic myelomatosis, a permeative pattern of bone destruction or a more discrete destructive lesion may be present.

*Orbital leukemia.* Leukemia is one of the most common childhood cancers. It is estimated that of approximately 7,100 cancers in children in the USA each year, 35% are leukemia. Leukemic disorders in children fall mainly into the lymphoid and myeloid groups. About 75% of cases are acute lymphoblastic leukemia, 20% are acute myelogenous leukemia, and 5% are chronic myelogenous leukemia. Chronic lymphocytic leukemia is a disease of adulthood and almost never affects children. The eye and its adnexae are not infrequently involved. Orbital involvement with leukemia is the result of direct infiltration of orbital bone or soft tissue by leukemic cells (Figure 10-34). Such infiltration most often occurs in the form of a granulocytic sarcoma in patients with acute myelogenous leukemia. A granulocytic sarcoma is commonly called a chloroma because the myeloperoxidase within the tumor imparts a green hue to it as seen on gross examination.

# Question 48

Concerning rhabdomyosarcoma of the orbit,

(A) it is the most common primary orbital cancer in children
(B) it arises from the pluripotential mesenchymal elements
(C) it commonly presents as a rapidly progressive unilateral proptosis
(D) it is resistant to both radiation therapy and chemotherapy

Rhabdomyosarcoma is the most common mesenchymal tumor of childhood, as well as the most common primary malignant tumor of the orbit in children **(Option (A) is true).** This tumor does not originate from preformed striated extraocular muscles, but rather from undifferentiated mesenchyme of the orbital soft tissues **(Option (B) is true).** The tumor is notorious for producing a rapidly developing unilateral proptosis **(Option (C) is true).** Any rapidly developing proptosis in childhood must presumptively be diagnosed as rhabdomyosarcoma (Figure 10-35). The differential diagnosis also includes leukemic and metastatic deposits, ruptured dermoid cyst, subperiosteal hematoma after trauma, and a chocolate cyst in a lymphangioma. Rhabdomyosarcomas are pleomorphic tumors, and the cells may be anaplastic. On the basis of their histopathologic characteristics, rhabdomyosarcomas are classified into one of the three histologic types: embryonal, differentiated, and alveolar. Differentiated rhabdomyosarcoma is the least frequent type and is rarely misdiagnosed, because cells with eosinophilic cytoplasmic fibrils that are usually cross-striated are used to identify the tumor. Embryonal rhabdomyosarcoma, the most common histologic subtype, is believed to arise from the primitive muscle cell since it is found in 7- to 10-week-old fetuses. The histologic differentiation of embryonal and alveolar rhabdomyosarcoma may be difficult. It has been estimated that up to 50% of proven cases of rhabdomyosarcoma are misdiagnosed on initial biopsy.

Rhabdomyosarcoma of the sinonasal tract and orbit often presents as a relatively innocuous problem (e.g., recurrent sinusitis, proptosis, or a small naso-orbital mass) (Figure 10-36). Secondary sinonasal tumors may arise from adjacent orbital spread of orbital rhabdomyosarcoma or pharyngeal rhabdomyosarcoma. Rhabdomyosarcomas are both aggressive bone-destroying lesions and bone-pushing lesions. Although rhabdomyosarcoma of the orbit is most often seen in children and in adults under 20 years of age, at times it affects older patients. Orbital pseudotumors in children may simulate orbital rhabdomyosarcoma. It is therefore important to attempt to do a biopsy if the CT and MR findings are not characteristic of pseudotumor. CT and MRI should be performed with

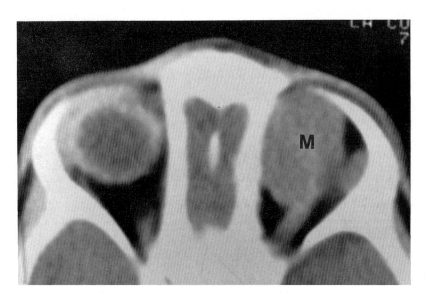

*Figure 10-35.* Rhabdomyosarcoma. Axial CT scan shows a large mass (M) in the superior medial portion of the left orbit. There is no bone erosion.

and without contrast enhancement, with particular attention to the presence of bone erosion and intracranial extension of the tumor (Figure 10-35). The initial surgical procedure should include biopsy of an adequate sample for confirmation, with complete excision of the tumor if possible without causing excessive morbidity. Chemotherapy has been very successful in treating primary tumors and controlling metastatic disease. Radiation therapy is used primarily for local control. In general, chemotherapy and radiation therapy are the primary treatment modalities for patients with rhabdomyosarcomas. Since the advent of combination therapy (surgery, chemotherapy, and radiation), there has been a significant and continuing improvement in survival of children with head and neck rhabdomyosarcomas **(Option (D) is false).**

*Mahmood F. Mafee, M.D.*

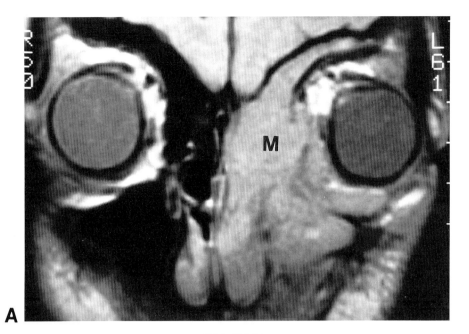

SE 2,300/20

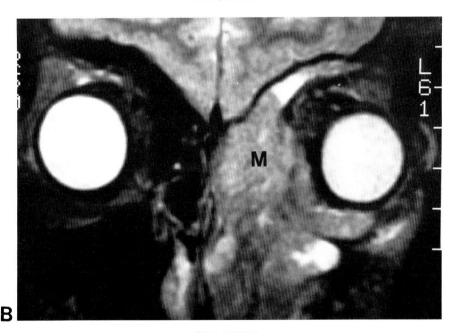

SE 2,300/80

*Figure 10-36.* Rhabdomyosarcoma. Coronal proton-density (A) and T2-weighted (B) MR scans show a large left ethmoid mass (M) invading the left orbit, left maxillary sinus, and left nasal cavity.

## PSEUDOTUMORS AND LYMPHOMAS

1. Blodi FC, Gas JD. Inflammatory pseudotumor of the orbit. Br J Ophthalmol 1968; 52:79–93
2. Curtin HD. Pseudotumor. Radiol Clin North Am 1987; 25:583–599
3. Flanders AE, Espinosa GA, Markiewicz DA, Howell DD. Orbital lymphoma. Role of CT and MRI. Radiol Clin North Am 1987; 25:601–613
4. Flanders AE, Mafee MF, Rao VM, Choi KH. CT characteristics of orbital pseudotumors and other orbital inflammatory processes. J Comput Assist Tomogr 1989; 13:40–47
5. Mafee MF, Putterman A, Valvassori GE, Campos M, Capek V. Orbital space-occupying lesions: role of computed tomography and magnetic resonance imaging. An analysis of 145 cases. Radiol Clin North Am 1987; 25:529–559
6. Mottow-Lippa L, Jakobiec FA, Smith M. Idiopathic inflammatory orbital pseudotumor in childhood. II. Results of diagnostic tests and biopsies. Ophthalmology 1981; 88:565–574

## DYSTHYROID ORBITOPATHY

7. Newton TH, Bilaniuk LT. Radiology of the eye and orbit. Philadelphia: Raven Press; 1990:550–556
8. Rootman J (ed). Diagnosis and management of orbital tumors. Philadelphia: WB Saunders; 1989:241–280
9. Rosen CE, Raikow RB, Burde RM, Kennerdell JS, Mosseri M, Scalise D. Immunohistochemical evidence for IgA1 involvement in Graves ophthalmopathy. Ophthalmology 1992; 99:146–152
10. Trokel SL, Hilal SK. Recognition and differential diagnosis of enlarged extraocular muscles in computed tomography. Am J Ophthalmol 1979; 87:503–512
11. Trokel SL, Jakobiec FA. Correlation of CT scanning and pathologic features of ophthalmic Graves' disease. Ophthalmology 1981; 88:553–564

## RHABDOMYOSARCOMA

12. Mafee MF. The orbit proper. In: Som PM, Bergeron RT (eds), Head and neck imaging. St. Louis: Mosby-Year Book; 1991:747–813
13. Rootman RT. Tumors. In: Rootman RT (ed), Diseases of the orbit. Philadelphia: JB Lippincott; 1988:281–480
14. Shields JA. Mycogenic tumors. In: Shields JA (ed), Diagnosis and management of orbital tumors. Philadelphia: WB Saunders; 1989:244–252
15. Vade A, Armstrong D. Orbital rhabdomyosarcoma in childhood. Radiol Clin North Am 1987; 25:701–714

*Notes*

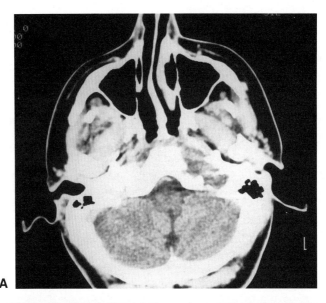

A

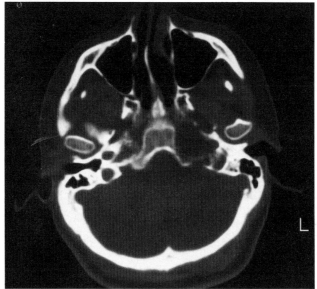

B

*Figure 11-1*
*Figures 11-1 through 11-4.* This 26-year-old woman presented with a headache and left-sixth-nerve palsy. You are shown a contrast-enhanced CT scan photographed at soft tissue (A) and bone (B) window settings (Figure 11-1), a coronal T1-weighted MR scan (Figure 11-2), an axial proton density MR scan (Figure 11-3), and two T1-weighted axial contrast-enhanced MR scans (Figure 11-4).

# Case 11:  Petrous Apex Chondrosarcoma

## Question 49

Which *one* of the following is the MOST likely diagnosis?

(A) Glomus jugulare tumor
(B) Cholesterol granuloma
(C) Intrapetrous carotid aneurysm
(D) Chondrosarcoma
(E) Intraosseous epidermoid tumor

Figures 11-1A and B are contrast-enhanced CT scans, photographed at soft tissue and bone-window settings, respectively, at the level of the base of the skull. These scans demonstrate a destructive mass of the left petrous apex centered at the petro-occipital suture (Figure 11-5, arrows). The mass is slightly medial to the jugular foramen and has relatively smooth margins, suggesting a slowly expansile process. On the coronal T1-weighted MR image (Figure 11-2), the mass has low signal intensity relative to brain and replaces the normally high signal intensity of the petrous apex marrow (see Figure 11-6). The signal intensity of the mass increases on the proton density sequence (Figure 11-3), and the lesion can be seen to extend down the medullary cavity of the basiocciput (see Figure 11-7). After gadolinium DTPA administration, the mass enhances homogeneously (Figure 11-4). There is no evidence of signal voids to suggest that the mass is hypervascular. The tumor displaces the prevertebral muscles anteriorly (open arrows, Figure 11-8), indicating that its origin is the skull base. In this example, the lesion in question is centered medial to the jugular foramen and has a homogeneous signal intensity on all imaging sequences. The findings are most characteristic of chondrosarcoma **(Option (D) is correct).**

Lesions of the skull base and petrous apex have a variable appearance on MR images. Glomus jugulare tumors (Option (A)), or paragangliomas, are benign hypervascular tumors arising from paraganglion cells. These cells occur throughout the body but are present in greatest concentration along the course of nerves within the carotid sheath and tympanic cavity. Glomus tumors most commonly occur at the carotid bifurcation (carotid

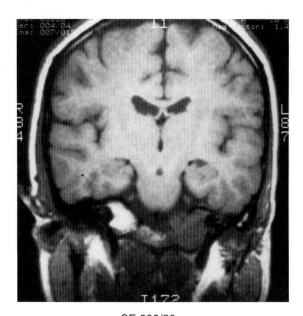

SE 600/20

*Figure 11-2*

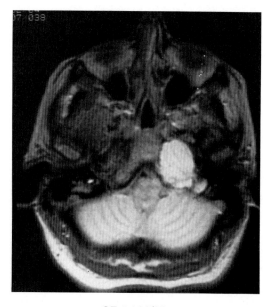

SE 2,000/35

*Figure 11-3*

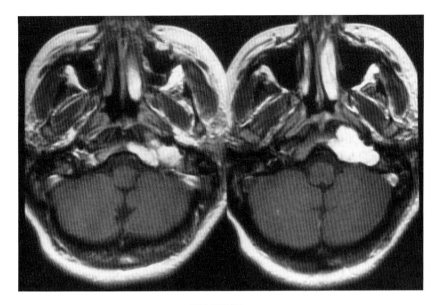

SE 600/20

*Figure 11-4*

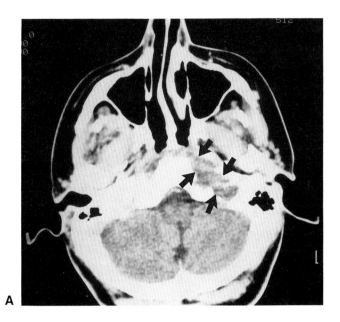

A

*Figure 11-5* (Same as Figure 11-1). Chondrosarcoma of the left petrous apex. Transaxial contrast-enhanced CT scan photographed at soft tissue (A) and bone (B) windows demonstrates an expansile mass in the left petrous apex with relatively smooth margins (arrows).

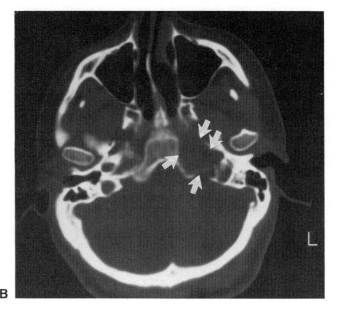

B

*Figure 11-5 (Continued)*

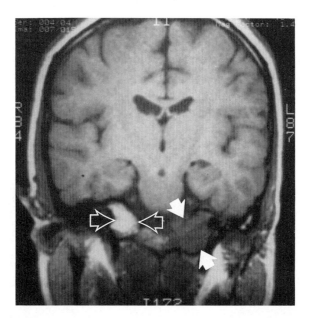

SE 600/20

*Figure 11-6* (Same as Figure 11-2). Chondrosarcoma of the left petrous apex. Coronal T1-weighted MR image demonstrates the soft tissue mass involving the left petrous apex (solid arrows). The mass replaces the normal high signal intensity of the marrow within the petrous apex, which is seen on the right (open arrows).

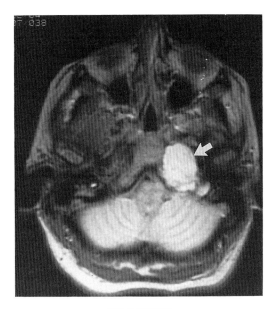

SE 2,000/35

*Figure 11-7* (Same as Figure 11-3). Chondrosarcoma of the left petrous apex. Proton density-weighted MR image. The mass (arrow) exhibits increased signal intensity by comparison with its appearance on the T1-weighted image and has some internal bands of linear hypointense signal, probably representing fibrous strands.

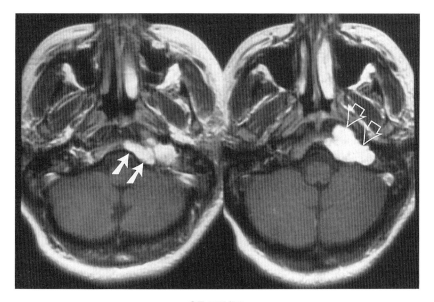

SE 600/20

*Figure 11-8* (Same as Figure 11-4). Chondrosarcoma of the left petrous apex. Contiguous contrast-enhanced axial T1-weighted MR scans. The solidly enhancing mass extends down into the medullary cavity of the clivus (solid arrows). In addition, it expands anteriorly to displace the prevertebral muscles (open arrows).

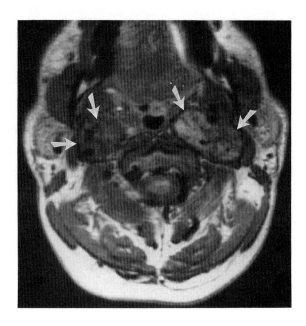

*Figure 11-9.* Bilateral paragangliomas of the carotid bodies. Axial T1-weighted MR image through the region of the oropharynx demonstrates bilateral inhomogeneous well-circumscribed masses centered at the carotid bifurcations (arrows). The internal signal of the masses is heterogeneous, and signal voids are present throughout the lesions; this appearance is consistent with the diagnosis of paraganglioma. The signal voids correspond to the rapid blood flow within the vessels supplying the tumors. On T2-weighted scans, areas of high signal intensity intermixed with the signal voids give these tumors a "salt-and-pepper" appearance.

body tumors), followed in descending order of frequency by tumors of the jugular fossa (glomus jugulare tumors), tympanic cavity (glomus tympanicum tumors), and the nodose ganglion of the vagus nerve (glomus vagale tumors). The glomus jugulare tumors generally present with neuropathies of the ninth to twelfth cranial nerves and with pulsatile tinnitus with or without hearing loss. Glomus jugulare tumors are centered at the jugular foramen, splaying the internal carotid artery anteriorly and the internal jugular vein posteriorly. On contrast CT, the glomus jugulare tumor typically compresses or invades the internal jugular vein and is visible as a hypervascular tumor that produces irregular bone erosion. On MR images, glomus tumors larger than 1 to 2 cm in diameter have an inhomogeneous signal intensity on T2-weighted sequences, which has been described as a "salt-and-pepper" appearance (Figure 11-9). Prominent signal voids and tumor enhancement are also

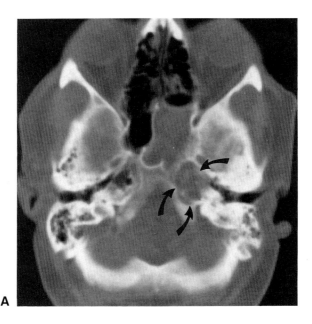

*Figure 11-10.* Cholesterol granuloma of the petrous apex. (A) Axial CT scan photographed at bone windows demonstrates an expansile left petrous apex mass (arrows). Note also the aeration of the right petrous apex. (B) Coronal CT scan photographed at bone windows demonstrates the expansile quality of the cholesterol granuloma (arrows), which has relatively smooth margins. (C) Axial T1-weighted MR scan. The cholesterol granuloma has a high signal intensity (solid arrows). This can be confused with normal marrow fat within the petrous apex as seen on the right side (open arrows). Incidentally noted is left sphenoid sinusitis. (D) Coronal proton density MR image through the skull base. The cholesterol granuloma remains high in signal intensity and is surrounded by a rim of low signal intensity (arrows). The fat within the marrow of the calvarium has decreased in signal intensity.

characteristics of glomus tumors. These typical features of a glomus jugulare tumor are not evident in the test images.

Cholesterol granuloma (Option (B)) is a non-neoplastic hemorrhagic cyst that develops as a result of obstruction of an air cell of the petrous apex. Although the CT appearance of cholesterol granuloma could be similar to that shown in the test images, a cholesterol granuloma typically demonstrates a high signal intensity on T1-weighted MR images as a result of the presence of methemoglobin (Figure 11-10). T2-weighted sequences usually demonstrate persistence of this high signal intensity, often with a peripheral hypointense rim, which most probably represents hemosiderin-laden macrophages. In addition, the cholesterol granuloma

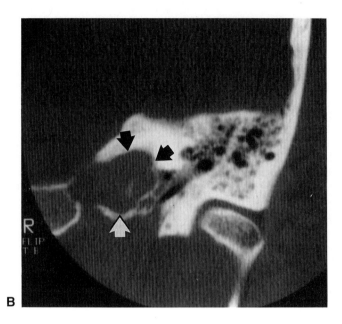

B

would not enhance, as does the lesion seen in the test images. Thus, the mass shown in the test images is not likely to be a cholesterol granuloma.

An intrapetrous carotid aneurysm (Option (C)) is a rare vascular lesion that can simulate a neoplasm of the petrous apex on CT. This aneurysm can usually be easily differentiated from a solid neoplasm on MR images (Figure 11-11). An aneurysm usually has variable signal intensities generated by the different blood products in the thrombosed portion of the aneurysm. Alternatively, if the aneurysm is patent and contains no thrombus, the MR studies show the characteristic signal void of rapidly flowing blood. In addition, a petrous carotid aneurysm would not be expected to enhance in a homogeneous fashion nor would it involve the medullary space of the basiocciput, in contrast to the findings in the test images.

Intraosseous epidermoid tumor (Option (E)) is a common lesion that occurs in the bones of the calvarium and skull base, and one of the more common sites in which this lesion develops is the petrous apex. However, the signal intensity of epidermoid tumors is usually similar to that of cerebrospinal fluid, being low on T1-weighted sequences and high on T2-weighted sequences (Figure 11-12). Importantly, these lesions do not enhance, and for this reason the test images are inconsistent with the diagnosis of an intraosseous epidermoid tumor.

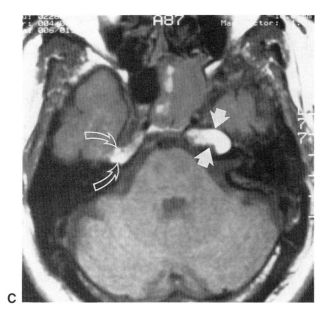

SE 600/20

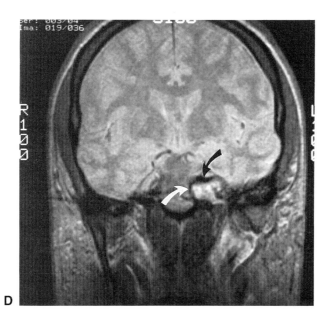

SE 2,800/35

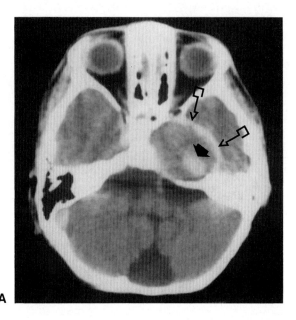

A

*Figure 11-11.* Aneurysm of the left petrous internal carotid artery. (A) Contrast-enhanced axial CT scan through the region of the left petrous apex demonstrating a mass of soft tissue density with peripheral enhancement (open arrows) and a solidly enhancing "nodule," which represents the lumen of the aneurysm (solid arrow). The majority of the mass has an attenuation similar to that of brain. Incidentally seen is opacification of the left mastoid air cells. This is due to serous fluid, which has accumulated because the caudal margin of the mass has obstructed the left eustachian tube. (B) Axial proton density MR image. The left petrous mass has a heterogeneous appearance that is due to the lamination of acute and chronic thrombus. There is also a signal void within the center of the mass (arrows), indicating flow within the patent portion of the aneurysm lumen. The serous fluid in the mastoid is seen to have high signal intensity. (C) Axial T2-weighted MR image at the same level as in panel B. The chronic thrombus has decreased further in signal intensity (arrows), whereas other areas have increased in signal intensity, indicating more subacute hemorrhagic constituents. The serous fluid in the left mastoid still has high signal intensity.

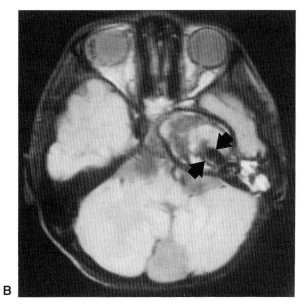

SE 2,000/35

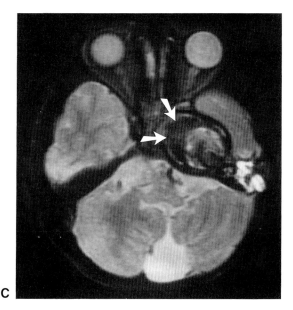

SE 2,800/80

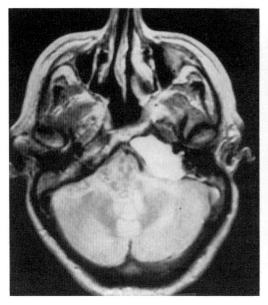
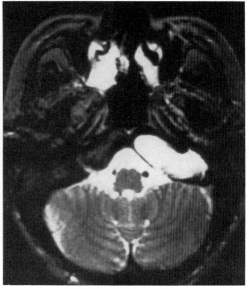

**A**

**B**

*Figure 11-12.* Epidermoid tumor. Axial proton density (A) and T2-weighted (B) MR images of a congenital epidermoid tumor. The mass has a signal intensity relatively similar to that of cerebrospinal fluid on the T2-weighted image; however, it is slightly brighter than cerebrospinal fluid on the proton density image. No contrast enhancement was visible after administration of gadolinium DTPA.

## Question 50

Concerning cholesterol granuloma,

- (A) it usually occurs in an obstructed air cell of the petrous apex
- (B) it occasionally occurs in the middle ear
- (C) it contains blood products
- (D) it typically causes third cranial nerve palsy
- (E) CT is as specific as MRI for the diagnosis

Cholesterol granuloma, or giant cholesterol cyst, is a distinct clinical entity, which should be in the differential diagnosis of lesions of the mid-cranial skull base or petrous apex. It is a benign cystic lesion that arises as a result of lack of aeration of air cells, and this commonly occurs within one of the air cells that may be present in the petrous apex **(Option (A) is true);** however, the process may also develop within an obstructed middle ear cavity **(Option (B) is true),** resulting in a "blue tympanic membrane" at otoscopy. The obstructed air cell develops a negative pressure, which initially causes a serous effusion. Presumably, repeated hemorrhage into the obstructed air cell occurs, with the subsequent development of an expansile mass that contains methemoglobin and cholesterol crystals, which are the breakdown products of hemoglobin and red blood cell membranes, respectively **(Option (C) is true).** The lining of the cyst wall is composed primarily of fibrous tissue and chronic inflammatory cells. Osteitis, bone erosion, and bone resorption have all been reported, but major bone destruction is rare. Headache and deficits of the fifth to eighth cranial nerves are the most common presenting symptoms **(Option (D) is false).** Deficits of the ninth to twelfth cranial nerves have also been described when the lesion becomes large enough to involve the jugular foramen. Cholesterol granuloma may occasionally be associated with Gradenigo's syndrome, which refers to fifth and sixth nerve palsies that are caused by an inflammation of the petrous apex. Specifically, as these cranial nerves pass over the petrous apex on their course into the cavernous sinus, they are either compressed or irritated by the adjacent petrous apex inflammation, which in this case is the result of a cholesterol granuloma.

The hemorrhagic nature of a cholesterol granuloma cannot be shown by CT. Although CT demonstrates an expansile mass with sharp bone margins that is centered at the apex of the petrous bone near the petro-occipital suture (Figure 11-10), the contents of the mass are of a soft tissue density, which cannot be easily differentiated from that of other masses that may occur in this region, such as congenital epidermoid tumors, chondrosarcomas, and neuromas. Intravenous administration of contrast agent may assist in this differentiation because cholesterol granulomas and congenital epidermoid tumors will not demonstrate enhancement, whereas other tumors will have some degree of contrast enhancement.

MRI is more specific than CT in the diagnosis of cholesterol granuloma **(Option (E) is false).** Cholesterol granulomas have a high signal intensity on T1-weighted MR sequences (Figure 11-10C). If the T1-weighted scans alone were obtained, this entity might be mistaken for the normal fatty marrow present in an unaerated petrous apex. However, unlike fat, which has a lower T2-weighted signal intensity, the signal intensity of a cholesterol granuloma is also high on T2-weighted sequences and does not decrease when fat-suppression sequences are used (Figure 11-10D and Table 11-1).

The treatment of cholesterol granuloma consists of drainage or marsupialization of the cyst, usually via a mastoid and middle-ear approach.

Table 11-1. Intensity of petrous apex lesions and marrow compared with adjacent brain

| Lesion | Relative intensity by: | | | Enhancement |
| | CT | MRI (T1) | MRI (T2) | |
| --- | --- | --- | --- | --- |
| Cholesteatoma | Decreased | Decreased | Increased | No |
| Cholesterol granuloma | Equal | Increased | Increased | No |
| Bone marrow | Equal | Increased | Decreased | Minimal |
| Neoplasm | Equal | Decreased | Increased | Yes |

Drainage can also be performed, depending on the position of the cyst, through a transsphenoidal, infralabyrinthine, transcochlear, or suboccipital route. After adequate decompression of the cyst, the signal intensity on T1-weighted sequences decreases.

## Question 51

Concerning intrapetrous carotid artery aneurysm,

(A) it is usually traumatic in origin
(B) CT is as specific as MRI for the diagnosis
(C) mature thrombus within the aneurysm has a decreased signal intensity relative to brain on T2-weighted images
(D) carotid occlusion is an accepted treatment

Aneurysms of the petrous portion of the internal carotid artery are rare lesions. The medical literature suggests that most of these aneurysms are congenital in origin **(Option (A) is false).** Other, less commonly reported etiologies include trauma, neurofibromatosis, and mycotic embolizations from the heart. These aneurysms can occur in patients of virtually all ages; however, one series gives the mean age as 30 years. Most aneurysms are fusiform in shape and contain chronic thrombus. The presenting symptoms may include pain, bruit, fifth to seventh cranial nerve dysfunction, epistaxis, and Horner's syndrome. Asymptomatic aneurysms have also been described.

The CT appearance of an aneurysm of the petrous carotid artery may be nonspecific. An expansile mass lesion involving the course of the carotid artery, with or without a definable enhancing lumen, is typical.

Chronic thrombus often occupies the majority of the lumen and has a soft tissue density on CT that may be confused with that of a neoplasm (Figure 11-11A). After contrast administration, the periphery of the aneurysm may enhance along with the remaining patent lumen (Figure 11-11A). Calcification in the wall of the aneurysm may also indicate its vascular nature. On MRI these lesions have a more specific appearance **(Option (B) is false).** The signal intensity of the aneurysm will vary depending on the amount of acute or chronic thrombus in its wall. If there is no thrombus formation and if rapid blood flow is present, the signal within the lumen of the aneurysm will be absent and misregistration artifact from the flowing blood may be detected along the plane of the phase-encoding gradient. As the aneurysm enlarges, layers of acute and chronic thrombus are laid down along the periphery of the lumen, resulting in an "onion skin" appearance with layers of different signal intensities ranging from high to low on T1- and T2-weighted sequences (Figure 11-11B and C). Generally, the signal intensity of mature thrombus decreases on T2-weighted sequences, reflecting the predominance of chronic blood products and fibrous tissue (Figure 11-11C) **(Option (C) is true).** A patent lumen is usually detected eccentrically within the thrombus (Figure 11-11B). Together, these features suggest the presence of an aneurysm and underscore the utility of MRI in assessing expansile petrous apex lesions.

Aneurysms of the petrous portion of the internal carotid artery can be treated effectively by either endovascular or surgical occlusive procedures **(Option (D) is true).** Owing to the anatomic position of the lesion, surgical clipping is rarely possible.

## Question 52

Concerning chondrosarcoma of the skull base,

- (A) it usually arises in the midline of the clivus
- (B) it is easily distinguished histologically from chordoma
- (C) it is a rapidly progressive lesion
- (D) enhancement on MRI is typical

Chondrosarcomas represent only about 8% of all malignant bone tumors, and they respond well to treatment. They tend to occur in older patients and often arise from a preexisting benign cartilaginous tumor. Most chondrosarcomas arise in the long bones, the pelvis, the sternum, or the ribs. Involvement of the skull and facial skeleton is rare. Nevertheless, when chondrosarcomas do occur in the head and neck, their most common sites include the paranasal sinuses, the skull base, and the parasellar region. The tumor is frequently positioned at a cartilaginous end plate or synchondrosis. In the skull base, the lesion most often occurs at the petro-occipital suture near the foramen lacerum **(Option (A) is false)**. Recognizing this location can help differentiate a chondrosarcoma from a chordoma, which most often arises in the midline of the clivus. However, chondrosarcoma can be otherwise difficult to differentiate from chordoma histologically and radiographically **(Option (B) is false)**. Although assessing the position of the lesion as determined by CT or MRI can be useful in making the correct diagnosis, differentiation of some chordomas and chondrosarcomas based on their location and sectional imaging appearance may be impossible. The growth rate of chondrosarcomas varies depending on the grade of malignancy. Most of these craniofacial lesions are low-grade malignancies that tend to run an indolent course **(Option (C) is false)**. CT features of chondrosarcoma include an irregularly destructive mass with internal calcifications centered off of the midline near the petro-occipital suture. Enhancement is typical.

On MRI, chondrosarcoma exhibits a homogeneous signal intensity, which is low on T1-weighted images and high on T2-weighted sequences. The lesion often has fairly well-circumscribed margins, which appear scalloped. These tumors have a tendency to erode into the medullary space of the clivus and may extend for a considerable distance within the clivus without breaking through its cortical margin (Figures 11-2 through 11-4). On MRI it is unusual to detect any calcified matrix in the chondrosarcoma, and enhancement of the tumor is usually homogeneous and intense (Figure 11-4) **(Option (D) is true)**. Chordoma may appear similar on T2-weighted images, but it is generally restricted to the midline and has a tendency to exhibit minimal contrast enhancement (Figure 11-13).

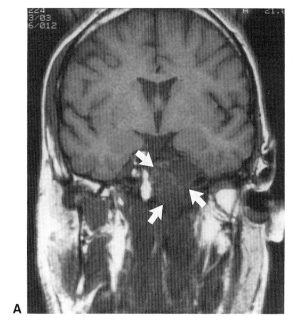

SE 600/20

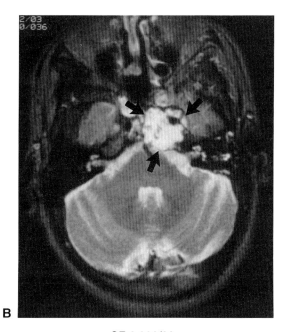

SE 2,800/80

*Figure 11-13.* Chordoma of the clivus. (A) Coronal T1-weighted image through the region of the clivus. A heterogeneous low-intensity mass (arrows) replaces the normal high signal intensity of the clivus marrow, which is seen along the right margin of the lesion. (B) T2-weighted image demonstrates increased signal intensity of the chordoma (arrows). Note its lobular but well-circumscribed configuration. Although primarily midline in position, it is slightly eccentric to the left side. The mass could conceivably be confused with a chondrosarcoma.

## Question 53

Concerning epidermoid tumor,

  (A)  it is a congenital tumor of epithelial tissue
  (B)  it usually arises in the mastoid antrum
  (C)  it frequently erodes into the middle ear
  (D)  it usually has low signal intensity on T2-weighted MR images

Epidermoid tumors result from the slow growth of epidermal inclusions that are trapped at the time of embryonic closure of the neural tube within otherwise normal tissue such as the middle ear, the calvarium, or the subarachnoid space **(Option (A) is true).** Epidermoid tumors, also referred to as congenital cholesteatomas, are histologically indistinguishable from acquired cholesteatomas of the middle ear. However, acquired cholesteatomas are usually associated with perforations of the tympanic membrane and chronic otitis media, whereas congenital ones are usually not infected and develop behind an intact tympanic membrane. The cholesteatoma grows as a result of normal squamous cell replication and desquamation, especially at the petrous apex. Such growth is usually clinically silent, allowing the tumor to become large. Most often, these tumors come to clinical attention only when they encroach on surrounding cranial nerves or the otic capsule. The most common location for epidermoid tumors is the petrous apex **(Option (B) is false),** followed in descending order by the middle ear and the facial canal. The mastoid is an unusual location for a congenital epidermoid tumor. Middle ear congenital epidermoid tumors usually result in conductive hearing loss. Although erosion into the middle ear may occur from petrous apex lesions, this is rather atypical **(Option (C) is false).**

Epidermoid tumors appear radiographically as expansile masses that generally demonstrate smooth margins because of their slow growth. On CT, the lesion generally has a low attenuation similar to that of fluid or soft tissue, with no calcifications or enhancement. Smooth, scalloped margins are typical (Figure 11-14). On MRI these tumors have a signal intensity almost identical to that of cerebrospinal fluid (Figure 11-12). Thus they exhibit low signal intensity on T1-weighted sequences and high signal intensity on T2-weighted sequences **(Option (D) is false).** The lack of contrast enhancement on MR images can be used to differentiate these lesions from tumors of the petrous apex (Figures 11-1 through 11-4; Table 11-1). Occasionally, epidermoid lesions may demonstrate a high signal intensity on T1-weighted images and a low signal intensity on T2-weighted sequences. This is believed to be secondary to

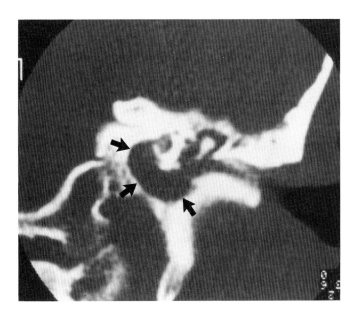

*Figure 11-14.* Congenital epidermoid tumor of the temporal bone. Coronal CT scan through the temporal bone demonstrates a well-marginated expansile mass that involves the left inferior petrous apex and extends into the middle ear (arrows). The mass is typical of a congenital epidermoid tumor.

the effect of a very high protein content, which acts to shorten the T1 and T2 relaxation times. They are readily differentiated from other mass lesions such as cholesterol granuloma, chordoma, and chondrosarcoma on MRI. Cholesterol granuloma has a high signal intensity on both T1- and T2-weighted sequences, chordoma is generally positioned in the midline, and chondrosarcoma enhances intensely. The only lesion that may be confused with an epidermoid tumor of the petrous apex is the rare petrous apex mucocele, which has a fluid density and does not enhance with gadolinium DTPA. The use of newer MR gradient-echo pulse sequences with spoiler pulses may be able to produce heavily T1-weighted images, which can assist in differentiating epidermoid tumors from fluid-filled cavities.

*William P. Dillon, M.D.*

SUGGESTED READINGS

## CHONDROSARCOMA

1. Burkey BB, Hoffman HT, Baker SR, Thornton AF, McClatchey KD. Chondrosarcoma of the head and neck. Laryngoscope 1990; 100:1301–1305
2. Coltrera MD, Googe PB, Harrist TJ, Hyams VJ, Schiller AL, Goodman ML. Chondrosarcoma of the temporal bone. Diagnosis and treatment of 13 cases and review of the literature. Cancer 1986; 58:2689–2696
3. Finn DG, Goepfert H, Batsakis JG. Chondrosarcoma of the head and neck. Laryngoscope 1984; 94:1539–1544
4. Gay I, Elidan J, Kopolovic J. Chondrosarcoma at the skull base. Ann Otol Rhinol Laryngol 1981; 90:53–55
5. Grossman RI, Davis KR. Cranial computed tomographic appearance of chondrosarcoma of the base of the skull. Radiology 1981; 141:403–408
6. Hassounah M, Al-Mefty O, Akhtar M, Jinkins JR, Fox JL. Primary cranial and intracranial chondrosarcoma. A survey. Acta Neurochir (Wien) 1985; 78:123–132
7. Kveton JF, Brackmann DE, Glasscock ME III, House WF, Hitselberger WE. Chondrosarcoma of the skull base. Otolaryngol Head Neck Surg 1986; 94:23–32
8. Long DM, Mattox DE. Tumors of the skull base. Md Med J 1990; 39:355–360
9. Oot RF, Melville GE, New PF, et al. The role of MR and CT in evaluating clival chordomas and chondrosarcomas. AJR 1988; 151:567–575
10. Russell EJ, Levy JM, Breit R, McMahan JT. Osteocartilaginous tumors in the parapharyngeal space arising from bone exostoses. AJNR 1990; 11:993–997
11. Sen CN, Sekhar LN, Schramm VL, Janecka IP. Chordoma and chondrosarcoma of the cranial base: an 8-year experience. Neurosurgery 1989; 25:931–940
12. Vener J, Rice DH, Newman AN. Osteosarcoma and chondrosarcoma of the head and neck. Laryngoscope 1984; 94:240–242

## CHOLESTEROL GRANULOMA

13. Amedee RG, Marks HW, Lyons GD. Cholesterol granuloma of the petrous apex. Am J Otol 1987; 8:48–55
14. Franklin DJ, Jenkins HA, Horowitz BL, Coker NJ. Management of petrous apex lesions. Arch Otolaryngol Head Neck Surg 1989; 115:1121–1125
15. Gherini SG, Brackmann DE, Lo WW, Solti-Bohman LG. Cholesterol granuloma of the petrous apex. Laryngoscope 1985; 95:659–664
16. Gray WC, Salcman M, Rao KC, Hafiz MA. Cholesterol granuloma of the petrous apex and sphenoidal sinus: a case report. Neurosurgery 1985; 17:67–69
17. Greenberg JJ, Oot RF, Wismer GL, et al. Cholesterol granuloma of the petrous apex: MR and CT evaluation. AJNR 1988; 9:1205–1214
18. Griffin C, DeLaPaz R, Enzmann D. MR and CT correlation of cholesterol cysts of the petrous bone. AJNR 1987; 8:825–829

19. Latack JT, Graham MD, Kemink JL, Knake JE. Giant cholesterol cysts of the petrous apex: radiologic features. AJNR 1985; 6:409–413

20. Lo WW, Solti-Bohman LG, Brackmann DE, Gruskin P. Cholesterol granuloma of the petrous apex: CT diagnosis. Radiology 1984; 153:705–711

21. Martin N, Sterkers O, Mompoint D, Julien N, Nahum H. Cholesterol granulomas of the middle ear cavities: MR imaging. Radiology 1989; 172:521–525

22. Nomura Y. Cholesterol metabolism in cholesteatoma and cholesterol granuloma. Ann Otol Rhinol Laryngol Suppl 1984; 112:129–132

23. Rosenberg RA, Hammerschlag PE, Cohen NL, Bergeron RT, Reede DL. Cholesteatoma vs. cholesterol granuloma of the petrous apex. Otolaryngol Head Neck Surg 1986; 94:322–327

24. Sataloff RT, Myers DL, Roberts BR, Feldman MD, Mayer DP, Choi HY. Giant cholesterol cysts of the petrous apex. Arch Otolaryngol Head Neck Surg 1988; 114:451–453

25. Smith PG, Leonetti JP, Kletzker GR. Differential clinical and radiographic features of cholesterol granulomas and cholesteatomas of the petrous apex. Ann Otol Rhinol Laryngol 1988; 97:599–604

26. Thedinger BA, Nadol JB Jr, Montgomery WW, Thedinger BS, Greenberg JJ. Radiographic diagnosis, surgical treatment, and long-term follow-up of cholesterol granulomas of the petrous apex. Laryngoscope 1989; 99:896–907

## INTRAPETROUS CAROTID ARTERY ANEURYSMS

27. Buckingham MJ, Crone KR, Ball WS, Tomsick TA, Berger TS, Tew JM Jr. Traumatic intracranial aneurysms in childhood: two cases and a review of the literature. Neurosurgery 1988; 22:398–408

28. Frank E, Brown BM, Wilson DF. Asymptomatic fusiform aneurysm of the petrous carotid artery in a patient with von Recklinghausen's neurofibromatosis. Surg Neurol 1989; 32:75–78

29. Gibson RD, Cowan IA. Giant aneurysm of the petrous carotid artery presenting with facial numbness. Neuroradiology 1989; 31:440–441

30. Glasscock ME III, Smith PG, Bond AG, Whitaker SR, Bartels LJ. Management of aneurysms of the petrous portion of the internal carotid artery by resection and primary anastomosis. Laryngoscope 1983; 93:1445–1453

31. Guha A, Montanera W, Hoffman HJ. Congenital aneurysmal dilatation of the petrous-cavernous carotid artery and vertebral basilar junction in a child. Neurosurgery 1990; 26:322–327

32. Halbach VV, Higashida RT, Hieshima GB, et al. Aneurysms of the petrous portion of the internal carotid artery: results of treatment with endovascular or surgical occlusion. AJNR 1990; 11:253–257

33. Kelly WM, Harsh GR IV. CT of petrous carotid aneurysms. AJNR 1985; 6:830–832

34. McGrail KM, Heros RC, Debrun G, Beyerl BD. Aneurysm of the ICA petrous segment treated by balloon entrapment after EC-IC bypass. Case report. J Neurosurg 1986; 65:249–252

35. Rawlinson J, Colquhoun IR. Aneurysms involving the intrapetrous internal

carotid artery: a rare cause of Horner's syndrome. Br J Radiol 1990; 63:69–72

36. Samuel J, Fernandes CM. Mycotic aneurysm of the petrous portion of the internal carotid artery. J Laryngol Otol 1989; 103:111–114

37. Willinsky R, Lasjaunias P, Pruvost P, Boucherat M. Petrous internal carotid aneurysm causing epistaxis: balloon embolization with preservation of the parent vessel. Neuroradiology 1987; 29:570–572


EPIDERMOID TUMOR

38. Brown RV, Sage MR, Brophy BP. CT and MR findings in patients with chordomas of the petrous apex. AJNR 1990; 11:121–124

39. DeSouza CE, Menezes CO, DeSouza RA, Ogale SB, Morris M, Desai AP. Profile of congenital cholesteatomas of the petrous apex. J Postgrad Med 1989; 35:93–97

40. Doyon D, Chan KY, Attia M, et al. Magnetic resonance investigations of non-acoustic petrous lesions. Arch Otorhinolaryngol 1989; 246:265–268

41. Frates MC, Oates E. Petrous apicitis: evaluation by bone SPECT and magnetic resonance imaging. Clin Nucl Med 1990; 15:293–294

42. Glasscock ME III, Woods CI III, Poe DS, Patterson AK, Welling DB. Petrous apex cholesteatoma. Otolaryngol Clin North Am 1989; 22:981–1002

43. King TT, Benjamin JC, Morrison AW. Epidermoid and cholesterol cysts in the apex of the petrous bone. Br J Neurosurg 1989; 3:451–461

44. Phelps PD, Wright A. Imaging cholesteatoma. Clin Radiol 1990; 41:156–162

*Notes*

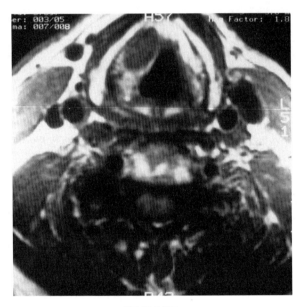

SE 600/25

*Figure 12-1.* This 77-year-old man presented with hoarseness. You are shown a T1-weighted axial MR image.

# Case 12: Obstructed Laryngocele

## Question 54

Which *one* of the following is the MOST likely diagnosis?

(A) Obstructed laryngocele
(B) Thyroglossal duct cyst
(C) Chondrosarcoma
(D) Squamous cell carcinoma
(E) Tuberculosis

The test image (Figure 12-1) shows a smooth-walled abnormality in the paraglottic space of the larynx (arrow, Figure 12-2). The image is at the false cord level of the supraglottic larynx, as evidenced by the bright signal of the paraglottic fat. The lesion has a homogeneous low-intensity signal on this T1-weighted image and is clearly separable from the mucosa. These findings are characteristic of an obstructed laryngocele or saccular cyst **(Option (A) is correct).**

The lesion in the test image is a submucosal abnormality. Squamous cell carcinoma (Option (D)), which is the most common tumor of the larynx, arises from the mucosa and therefore is not separable from the mucosal surface on imaging. An obstructed laryngocele can be caused by a carcinoma at the level of the ventricle, but the test image does not show this level. In fact the test patient did have a small laryngeal cancer, which was readily apparent on a more caudal scan (Figure 12-3). However, the test image did not demonstrate this carcinoma. Moreover, obstructed laryngocele is more commonly a result of inflammatory disease than of carcinoma. Thus, squamous cell carcinoma is not the most likely diagnosis.

A chondrosarcoma (Option (C)) can present as a submucosal mass, but it has a clear connection to the laryngeal cartilage from which it arises.

---

Figures 12-1 and 12-2 are reprinted with permission from Curtin [2].

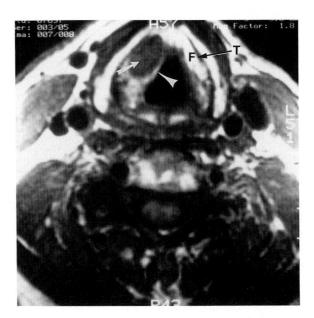

SE 600/25

*Figure 12-2* (Same as Figure 12-1). Obstructed laryngocele (saccular cyst). The T1-weighted MR image through the supraglottic larynx shows a smoothly marginated oval abnormality (arrow) of intermediate signal intensity. This represents the fluid-filled saccular cyst or obstructed laryngocele. Note the intact mucosa (arrowhead) over the cyst. The cyst is in the paraglottic space. Note the bright signal of the fat (F) in the paraglottic space on the normal side, which indicates that this slice is at the supraglottic level. The inner cortex of the thyroid cartilage (T) is also indicated.

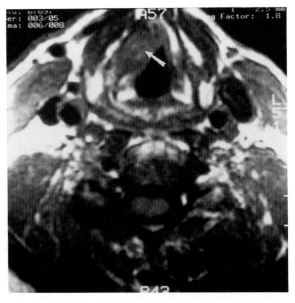

SE 600/25

*Figure 12-3.* Same patient as in Figures 12-1 and 12-2. Obstructed laryngocele. Slightly lower slice shows a more irregular abnormality (arrow) close to the ventricle. This represents a small carcinoma, which is actually causing the obstruction of the laryngeal appendix.

The lesion in the test case has no connection to any of the laryngeal cartilages. Although a chondrosarcoma can extend within the soft tissues, such an extension is unlikely to give the appearance of a sharply marginated abnormality totally within the paraglottic space.

The position of the abnormality in the test image is inappropriate for a thyroglossal duct cyst (Option (B)), which is almost always situated outside the larynx. Tuberculosis (Option (E)) rarely affects the larynx; when it does, it primarily involves the mucosa.

## Question 55

An obstructed laryngocele:

   (A) leaves the larynx via the thyroid notch
   (B) passes through the thyrohyoid membrane
   (C) frequently involves the true cord
   (D) ascends in the paraglottic space
   (E) arises from the laryngeal ventricular saccule (appendix)

The appendix or saccule of the laryngeal ventricle arises anterolaterally from the depths of the ventricle and extends superiorly in the paraglottic space of the supraglottic larynx (Figure 12-4). The ventricular appendix is lined with mucosa, and if it becomes obstructed, a fluid-filled cyst forms. This cyst is called a saccular cyst or an obstructed laryngocele **(Option (E) is true).** Such a saccular cyst is benign, and the obstruction is most often the result of mucosal inflammatory disease. However, it may also be the result of a carcinoma either at the level of the true vocal cord or arising within the ventricle. To cause such a cyst, the tumor must obstruct the narrow outlet or opening of the laryngeal appendix.

Most authors refer to a dilated air-filled appendix as a laryngocele and call an obstructed fluid-filled dilated appendix a saccular cyst. Other authors use the term "laryngocele" to refer to either a dilated air-filled or a fluid-filled appendix.

An enlarging cyst initially follows the path of the laryngeal appendix. First the cyst enlarges into the paraglottic space at the false cord level (Figure 12-5) **(Option (D) is true).** With further enlargement the obstructed laryngocele can pass over the thyroid cartilage and through the thyrohyoid membrane, developing an extralaryngeal component (Figures 12-5 and 12-6). The laryngocele or saccular cyst passes through the thyrohyoid membrane laterally **(Option (B) is true)** rather than

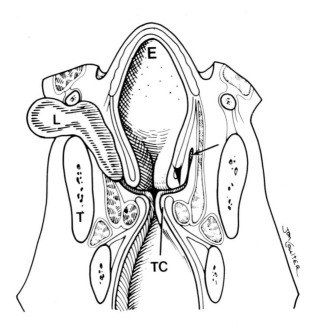

*Figure 12-4.* Diagram of the larynx in coronal section showing the ventricle and a laryngocele. The laryngeal appendix (arrow) extends superiorly from the laryngeal ventricle (arrowhead) into the paraglottic space at the level of the false cord. Obstruction with dilatation causes a cystic accumulation called a laryngocele (L) or saccular cyst. T = thyroid cartilage; E = epiglottis; TC = true cord.

through the notch of the thyroid cartilage **(Option (A) is false).** Actually, the saccular cyst or laryngocele can be totally within the larynx (internal) or have its main mass outside the larynx (external). However, all lesions that have an external component also have an internal component and are probably more accurately referred to as mixed or combined laryngoceles.

The ventricular appendix extends cranially from the ventricle toward the false cord level rather than caudally to the true cord level. Similarly, a laryngocele or saccular cyst does not extend caudally to the true cord **(Option (C) is false).** The true cord level should be normal on imaging.

Laryngoceles or saccular cysts usually present as a swelling in the upper larynx. If mass effect is large enough, the patient may present with difficulty breathing. Occasionally the external component of the laryngocele can be so large that the patient presents with a swelling in the neck.

Larger symptomatic laryngoceles are removed surgically. The role of the radiologist is to establish the diagnosis and to look for a lesion at the

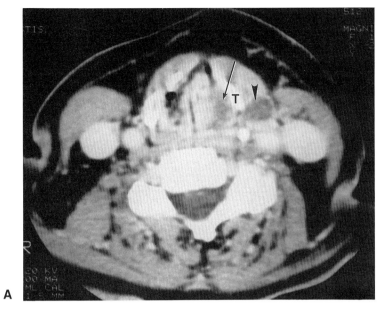

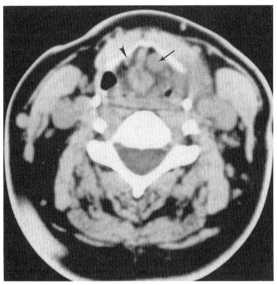

*Figure 12-5.* Laryngocele (saccular cyst). (A) CT scan at the supraglottic level showing both an intralaryngeal (arrow) and an extralaryngeal (arrowhead) component of this saccular cyst. At this point the cyst is just passing over the upper edge of the thyroid cartilage (T). The extralaryngeal component is in the posterior part of the strap muscle. Note the fat in the paraglottic space on the normal side indicating that the image is at the level of the supraglottic larynx. (B) CT scan at a slightly lower level showing the dilated lower portion of the saccular cyst (arrow) extending through the paraglottic fat. Note the nondilated ventricular appendix (arrowhead) on the normal side. The abnormality could be followed down to the level of the ventricle. The level of the true cord was normal. (Reprinted with permission from Curtin [3].)

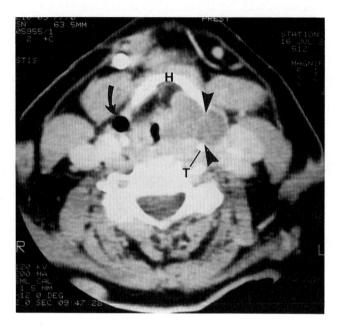

*Figure 12-6.* Laryngocele (saccular cyst). CT scan at the level of the hyoid bone (H) showing the laryngocele passing below the hyoid bone through the thyrohyoid membrane, which would be located between the arrowheads. T = upper horn of the thyroid cartilage. A small air-filled laryngocele is seen on the opposite side (arrow).

level of the ventricle. Although carcinoma may be identified at imaging, neither CT nor MRI can completely exclude a small lesion. For this reason, these patients undergo endoscopy with special attention to the ventricle and upper true cord.

## Question 56

Concerning thyroglossal duct cysts,

(A) a prominent intralaryngeal component is usually present
(B) when surgically excised, a portion of the hyoid bone is removed
(C) when infrahyoid, they have an intimate association with the strap muscles
(D) malignant lesions related to thyroglossal duct remnants are usually carcinomas

The thyroglossal duct is the embryonic pathway along which the thyroid gland descends from its origin in the floor of the embryonic

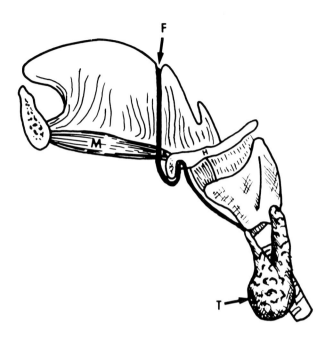

*Figure 12-7.* Diagram of the pathway of the thyroglossal duct. The thyroglossal duct remnant can extend from the foramen cecum (F) in the posterior part of the tongue inferiorly through the mylohyoid muscle (M) to the level of the hyoid bone (H). Here it wraps around the posterior aspect of the body of the hyoid bone. The infrahyoid portions extend inferiorly, following the strap muscle to the level of the pyramidal process of the thyroid gland (T). (Reprinted with permission from Reede et al. [6].)

pharynx to its final location in the lower neck (Figure 12-7). Its route begins in the base of the tongue at the foraman cecum and continues through the tongue to the upper neck just anterior to the hyoid bone. The duct then passes around the inferior margin of the hyoid bone before attaching to the posterior surface of the body of this bone. From here it descends caudally in the neck to the level of the adult thyroid gland. A thyroglossal duct cyst can form at any point along the course of this duct (or its remnant). Thyroglossal duct cysts are usually classified as being suprahyoid or infrahyoid depending on their location in the neck.

The infrahyoid thyroglossal duct does not actually enter the larynx. Rather, it passes external to the thyroid cartilage and the thyrohyoid membrane. An enlarging thyroglossal duct cyst at this level can bulge over the superior edge of the anterior thyroid cartilage and cause a posterior indentation of the thyrohyoid membrane into the pre-epiglottic

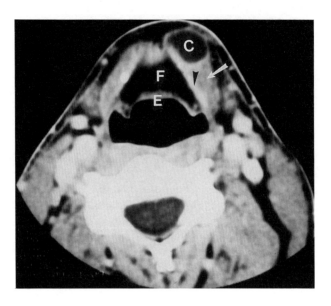

*Figure 12-8.* Thyroglossal duct cyst. CT scan at the level of the epiglottis (E). The cyst (C) is seen within the strap muscles (arrow) external to the lamina of the thyroid cartilage (arrowhead). This is at the level of the pre-epiglottic fat (F). (Reprinted with permission from Curtin [3].)

fat. This apparent intralaryngeal component is usually quite small **(Option (A) is false).**

Most infrahyoid thyroglossal duct cysts are close to, but slightly off, the midline and are embedded in or immediately deep to the strap muscles, which pass along the anterolateral aspect of the thyroid cartilage (Figure 12-8) **(Option (C) is true).**

At surgery, an attempt is made to remove all of the identifiable thyroglossal duct in order to reduce recurrences. This includes the central body of the hyoid bone because of the attachment of the duct to its posterior surface **(Option (B) is true).** The duct can often be followed well up into the base of the tongue.

Cysts and fistulas are the most common abnormalities associated with a thyroglossal duct remnant, and these entities most often present clinically as a draining sinus or a painless swelling in the anterior neck (usually midline). The cyst or fistula may become infected and present as an apparent anterior neck abscess. Rarely, a malignant lesion arises in the duct (Figure 12-9). The duct is lined with epithelial tissue, so the lesion is usually a papillary or papillary-follicular thyroid carcinoma **(Option (D) is true).**

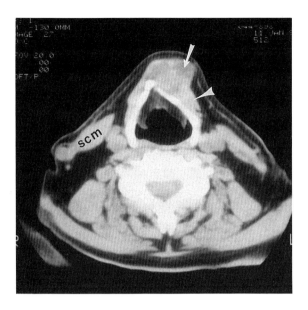

*Figure 12-9.* Papillary carcinoma arising in a thyroglossal duct remnant. The irregular inhomogeneous mass (arrow) presented as a hard lump in the anterior neck. Note that the lesion is in the anterior part of the strap muscles (arrowhead). The strap muscles consist of the sternohyoid, sternothyroid, and thyrohyoid muscles. scm = sternocleidomastoid muscle.

Thyroglossal duct cysts can be diagnosed by either CT or ultrasonography. The radiologist should attempt to identify any additional abnormality along the course of the thyroglossal duct remnant, especially in the base of the tongue. There should also be documentation that there is normal thyroid tissue, which is in its normal position in the lower neck and which is separate from the abnormality. Occasionally, a mass thought to be a thyroglossal duct cyst actually represents the patient's only functioning thyroid tissue.

## Question 57

Concerning laryngeal chondrosarcomas,

  (A) most arise from the epiglottic cartilage
  (B) the involved cartilage is expanded
  (C) metastasis is common
  (D) when they involve the thyroid cartilage, a total laryngectomy is usually required

Cartilaginous tumors of the larynx are rare. They usually present as a submucosal mass in the larynx. They may be benign or malignant, although the distinction is often difficult, even by pathologic examination. Metastasis is rare even when the histologic examination indicates a malignant variant **(Option (C) is false)**.

More than 70% of chondroid lesions of the larynx arise in the cricoid cartilage (Figure 12-10) **(Option (A) is false)**. An epiglottic origin is extremely rare. When the lesion arises in the cricoid or the thyroid cartilage, a degree of cartilage expansion often occurs **(Option (B) is true)**. At imaging the tumor appears to arise from within and then break out of the cartilage rather than erode into the cartilage from the outside (as would occur in squamous cell carcinoma). In addition, cartilaginous tumors frequently calcify (Figure 12-11). These calcifications, which are more easily seen on CT than on MRI, are a strong indication of the cartilaginous nature of the tumor.

When the tumor does involve the cricoid cartilage, resection of the cartilage is often required. It is difficult to remove the tumor and leave enough of the cricoid to allow adequate reconstruction of the larynx. For this reason a total laryngectomy is often done, even if the tumor is considered benign. If the tumor arises in and is limited to the thyroid cartilage, a partial laryngectomy is usually possible, and thus speech can be preserved **(Option (D) is false)**.

*Hugh D. Curtin, M.D.*

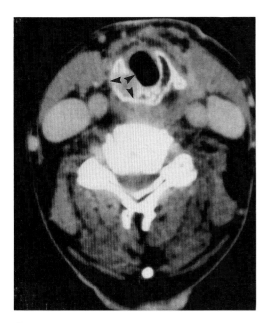
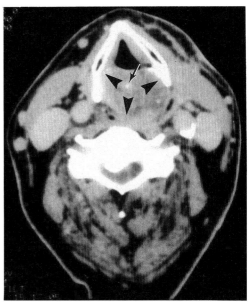

**A**                                                               **B**

*Figure 12-10.* Chondrosarcoma arising in the cricoid cartilage. (A) CT scan through the cricoid cartilage showing a lesion arising in the medullary cavity of the cricoid and expanding outward (arrowheads). This is typical for a chondrosarcoma. (B) Slightly higher slice showing the bulk of this tumor (arrowheads) as well as some small calcifications (arrow).

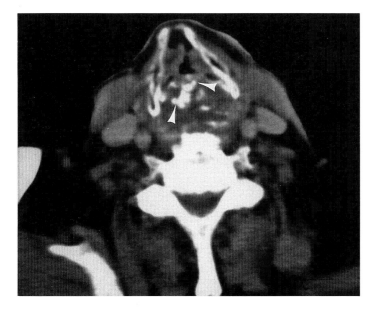

*Figure 12-11.* Chondrosarcoma of the larynx. CT scan shows this expanding tumor arising in the posterior larynx. The calcifications (arrowheads) indicate the cartilaginous origin of the tumor.

# SUGGESTED READINGS

### LARYNGOCELE

1. Barnes L, Gnepp DR. Disease of the larynx, hypopharynx, and esophagus. In: Barnes L (ed), Surgical pathology of the head and neck. New York: Marcel Dekker; 1985:145–148
2. Curtin HD. Imaging of the larynx: current concepts. Radiology 1989; 173:1–11
3. Curtin HD. The larynx. In: Som PM, Bergeron RT (eds), Head and neck imaging, 2nd ed. Chicago: Mosby-Year Book; 1991:593–692
4. Glazer HS, Mauro MA, Aronberg DJ, Lee JK, Johnston DE, Sagel SS. Computed tomography of laryngoceles. AJR 1983; 140:549–552
5. Hubbard C. Laryngocele—a study of five cases with reference to the radiologic features. Clin Radiol 1987; 38:639–643

### THYROGLOSSAL DUCT CYSTS

6. Reede DL, Bergeron RT, Som PM. CT of thyroglossal duct cysts. Radiology 1985; 157:121–125
7. Smoker WRK, Harnsberger HR, Reede DL, Holliday RA, Som PM, Bergeron RT. The neck. In: Som PM, Bergeron RT (eds), Head and neck imaging, 2nd ed. Chicago: Mosby-Year Book; 1991:497–592

### CHONDROSARCOMA

8. Barnes L, Peel RL, Verbin RS, Goodman MA, Appel BN. Disease of the bones and joints. In: Barnes L (ed), Surgical pathology of the head and neck. New York: Marcel Dekker; 1985:957–960
9. Burggraaf BA, Weinstein GS. Chondrosarcoma of the larynx. Ann Otol Rhinol Laryngol 1992; 101:183–184
10. Neis PR, McMahon MF, Norris CW. Cartilaginous tumors of the trachea and larynx. Ann Otol Rhinol Laryngol 1989; 98:31–36
11. Pilch BZ, Brodsky GL, Goodman ML. Pathology of laryngeal malignancies. In: Fried MP (ed), The larynx: a multidisciplinary approach. Boston: Little, Brown; 1988:446–448

*Notes*

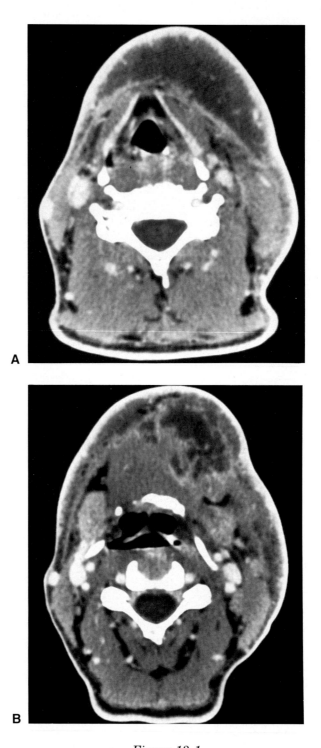

*Figure 13-1*

*Figures 13-1 and 13-2.* This 46-year-old man has submandibular pain and swelling. You are shown a series of postcontrast axial CT scans (Figure 13-1) and a bone-window axial image of the most superior section in the series (Figure 13-2).

# Case 13: Submandibular Space Abscess

## Question 58

Which *one* of the following is the MOST likely diagnosis?

(A) Squamous cell carcinoma
(B) Plunging ranula
(C) Epidermoid cyst
(D) Abscess
(E) Cystic hygroma

The postcontrast axial CT test images (Figure 13-1) show diffuse enhancement of the skin and subcutaneous tissues adjacent to the left side of the mandible (see Figure 13-3). There is a focal fluid collection with a well-defined wall adjacent to an extraction socket of the left canine tooth (see Figure 13-4). This fluid collection extends between the skin and superficial musculature below the mandible into the upper neck. The most caudal image (Figures 13-1A and 13-3A) documents a large subcutaneous collection extending down to the level of the thyroid cartilage of the larynx. There is early osteomyelitis with destruction of the lingual cortex of the mandible at the extraction socket of the left canine tooth, visible in the bone-window image (Figures 13-2 and 13-4). These findings are characteristic of a submandibular space abscess with cellulitis of the left neck secondary to an odontogenic infection **(Option (D) is correct).**

The oral portion of the upper aerodigestive tract is located between the palate and the valleculae. This portion of the aerodigestive tract has two components: the oral cavity and the oropharynx. A ring of structures comprising the soft palate, the anterior tonsillar pillars, and the circumvallate papillae separates the oral cavity anteriorly from the oropharynx posteriorly. The cranial or superior boundary of the oral cavity is formed by the hard palate, the superior alveolar ridge, and the maxillary teeth. The caudal or inferior limit is formed by the mucosa of the floor of the mouth and the inferior alveolar ridge and mandibular teeth. The lateral

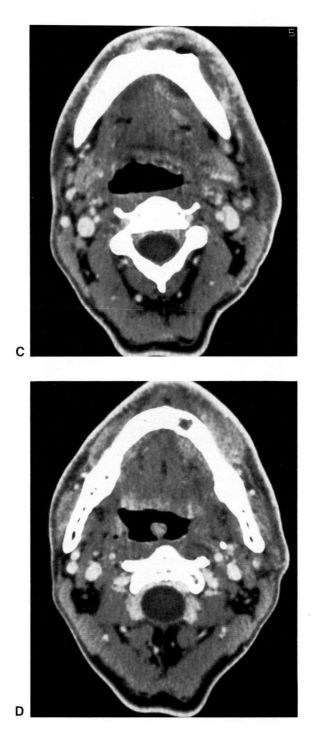

*Figure 13-1 (Continued)*

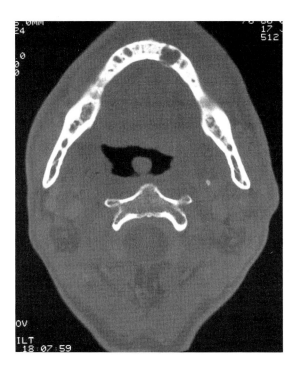

*Figure 13-2*

boundaries are the cheeks, while the anterior tonsillar pillars and circumvallate papillae limit the oral cavity posteriorly.

The oral cavity contains the oral tongue (i.e., the mobile portion of the tongue or the anterior two-thirds of the tongue situated anterior to the circumvallate papillae) and the floor of the mouth. The floor of the mouth is formed above by the mucosa and below by the mylohyoid muscle, which is a muscular sling or tent that attaches to the lingual aspect of each mandibular body and divides the floor of the mouth into a superior sublingual space and an inferior submandibular space. These two spaces connect posteriorly over the free edge of the mylohyoid muscle and are sometimes referred to jointly as the submaxillary space. The sublingual space is separated by the lingual septum and the midline tongue muscles.

The superficial margins of the submandibular space are cranially the lower margin of the mandibular body and caudally the posterior and anterior bellies of the digastric muscle. Posteriorly, there is free communication with the posterior aspect of the sublingual space and possibly the inferior aspect of the parapharyngeal space. The superficial layer of deep cervical fascia covers the superficial surface of this space by

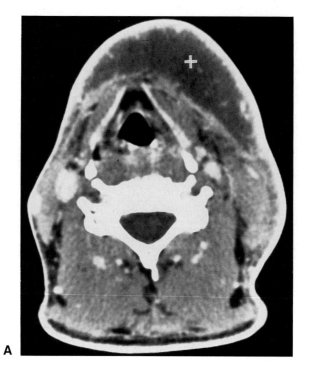

**A**

*Figure 13-3* (Same as Figure 13-1). Axial postcontrast CT scans of sub-mandibular space abscess with osteomyelitis. (A) There is a large subcutaneous fluid collection (+) centered on the left side of the upper neck but extending across the midline in front of the larynx. (B) In the submandibular region, the lesion demonstrates irregular enhancing margins around a necrotic center (+). (C) An abscess cavity (arrows) containing a small amount of air (open arrow) is seen near the inferior surface of the left hemimandible. (D) There is destruction of a portion of the body of the mandible (arrow) around an extraction socket.

extending between the mandible and the digastric muscle. The floor or medial margin of this space is the external surface of the mylohyoid muscle. The submandibular space contains the superficial portion (which represents the major bulk) of the submandibular gland and the submandibular lymph nodes (Figure 13-5).

Disruption of the soft tissue planes separating the extrinsic tongue muscles and involvement of contiguous anatomic spaces are features of both infections and invasive neoplasms such as squamous cell carcinomas (Option (A)). However, the presence of cellulitis of the subcutaneous soft tissues and of the platysma allows distinction between these two entities. Diffuse swelling and irregular contrast enhancement, as seen in the test

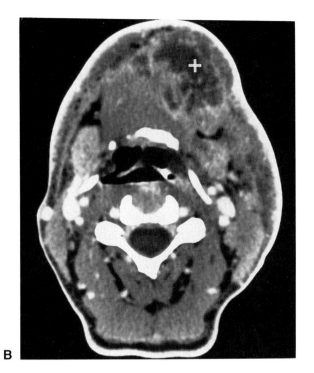

**B**

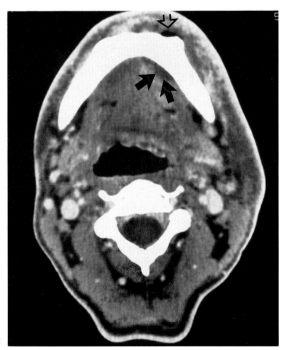

**C**

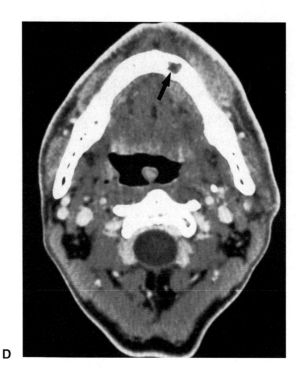

**D**

images, suggest cellulitis, and the presence of a fluid collection with thickened irregular walls indicates an abscess.

A ranula is a mucocele, usually of a sublingual gland and rarely of a minor salivary gland. When the wall of a ranula ruptures, the mucoid secretions drain into the floor of the mouth. Such a ruptured ranula is referred to as a deep or plunging ranula (Option (B)). The drainage from a plunging ranula may penetrate through the mylohyoid muscle to involve the submandibular space. However, there is typically a small tail of secretions lingering in the sublingual space (Figure 13-6), a finding not present in the test patient. Clinically, a plunging ranula presents as a painless mass in the submandibular region, unlike the clinical situation in the test case. Similarly, an epidermoid cyst (Option (C)) usually presents clinically as a painless solid mass or cyst with no involvement or thickening of the adjacent subcutaneous structures. On CT, such a cyst is ovoid and well defined, unlike the irregular lesion in the test case.

A cystic hygroma or cystic lymphangioma (Option (E)) may present as a cystic lesion in the submandibular space. CT examination will reveal a unilocular or multilocular cystic mass, with each cyst demonstrating

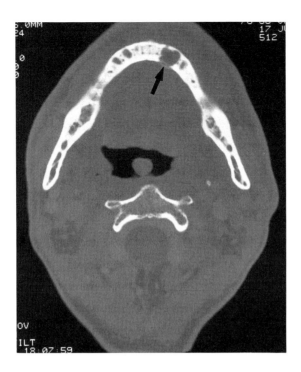

*Figure 13-4* (Same as Figure 13-2). Submandibular space abscess with osteomyelitis. Bone-window axial image of same CT section shown in Figure 13-3D. The expansion of the extraction socket for the left canine tooth is evident. Note the early destruction of the posterior surface of the body of the mandible (arrow).

very thin, nearly unidentifiable walls (Figure 13-7). There is homogeneous water-density fluid within these cysts, unless there has been hemorrhage into the lesion, in which case there would be areas of higher density. Thickening and enhancement of the cyst wall and adjacent soft tissues suggest a superimposed infectious process. The test patient's lesion could represent an infected cystic hygroma; however, the presence of osteomyelitis in the tooth socket suggests that the cystic collection is most probably an abscess secondary to mandibular osteomyelitis. In addition, most cystic hygromas are diagnosed in patients younger than 2 years of age.

Surgery on the test patient documented the presence of a submandibular space abscess. There was necrotic tissue occupying the left side of the lower mandible, including necrosis of the left anterior belly of the digastric muscle (Figure 13-1B).

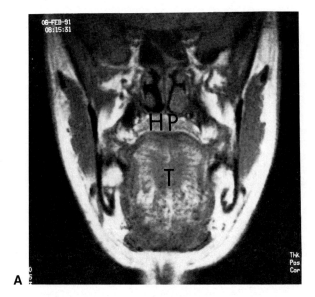

SE 600/15

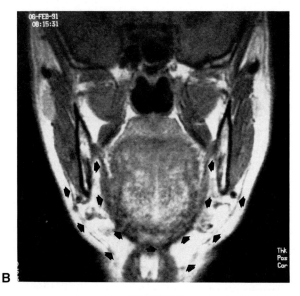

SE 600/15

*Figure 13-5.* Coronal T1-weighted MR images demonstrate normal anatomy of the oral cavity and submandibular spaces. (A) The oral cavity contains the oral tongue (T) beneath the hard palate (HP). (B) The floor of the mouth is formed by the mylohyoid muscle, which attaches to the medial aspect of the mandibular bodies (inner row of arrows). The submandibular spaces are beneath the mylohyoid muscle and are located within the platysma (outer row of arrows). (C) Note the bilateral submandibular glands (SG) adjacent to the flow voids of the facial veins and facial arteries. The soft palate (SP) separates the nasopharynx superiorly from the oropharynx inferiorly.

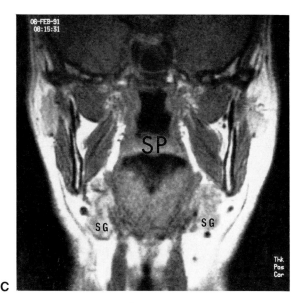

SE 600/15

Infections related to the mandibular molar teeth account for about 90% of cases of abscesses of the floor of the mouth. The relationship of the apices of the mandibular teeth to the mandibular attachment of the mylohyoid muscle plays a role in determining the primary space of involvement. As a general rule, dental infections anterior to the second molar teeth tend to involve the sublingual space (superior to the mylohyoid muscle) first, whereas infections of the second and third molars tend to involve the submandibular space directly (since the roots extend beneath the mylohyoid ridge). However, as in the test case, infections of the anterior teeth can also spread directly into the submandibular space. Other causes of floor of the mouth abscesses are laceration, peritonsillar abscess, otitis media, osteomyelitis, and mandibular fractures. *Streptococcus* and *Staphylococcus* species are often the offending agents. The patient is usually between 20 and 60 years of age.

Clinically, a patient with a floor of the mouth abscess has severe neck pain and an inferiorly bulging, indurated submandibular triangle whenever the submandibular space is involved. Disease in the sublingual space results in elevation and posterior displacement of the tongue with compromise of the airway. Pain is usually relieved when the patient is in a semierect position. Other common symptoms include trismus and restricted neck mobility. Swelling and displacement of the tongue may

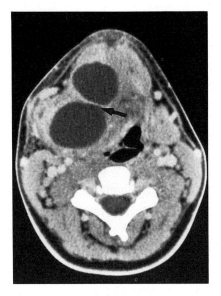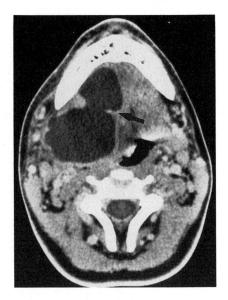

*Figure 13-6.* Plunging ranula in the right sublingual and submandibular spaces. Postcontrast axial CT scans show a bicompartmentalized cystic lesion in the right side of the floor of the mouth and submandibular space. The anterior superior compartment lies within the sublingual space and represents the original site of the ranula. As the lesion expanded, it penetrated through the right mylohyoid muscle, where a waistlike narrowing is evident in the middle of the lesion (arrow). A larger portion of the cystic mass lies posterolaterally within the submandibular space.

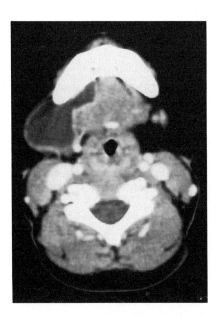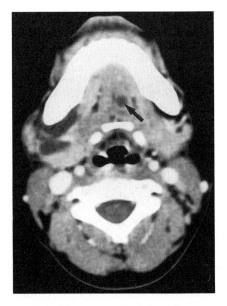

*Figure 13-7.* Cystic hygroma. Postcontrast axial CT scans demonstrate a cystic lesion with thin walls in the right submandibular space. The cystic lesion surrounds the right side of the body of the mandible and extends minimally into the right floor of the mouth. There is a small, sharply defined cystic lesion on the left side of the floor of the mouth (arrow). This may represent a simple ranula or a separate portion of the cystic hygroma.

result in dysphagia, dysphonia, odynophagia, or drooling. Tachycardia, fever, dyspnea, and stridor may also be present.

Before the advent of antibiotics, the infection often spread to the parapharyngeal, retropharyngeal, or visceral space. Dissection of the process into the mediastinum causes substernal chest pain, which may simulate angina pectoris.

In patients with a suspected abscess of the floor of the mouth, CT is currently used to search for a drainable collection of pus and to determine on which side of the neck an attempted drainage should be made. The identification of a fluid collection with respect to the mylohyoid muscle is crucial in determining the surgical approach—intraoral for the sublingual space and submandibular for the submandibular space.

## Question 59

Concerning ranulas,

  (A) they most commonly originate in the sublingual glands
  (B) the plunging variety usually extend into the masticator space
  (C) a location medial to the mylohyoid muscle is typical
  (D) they are common in trumpet players

Ranulas are uncommon acquired mucoceles or cystic lesions usually originating in the sublingual glands or occasionally in the minor salivary glands of the sublingual space **(Option (A) is true).** There are two forms of ranula: simple ranula and plunging ranula. A simple ranula is a true epithelium-lined retention cyst that is due to partial obstruction of a salivary gland duct. A simple ranula of the floor of the mouth is confined to the sublingual space and presents as an intraoral mass located off the midline. It usually causes a bluish discoloration of the elevated mucosa of the floor of the mouth.

A deep or plunging ranula results from the rupture of the wall of a simple ranula. The lesion is not caused by increases in intraoral pressure or by performing the Valsalva maneuver. Neither plunging ranula nor simple ranula is more common in individuals with occupationally increased intraoral pressures (trumpeters, glassblowers, etc.) **(Option (D) is false).** The mucus extravasating into the surrounding soft tissues forms mucus-filled pseudocysts with no epithelial lining. These lesions may dissect down between the facial planes into the neck or, more rarely, across the midline. A plunging ranula may herniate through a dehiscence in the mylohyoid muscle or posterior to the mylohyoid muscle to involve the submandibular space (Figure 13-6) or, rarely, the inferior para-pharyngeal space. Extension into the masticator space is extremely rare **(Option (B) is false).** The bulk of a plunging ranula is in the subman-dibular space. A small collection of mucoid tissue remains in the sub-lingual space. If the tail is lacking, the lesion must be seen to abut the sublingual space in order to diagnose a plunging ranula. A plunging ranula presents clinically as a painless mass in the submandibular or submental triangle of the neck, with or without an associated mass in the floor of the mouth.

In the absence of previous surgery or infection, a ranula is a sharply marginated, unilocular cystic lesion with imperceptibly thin walls. The content of a ranula is homogeneous, with a low (0- to 20-HU) central attenuation. A ranula typically involves the sublingual space; therefore, it is located lateral to the genioglossus muscle and superomedial to the mylohyoid muscle **(Option (C) is true).** The simple ranula is entirely confined to the sublingual space, whereas the plunging variety either extends into the submandibular space or abuts the submandibular space posteriorly.

The differential diagnosis of a simple ranula based on location of the lesion includes lateral epidermoid or dermoid cysts, lipomas, and salivary gland tumors. Lipomas are thin-walled, encapsulated fatty lesions that may occur anywhere and may resemble cysts if wide CT windows are used. CT density measurements below –20 HU help differentiate a lipoma from a ranula. Dermoid cysts in the sublingual space may be distinguished from ranulas by their internal architecture, which consists of focal collections of cholesterol and oily sebaceous or sweat gland secretions. There may be subtle heterogeneity within the central fluid of a dermoid cyst as a result of the presence of several different skin elements with different densities. An epidermoid cyst in the sublingual space may not be distinguishable from a simple ranula by CT or by MRI (Figure 13-8). However, the differentiation is not crucial since the surgical approach is the same for both lesions.

Treatment of a simple ranula in the floor of the mouth consists of excision or marsupialization of the cyst wall. A plunging ranula is treated by meticulous dissection of the pseudocyst and, to prevent recurrence, an "en bloc" excision with the sublingual-space salivary gland of origin.

The radiologic differential diagnosis of a plunging ranula by location includes lateral dermoid or epidermoid cysts, cystic hygromas, second branchial cleft cysts, suprahyoid thyroglossal duct cysts, and (less likely) reactive or malignant adenopathy. Differentiation among these is made

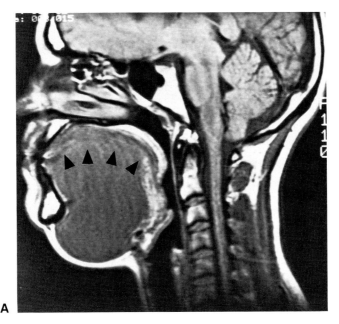

SE 600/15

*Figure 13-8.* Midline epidermoid inclusion cyst in the floor of the mouth. (A) Sagittal T1-weighted MR image shows a cystic lesion in the floor of the mouth above the mylohyoid muscle and beneath the elevated tongue. The superior margin of the cyst is denoted by arrowheads. The signal characteristics are those of pure fluid. (B) Axial T2-weighted MR image shows high signal intensity in the purely cystic lesion. There is marked displacement of the central structures of the floor of the mouth but no extension of the lesion into the surrounding soft tissues.

on the basis of morphology, location, and CT density or MR signal intensity. Cystic hygromas are mostly multilocular thin-walled cystic masses, which are usually located in the submandibular space or posterior triangle of the neck (Figure 13-7). They may cross the midline into the opposite submandibular space. They usually are not infected, and so they have a barely perceptible wall. A rare cystic hygroma involving both the submandibular and sublingual spaces may not be distinguishable by imaging methods from a plunging ranula. However, in most cases the lack of association with the sublingual space and the multilocularity of the lesion permit differentiation from a ranula.

Second branchial cleft cysts typically occur at the level of the mandibular angle, medial to the anterior border of the sternocleidomastoid muscle and lateral to the carotid sheath. The typical location and the lack of association with the sublingual space allow a distinction from ranulas.

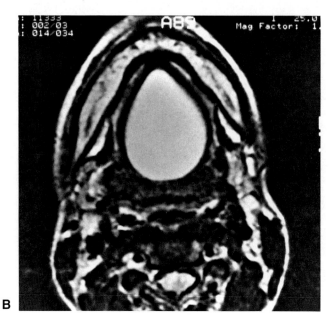

B

SE 2,000/80

About 20% of thyroglossal duct cysts are suprahyoid cysts. Approximately 75% of thyroglossal duct cysts are located in the anterior midline of the neck; the other 25% are in a paramedian location. A midline and juxtahyoid location makes differentiation of a thyroglossal duct cyst from a ranula relatively easy. A rare suprahyoid paramedian thyroglossal duct cyst may be indistinguishable from a plunging ranula. However, in such cases the thyroglossal duct cyst usually touches the hyoid bone, a differentiating point from a ranula.

A reactive or malignant lymph node (or nodes) in the submandibular space usually displays thick, irregular walls with associated central necrosis and irregular enhancement of the walls (Figure 13-9). In the case of a tumor, there is usually an associated primary lesion in the oral cavity. Infections in the oral cavity (including odontogenic infections) usually cause submandibular adenopathy.

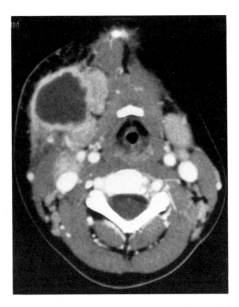

*Figure 13-9.* Necrotic nodal mass in the right submandibular space. Postcontrast axial CT scan shows a centrally necrotic mass in the right submandibular space, located within a group of large reactive lymph nodes. There is thickening of the overlying facial planes and fat, suggesting an inflammatory process. At surgery, a group of enlarged necrotic nodes was identified. Drainage of the central cystic portion documented an abscess cavity.

## Question 60

Concerning epidermoid cysts of the head and neck,

    (A) they represent ectodermal inclusions
    (B) they occur along the lines of embryologic fusion
    (C) they contain skin appendages
    (D) they are attached to the tongue and hyoid bone

Epidermoid cysts (epidermoidomas) represent the most common of the developmental lesions (epidermoids, dermoids, and teratomas) that occur in the head and neck region. They result from the congenital inclusion of ectodermal tissues along lines of embryologic fusion **(Option (A) is true).** This results in the accumulation of desquamated epithelial debris. Epidermoid cysts are variously estimated to account for 0.2 to 1.0% of all head and neck masses. Most lesions are detected in the fourth through sixth decades of life, and there is a slight male predominance. The symptoms depend on the location of the mass. Epidermoids occurring in the soft tissues of the head and neck present as painless masses, growing along the lines of embryologic fusion of the facial bones **(Option (B) is true)**. There is no predilection for involvement of a particular organ or structure; these lesions are not attached to the tongue and the hyoid bone **(Option (D) is false).**

Epidermoid cysts vary greatly in size but are consistently circum-scribed by a smooth capsule that sometimes has a striking mother-of-pearl sheen on gross pathologic inspection. There may be foci of calcifica-tion in the capsule. The interior of the cyst is characteristically filled with soft, white material that is rich in cholesterol crystals. The source of the cholesterol crystals is unclear. Some investigators believe that the crystals form as a result of the progressive desquamation and breakdown of keratin from the epithelial lining of the cyst. Others claim that the cholesterol derives from the products of antecedent hemorrhage.

The lining of an epidermoid cyst is composed of a simple stratified squamous epithelial layer supported by an outer layer of collagenous tissue. Progressive exfoliation of keratinous material toward the interior of the cyst produces the layered character of the contents and leads to slow expansion of the lesion.

Grossly, an epidermoid cyst may be cystic or solid, depending on what becomes trapped within the lesion. The solid form of an epidermoid cyst gives rise to the classic glistening pearly white mass that has white, cheesy central contents. It is important to note that although evidence of fat may be suggested on CT or MRI, a true epidermoid cyst contains no fat. The breakdown products of sweat and sebaceous glands (skin appendages) are present in a dermoid cyst but not in an epidermoid lesion **(Option (C) is false).** The presence of true fat, a tissue of mesodermal origin, reclassifies the lesion as a teratoma. Epidermoid cysts are usually entirely benign histologically. Their growth rate is linear; i.e., it approxi-mates that of normal skin rather than the exponential growth demon-strated by some neoplasms. If incompletely removed, the lesions will gradually recur.

# Question 61

A midline mass in the floor of the mouth is MOST likely to represent:

(A) an epidermoid cyst
(B) a ranula
(C) a salivary duct stone
(D) an odontogenic cyst
(E) an enlarged lymph node

Of the options listed, only epidermoid cyst is typically a midline lesion **(Option (A) is correct).** An epidermoid cyst is one of the three varieties of germ cell cysts (the other two being dermoid cyst and teratoid cyst), and these cysts almost always occur in the midline of the floor of the mouth, even though they may extend laterally or inferiorly as they enlarge (Figure 13-8). Epidermoid cysts are lined by simple squamous epithelium, while dermoid cysts contain skin appendages, including hair follicles and sebaceous glands, within the epithelial lining of their walls.

A ranula (Option (B)) is not the correct choice since ranulas typically occur off the midline, in the area of the sublingual glands (Figure 13-6). Both simple and plunging ranulas occur off the midline in the submandibular, sublingual, or inferior parapharyngeal space.

A salivary duct stone (Option (C)) is not the correct choice since such stones in the floor of the mouth are located primarily along the path of the submandibular gland duct (Wharton's duct), which is located off the midline along its course from anteriorly to posteriorly where it joins the submandibular gland. The sublingual glands rarely have stones, and these glands are located on either side of the midline.

The lymph nodes (Option (E)) that drain the floor of the mouth are located primarily in the submandibular and submental regions. Some lymph tissue is also scattered in the sublingual regions. A squamous cell carcinoma of the floor of the mouth or the oral portion of the tongue may spread to these nodes. The submental lymph nodes are located in the midline between the anterior bellies of the digastric muscles and represent one of the main sites of spread of a squamous cell carcinoma of the lips or oral tongue. However, these nodes are caudal to the mylohyoid muscle and thus are not strictly in the floor of the mouth. Clinically, such nodes present as a submental mass rather than as a mass in the floor of the mouth. In addition, when such nodes are present, the primary tumor is also visualized. In either case, an enlarged lymph node is not the most likely cause of a midline lesion in the floor of the mouth.

An odontogenic cyst (Option (D)) arises from tooth derivatives and is located in the mandible or maxilla. Although such a mass arising from the mandible may encroach into the floor of the mouth, the main component of an odontogenic cyst is not located there. Odontogenic cysts can be subdivided on the basis of the histology of their epithelial layers, the associated clinical findings, and their relationship to the involved tooth. Periodontal or radicular cysts are the most common types of odontogenic cysts and are most often associated with untreated, carious teeth. They present as well-circumscribed radiolucencies, usually surrounded by a thin rim of cortical bone, at the apex of a tooth. Expansion of the cyst may cause displacement of the teeth. A dentigerous or follicular cyst is the second most common type of cyst; it develops around the crown of an unerupted tooth. Radiographically, a circumscribed, radiolucent, usually unilocular cyst is seen with the unerupted tooth at the margin of the cyst wall (Figure 13-10). Approximately 75% of dentigerous cysts are located in the mandible, and 25% arise in the maxilla.

*Anton N. Hasso, M.D.*
*Thu-Anh Hoang, M.D.*
*Monika L. Kief-Garcia, M.D.*

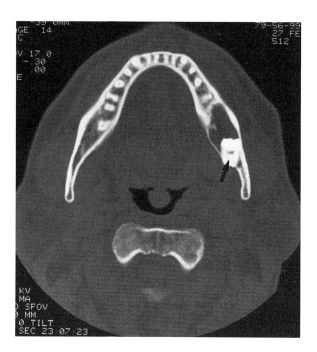

*Figure 13-10.* Dentigerous cyst of the mandible. Axial bone-window CT image demonstrates a unilocular cyst in the left side of the mandible. The cyst originated from the crown of an unerupted molar tooth (arrow), which is displaced by the cyst.

## SUGGESTED READINGS

### ORAL CAVITY: SUBMANDIBULAR AND SUBLINGUAL SPACES

1. Dillon WP. The pharynx and oral cavity. In: Som PM, Bergeron RT (eds), Head and neck imaging, 2nd ed. St. Louis: CV Mosby; 1991:407–466
2. Dillon WP, Mancuso AA. The oropharynx and nasopharynx. In: Newton TH, Hasso AN, Dillon WP (eds), Computed tomography of the head and neck. New York: Raven Press; 1988:10.1–10.68
3. Hardin CW, Harnsberger HR, Osborn AG, Smoker WR. CT in the evaluation of the normal and diseased oral cavity and oropharynx. Semin US CT MR 1986; 7:131–153
4. Harnsberger HR. The oral cavity: the sublingual and submandibular spaces. In: Handbooks in radiology—head and neck imaging. Chicago: Mosby-Year Book; 1990:112–137
5. Nguyen VD, Potter JL, Hersh-Schick MR. Ludwig angina: an uncommon and potentially lethal neck infection. AJNR 1992; 13:215–219

## RANULA AND NECK CYSTS

6. Charnoff SK, Carter BL. Plunging ranula: CT diagnosis. Radiology 1986; 158:467–468

7. Coit WE, Harnsberger HR, Osborn AG, Smoker WR, Stevens MH, Lufkin RB. Ranulas and their mimics: CT evaluation. Radiology 1987; 163:211–216

8. Harnsberger HR, Mancuso AA, Muraki AS, et al. Branchial cleft anomalies and their mimics: computed tomographic evaluation. Radiology 1984; 152:739–748

9. Reede DL, Bergeron RT, Som PM. CT of thyroglossal duct cysts. Radiology 1985; 157:121–125

10. Salazar JE, Duke RA, Ellis JV. Second branchial cleft cyst: unusual location and a new CT diagnostic sign. AJR 1985; 145:965–966

11. Smoker WR, Harnsberger HR. Normal anatomy of the neck. In: Som PM, Bergeron RT (eds), Head and neck imaging, 2nd ed. St. Louis: CV Mosby; 1991:498–530

12. Som PM, Sacher M, Lanzieri CF, et al. Parenchymal cysts of the lower neck. Radiology 1985; 157:399–406

## EPIDERMOID AND DERMOID CYSTS

13. Guidetti B, Gagliardi FM. Epidermoid and dermoid cysts. Clinical evaluation and late surgical results. J Neurosurg 1977; 47:12–18

14. Hasso AN, Smith DS. The cerebellopontine angle. Semin US CT MR 1989; 10:280–301

15. Hunter TB, Paplanus SH, Chernin MM, Coulthard SW. Dermoid cyst of the floor of the mouth: CT appearance. AJR 1983; 141:1239–1240

16. Panagopoulos KP, el-Azouzi M, Chisholm HL, Jolesz FA, Black PM. Intracranial epidermoid tumors. A continuing diagnostic challenge. Arch Neurol 1990; 47:813–816

17. Russell DS, Rubinstein LJ. Pathology of tumours of the nervous system, 5th ed. Baltimore: Williams & Wilkins; 1989:690–695

18. Steffey DJ, DeFilipp GJ, Spera T, Gabrielsen TO. MR imaging of primary epidermoid tumors. J Comput Assist Tomogr 1988; 12:438–440

19. Tampieri D, Melanson D, Ethier R. MR imaging of epidermoid cysts. AJNR 1989; 10:351–356

*Notes*

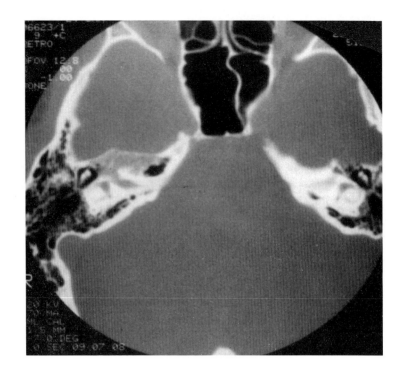

*Figure 14-1*

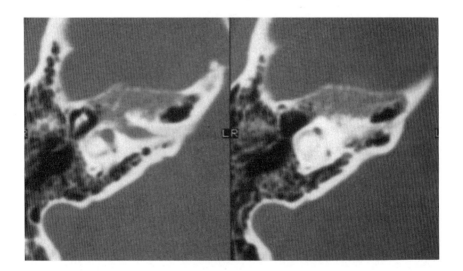

*Figure 14-2*
*Figures 14-1 and 14-2.* This 19-year-old woman has recurrent episodes
of right facial palsy. You are shown two bone-algorithm axial CT scans
through the temporal bones.

# Case 14: Temporal Bone Hemangioma

## Question 62

Which *one* of the following is the MOST likely diagnosis?

(A) Facial nerve schwannoma
(B) Perineural extension of adenoid cystic carcinoma
(C) Hemangioma
(D) Glomus faciale tumor
(E) Cholesteatoma

The facial nerve (cranial nerve VII) follows a narrow bony canal through the temporal bone from the internal auditory canal to the stylomastoid foramen. Any abnormalities that involve the facial nerve in this confined space can cause a facial paralysis. The lesion can develop from the nerve itself or can grow from outside into the canal. Paralysis results when the nerve is invaded by tumor or when a mass causes pressure on the nerve, perhaps compromising its blood supply. Thus, in cases of facial nerve paralysis, the CT findings can be very helpful in determining the diagnosis.

The test images show an irregular lesion involving the bone in the region of the geniculate ganglion and first genu or turn of the facial nerve canal (Figures 14-1 and 14-2). The bone is abnormal outside of the canal, and the canal itself is indistinct and slightly enlarged (Figure 14-3, arrow). Fine calcifications or ossifications seen within the lesion in the axial magnified views (see Figure 14-4) are very suggestive of hemangioma (ossifying hemangioma) **(Option (C) is correct).**

Recent reports have indicated that hemangiomas involving the facial nerve are more common than previously realized. Most series, however, have found that the schwannoma (also known as facial neuroma or facial neurinoma) (Option (A)) is still the predominant lesion. Schwannomas

Figure 14-1 was reprinted with permission from Curtin et al. [3].

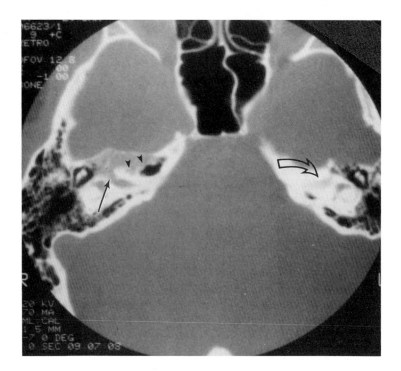

*Figure 14-3* (Same as Figure 14-1).   Ossifying hemangioma of the temporal bone. An irregular lesion involves the bone in the area of the geniculate turn of the facial nerve. The abnormality extends toward the petrous apex and has an irregular margin (arrowheads). The labyrinthine segment of the facial nerve canal is enlarged (straight arrow). Compare with the normal facial nerve canal (curved arrow) on opposite side. (Adapted with permission from Curtin et al. [3].)

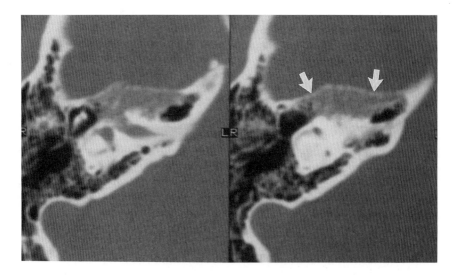

*Figure 14-4* (Same as Figure 14-2).   Axial CT scans at cranial (right image) and slightly more caudal (left image) levels through the petrous portion of the temporal bone. There is an irregular lesion within the bone (arrows) that involves the geniculate ganglion and first genu of the focal nerve. The bone outside of the canal is abnormal and there are fine calcifications or ossifications within the lesion that are suggestive of a hemangioma.

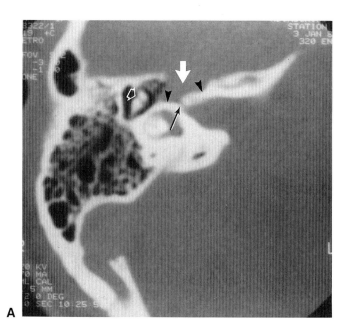

**A**

*Figure 14-5.* Facial neuromas (schwannomas) in three different patients. (A) Axial CT scan shows an expansile lesion in the region of the geniculate turn. Note the sharp margins (arrowheads) where the lesion abuts the bone. The anterior margin of the tumor is not seen on this bone-algorithm scan but is approximately at the white arrow. The labyrinthine segment (black arrow) is normal. The malleus and incus (open arrow) are normal in the attic region. (B) Axial CT scan shows a neuroma in the region of the pyramidal process. Note the well-corticated margin, which represents the bony wall of the expanded facial nerve canal (arrowheads). The lesion arose within the canal and gradually expanded it. (C) Coronal CT scan shows a facial neuroma extending along the vertical segment of the facial nerve canal (arrow). Again, there is smooth enlargement of the canal itself.

arise from the sheath of the facial nerve and therefore develop within the facial nerve canal. These facial nerve sheath tumors grow slowly and tend to cause expansion rather than destruction of the bony canal (Figure 14-5). There is often concentric enlargement of the canal, and segments of the expanded bony wall remain intact and sharp. The irregular appearance of the bone both along the canal wall and outside the canal, as shown in the test images, is not characteristic of a schwannoma. Further, the presence of calcifications suggests that a schwannoma is not the correct diagnosis, since such calcifications are distinctly unusual in nerve sheath tumors.

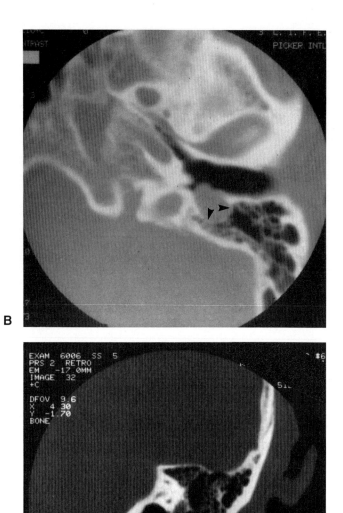

B

C

Concentric enlargement of the facial canal is typical of, but not specific for, facial nerve sheath tumor (schwannoma). Cancers can use the facial nerve canal as a conduit to extend into and even through the temporal

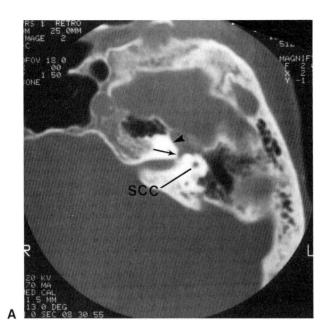

*Figure 14-6.* Perineural tumor extension along the facial nerve from an adenoid cystic carcinoma of the parotid gland. (A) Axial CT scan through the geniculate ganglion shows an expanded bony facial canal in the region of the geniculate ganglion. The cortical margins of the canal are smooth (arrowhead), suggesting gradual enlargement of the canal. The labyrinthine segment (arrow) is normal. The superior semicircular canal (SCC) in indicated. (B) Coronal CT scan through the tympanic segment of the canal. There is obvious enlargement (arrowhead) of the tympanic segment of the facial canal as the tumor extends along it. Though enlarged by the tumor, the cortical margin remains intact. The oval window (arrow) is indicated. (C) Axial CT scan through the parotid gland shows a large tumor (T) of this gland. This image was taken during a CT sialogram, and the sialographic contrast (arrow) is seen in the margin of the gland.

bone (Figure 14-6). Such perineural tumor spread usually originates from a tumor in the parotid gland and can follow the facial nerve canal to the geniculate turn or even into the internal auditory canal. Such a tumor is usually an adenoid cystic carcinoma (Option (B)), which, although malignant, can grow slowly enough that the canal is gradually and concentrically enlarged, mimicking the appearance of a benign schwannoma at imaging. However, diagnostic confusion is unlikely, since the primary carcinoma in the parotid gland is usually obvious both clinically and radiographically. Because this type of tumor spread can occur, the

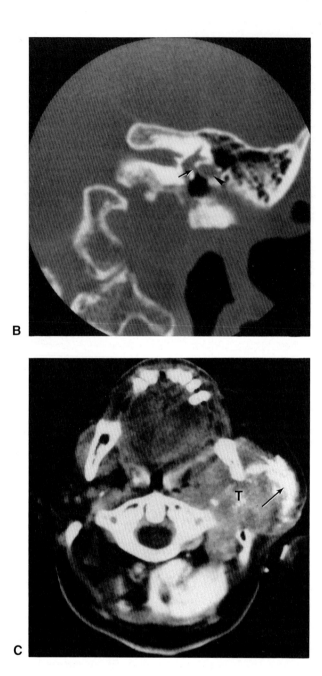

B

C

entire course of the facial nerve in any patient with a parotid tumor should be carefully examined, especially if there is paralysis of the seventh nerve.

Glomus tumors (paragangliomas) can occur wherever there are paraganglion cells. In the temporal bone, most of these tumors arise in the medial wall of the middle ear or in the lateral wall of the jugular canal. However, there are such paraganglion cells that can give rise to paragangliomas in other locations. Indeed, small islands are found along the facial nerve canal, and a lesion developing from these cells can be referred to as a glomus faciale tumor (Option (D)). Such tumors have been reported to occur in the geniculate ganglion region, but they can occur in other parts of the canal as well. A glomus tumor may have an irregular pattern of bone destruction very similar to a hemangioma, or it may cause facial canal expansion with an appearance not unlike that of a facial schwannoma. However, because this type of tumor is exceedingly rare, it is not the most likely diagnosis in the test case.

Similarly, a meningioma can also occur in the region of the facial canal, and this tumor may have calcifications. Even though this type of tumor should be included in the radiographic differential diagnosis of such a lesion, a meningioma in this location is rare. Certainly meningiomas can involve the floor of the middle cranial fossa, but the lesion in the test images appears to arise within the temporal bone itself.

Most cholesteatomas (Option (E)) occur in the middle ear and are associated with chronic middle ear disease and perforation of the tympanic membrane. They can erode into the facial nerve canal, but facial nerve paralysis is uncommon. Therefore, the radiologist should carefully examine the facial nerve canal for erosions even when there is no clinical evidence of paralysis. If a cholesteatoma has eroded into the facial nerve canal, there is an increased risk of nerve damage at the time of surgery. There is also an uncommon entity called invasive cholesteatoma, which usually involves the labyrinth and petrous apex and may cause facial paralysis (Figure 14-7). It can be lobulated and can enlarge the facial canal, but characteristically there is a smooth, sharply defined margin, unlike the appearance in the test images.

Finally, although the test images are very typical of an ossifying hemangioma, not all hemangiomas have this appearance. Uncommonly, some hemangiomas that arise in the facial canal will gradually expand the canal and will not contain small flecks of calcium (Figure 14-8). In such cases, the lesion can appear identical to a facial nerve sheath tumor on a CT scan.

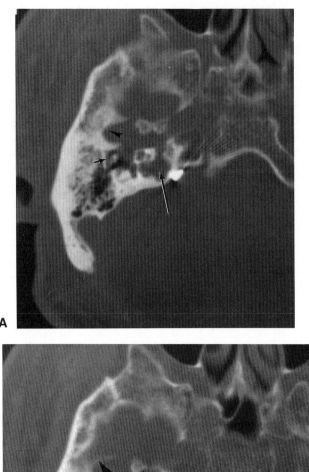

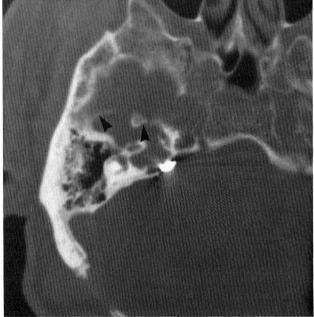

*Figure 14-7.* Invasive cholesteatoma. (A) An axial CT scan shows a large expansile lesion extending from the internal auditory canal (IAC) (long arrow) past the geniculate ganglion area and out into the more lateral temporal bone (arrowhead). Note the sharp margin of the lesion. The attic and the ossicles (short arrow) are relatively uninvolved. The patient had a history of exploration of the cerebellopontine angle via a retromastoid approach 20 years ago. No abnormality had been found. (B) Slightly higher axial scan shows the well-corticated smooth margins of the lesion (arrowheads). A clip in the region of the IAC is from the previous surgery.

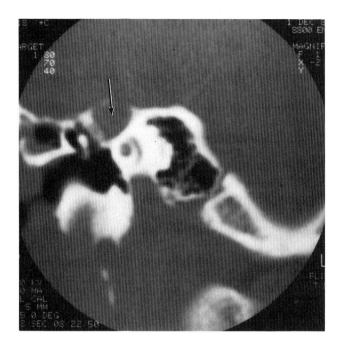

*Figure 14-8.* Hemangioma. Coronal CT scan shows a hemangioma of the geniculate ganglion region (nonossifying). The expansile lesion (arrow) does not show central calcification and replaces both the labyrinthine and tympanic segments of the facial nerve canal. It would be difficult to differentiate this lesion from a facial nerve neuroma.

## Question 63

An acute onset of facial nerve paralysis is MOST commonly due to:

(A) facial nerve schwannoma
(B) hemangioma of the temporal bone
(C) meningioma of the facial canal
(D) acute otitis media
(E) Bell's palsy

The term Bell's palsy is used to describe "idiopathic" facial nerve paralysis, i.e., a facial paralysis for which no obvious etiology is found. No tumor or severe infection is demonstrable by physical examination or by imaging. Many current investigators believe that idiopathic Bell's palsy has a viral etiology.

Typical Bell's palsy has a very characteristic clinical course, and many clinicians do not believe that imaging of these patients is warranted. The paralysis has a very rapid onset, often developing overnight or in a matter of hours, and does not progress. Almost all patients with Bell's palsy show some improvement within several weeks. The improvement can be partial with significant residual paralysis, or recovery can be complete. A second episode of paralysis is distinctly uncommon.

A tumor, such as facial nerve schwannoma (Option (A)), temporal bone hemangioma (Option (B)), or facial canal meningioma (Option (C)), should be suspected when there is a significant deviation from the typical clinical pattern of Bell's palsy. When this occurs, most of the patients are referred for imaging. If, as an example, there is a slowly progressive paralysis that continues to worsen over several days or weeks, a tumor should be suspected. Other situations that suggest a tumor are a failure to show any improvement, recurrent paralysis, or bilateral paralysis. Certainly some tumors present with a rapid-onset acute paralysis, but this is distinctly unusual. Even if the differing presentations are not taken into account, Bell's palsy is far more common than facial paralysis secondary to tumor **(Option (E) is correct)**.

Acute otitis media (Option (D)) can cause a facial nerve paralysis. However, in these patients the diagnosis of acute otitis media is obvious clinically. It is estimated that about 5% of facial nerve paralysis is caused by acute otitis media, and therefore it is a far less common cause of facial paralysis than is Bell's palsy.

## Question 64

Concerning the course of the facial nerve canal through the normal temporal bone,

  (A) the labyrinthine segment passes superior to the cochlea
  (B) the tympanic segment passes superior to the horizontal semicircular canal
  (C) the tympanic segment passes inferior to the oval window
  (D) the second or pyramidal turn is more posterior than the geniculate turn

The facial nerve exits the brain stem at the pontomedullary junction and then crosses the cerebellopontine angle cistern before entering the internal auditory canal (IAC). The nerve travels the length of the canal and then exits the IAC into the facial nerve canal (fallopian canal) at the anterosuperior position of the lateral limit of the IAC. From this point the nerve winds through the temporal bone (Figure 14-9), eventually

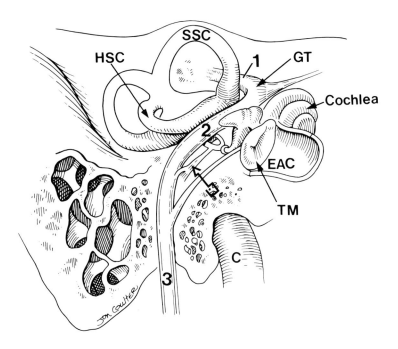

*Figure 14-9.* Diagram of the facial nerve. The labyrinthine segment (1) passes close to the cochlea and semicircular canals. This segment connects the IAC (not shown) with the geniculate area. The tympanic segment (2) extends along the medial wall of the middle ear. The mastoid or vertical segment (3) travels through the mastoid region to the stylomastoid foramen. The stapedial muscle (arrow) marks the position of the pyramidal process. C = carotid artery; EAC = external auditory canal; GT = geniculate turn; HSC and SSC = horizontal and superior semicircular canals; TM = tympanic membrane.

reaching the stylomastoid foramen, where it leaves the bone and then enters the parotid gland.

The facial nerve canal has three segments or regions. The first segment is called the labyrinthine segment because of its close relationship to the otic labyrinth. This segment passes from the IAC to the geniculate turn (often called the first genu) in the region of the geniculate ganglion. Here the canal is just anterior to the superior semicircular canal and just superior to the cochlea (Figures 14-9 and 14-10A) **(Option (A) is true).**

At the geniculate turn, the nerve makes a 90° bend and continues as the second or tympanic segment, so called because the nerve passes along the medial wall of the middle ear or tympanic cavity. This segment passes just inferior to the horizontal semicircular canal and close to the superior

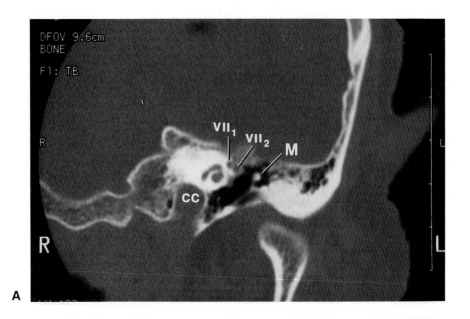

A

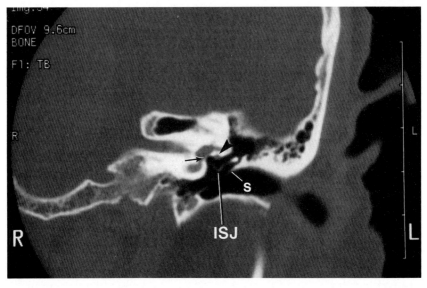

B

*Figure 14-10.* Facial nerve relationships. (A) Coronal bone-algorithm CT image through the temporal bone. The facial nerve canal is seen just above the cochlea. The labyrinthine segment (VII$_1$), tympanic segment (VII$_2$), carotid canal (cc), and malleus (M) are indicated. (B) A slightly posterior coronal scan shows the facial nerve (arrowhead) just inferior to the horizontal semicircular canal, oval window (arrow), incudostapedial joint (ISJ), and scutum (s).

edge of the oval window (Figure 14-10B) **(Options (B) and (C) are false)**.

At the posterior extreme of the tympanic segment of the facial nerve canal there is a second turn (or genu), which carries the nerve into the canal as the third or mastoid segment (vertical portion). This second turn, like the geniculate turn, is approximately 90° and has been called the pyramidal turn because of the proximity to the pyramidal eminence. The pyramidal eminence is the small point of bone from which the stapedius muscle emerges into the middle ear. The pyramidal turn is posterior to the geniculate turn **(Option (D) is true)**.

## Question 65

Concerning cholesteatoma,

    (A) the most common location is in the inferior tympanic cavity
    (B) the posterior semicircular canal is the most likely canal to be eroded
    (C) an automastoidectomy is the defect left when a cholesteatoma evacuates into the external canal
    (D) a normal scutum excludes this diagnosis
    (E) it usually has low signal intensity on T1-weighted MR images
    (F) the central portion enhances on MRI with gadolinium DTPA

Keratinous debris shed by the squamous epithelium of the external auditory canal (EAC) is usually eliminated from the canal. If squamous epithelium is trapped in the middle ear so that this keratinous debris cannot evacuate along normal pathways, a cholesteatoma will result. The cholesteatoma is simply a saclike collection of this keratinous debris. The wall will contain keratinizing squamous epithelium as well as some fibrous supporting structure. The cholesteatoma grows as more and more keratin is produced and trapped inside the closed sac.

There are many different classification systems used to categorize cholesteatomas. Most otologists separate these lesions into congenital and acquired types. Congenital cholesteatomas are thought to arise from embryonic epithelial rests and therefore can occur anywhere in the temporal bone. The usual simple description is that of a lesion behind an intact tympanic membrane.

Acquired cholesteatomas are associated with chronic middle ear disease and perforation or retraction of the tympanic membrane. A perforation allows migration of the EAC epithelium into the middle ear (Figure 14-11). Scarring and retraction of a part of the tympanic mem-

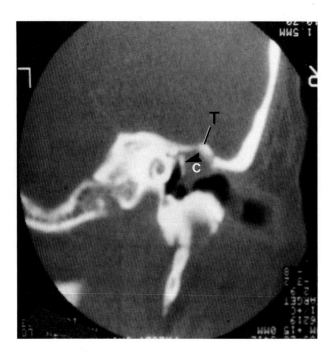

*Figure 14-11.* Cholesteatoma of the attic. Coronal CT scan shows a lesion (c) in the attic that displaces the malleus (arrowhead) medially. This lesion, having eroded the scutum, would be visible through the external auditory canal. T = tegmen tympani.

brane can actually pull this epithelium into the attic (the upper middle ear just lateral to the head of the malleus); the retraction pocket then closes off, trapping the epithelium and creating the cholesteatoma.

Most acquired cholesteatomas are found in the upper part of the tympanic membrane (pars flaccida) and contiguous attic of the upper middle ear cleft **(Option (A) is false).** The lower middle ear is an unusual location for a cholesteatoma.

As the cholesteatoma grows, bone is eroded as a result of at least two factors. First, the bone is under pressure from the mass, which enlarges as more keratin is produced. Second, the wall of the cholesteatoma may release enzymes that can potentiate this bone erosion. The bone most frequently eroded is the scutum (lateral attic spur), which is the junction line where the roof of the EAC meets the lateral wall of the attic of the middle ear. However, small cholesteatomas may not cause erosion and not all cholesteatomas arise in this location, so a normal scutum does not exclude the diagnosis of cholesteatoma **(Option (D) is false).** For instance, a cholesteatoma arising in the inferior part of the tympanic membrane or middle ear would not be expected to erode the scutum.

Although the scutum is the most frequently eroded structure, other sites can be affected and are often more clinically significant. The cholesteatoma can erode into the bony labyrinth; by itself, this may cause no symptoms relating to the labyrinth because the proceeds gradually with the cholesteatoma tamponading the hole in the bone, thereby protecting the vestibular system. However, even a small erosion can be very significant if the patient undergoes surgery. In removing the wall of the cholesteatoma, the surgeon can injure the membranous labyrinth and cause not only a deterioration in vestibular function, but also complete hearing loss. Therefore, the radiologist must carefully inspect the integrity of the bony walls of the semicircular canals. The horizontal or lateral semicircular canal forms part of the medial wall of the attic and is therefore the most likely semicircular canal to be eroded (Figure 14-12) **(Option (B) is false).** The posterior canal is almost never involved in this way.

A growing cholesteatoma can also erode other regions of the temporal bone. Superior extension of the mass involves the tegmen tympani (roof of the middle ear). This can lead to intracranial extension of either the cholesteatoma or a concurrent infection. If such a cholesteatoma is surgically removed, a postsurgical encephalocele can develop through the weakened or destroyed bone, with part of the inferior temporal lobe herniating into either the middle ear or the mastoid (Figure 14-13).

The early erosion of the scutum by a cholesteatoma can, with continued growth, progress to include more of the roof of the EAC. Occasionally, the membranous wall of the cholesteatoma will rupture into the EAC and the keratinous debris will drain spontaneously. Usually, by the time this happens, there has already been significant bone erosion in the mastoid region and the evacuated debris leaves a fairly large air-filled cavity, which represents the prior extent of the cholesteatoma. This defect is lined with keratinizing squamous epithelium. However, the desquamated keratinous debris is no longer trapped and can drain along the reestablished communication with the external auditory canal. This resulting defect does have some of the characteristics of a mastoidectomy cavity and so has been referred to as an automastoidectomy (Figure 14-14) **(Option (C) is true).** On imaging, the characteristic defect in the lateral wall of the mastoid seen as a result of the mastoidectomy approach is not present if the defect is a result of an automastoidectomy.

On CT, a cholesteatoma is visualized as abnormal soft tissue that replaces the air that usually fills the middle ear and mastoid cells. Bone

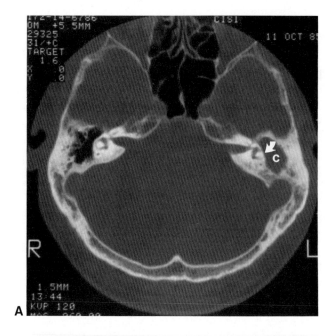

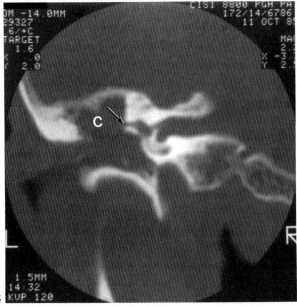

*Figure 14-12.* (A) Cholesteatoma with a fistula to the horizontal semi-circular canal. Axial CT scan shows the lesion in the attic and antrum (C). There is scalloping (arrow) of the outer bony wall of the horizontal semicircular canal, which has lost its smooth lateral curve and the thin white line of the otic capsule over its lateral aspect. Compare with the opposite side. (B) Coronal CT scan shows the lesion (C) filling the antrum and eroding the scutum. Compare to Figure 14-10B, where the scutum is indicated. The fistula is identified as a defect in the lateral cortical margin of the horizontal canal (arrow).

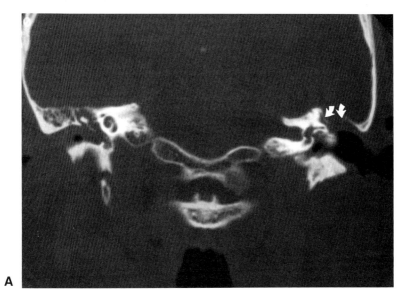

A

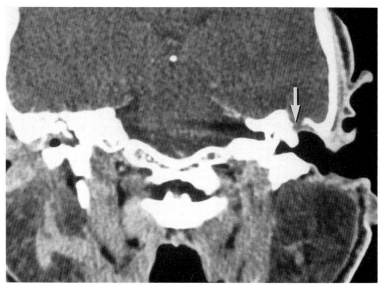

B

*Figure 14-13.* Postsurgical encephalocele. (A) Bone-algorithm coronal CT image shows a mastoidectomy defect on the left side. Small pieces of cortical bone (arrows) represent the fragments of the tegmen tympani, which has "fractured" down into the mastoidectomy defect. (B) Coronal soft-tissue-algorithm CT image shows that a small amount of the temporal lobe (arrow) protrudes into this defect. Characterization of this tissue and demonstration of the inferior surface of the temporal lobe would be easier by MRI, but the small cortical bones are better visualized by CT.

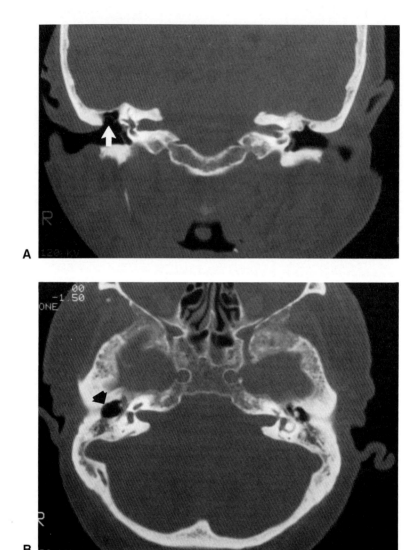

*Figure 14-14.* Automastoidectomy. (A) Coronal CT image shows a defect in the roof of the external auditory canal extending into the mastoid antrum (arrow). The ossicles are not present. The patient had not had surgery on that ear. This represents a cholesteatoma that had evacuated into the external auditory canal. (B) Axial CT image of the same patient shows a characteristic defect (arrow) with the rounded erosion and expansion of the attic. A cholesteatoma would have a similar appearance but would be filled with soft tissue density material.

SE 800/30

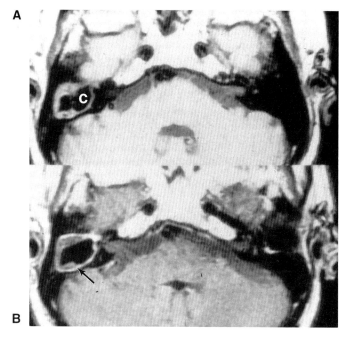

SE 800/30
Postcontrast

*Figure 14-15.* Cholesteatoma. (A) Axial T1-weighted MR image shows a cholesteatoma in the attic. The lesion (c) fills the attic and the antrum. Note the extremely low signal intensity of the central mass. (B) With injection of gadolinium DTPA, the wall and surrounding inflamed mucosa enhance (arrow) but the central portion of the lesion does not. (Courtesy of Mahmood F. Mafee, M.D., University of Illinois Hospital, Chicago.)

erosion is important in making the CT diagnosis of a cholesteatoma, because the presence of soft tissue filling the attic and middle ear is a nonspecific finding that can represent granulation tissue resulting from chronic inflammation or serous or mucoid secretions. Only when the typical bone erosion is present can the diagnosis confidently be made by CT.

Recently there has been some interest in the use of MRI in differentiating cholesteatoma from other inflammatory changes (Figure 14-15). The central part of a cholesteatoma usually has a fairly low signal intensity on T1-weighted sequences **(Option (E) is true).** However, this appearance does not consistently distinguish cholesteatoma from retained fluid secretions secondary to an obstruction, which may have a low signal intensity on T1-weighted sequences. Inflammatory tissues such as granulation tissues and inflamed mucosa enhance after gadolinium DTPA administration. Although the wall of a cholesteatoma may enhance, the keratin-filled central portion of the cyst is avascular and does not **(Option (F) is false).** Therefore, according to preliminary reports, MRI can help distinguish between cholesteatoma and other chronic middle ear inflammatory disease.

*Hugh D. Curtin, M.D.*

SUGGESTED READINGS

1. Bergeron RT, Lo WW, Swartz JD, et al. The temporal bone. In: Som PM, Bergeron RT (eds), Head and neck imaging. Chicago: Mosby-Year Book; 1991:925–1115
2. Chakeres DW, Kapila A. Normal and pathologic radiographic anatomy of the motor innervation of the face. AJNR 1984; 5:591–597
3. Curtin HD, Jensen JE, Barnes L Jr, May M. "Ossifying" hemangiomas of the temporal bone: evaluation with CT. Radiology 1987; 164:831–835
4. Lo WW, Horn KL, Carberry JN, et al. Intratemporal vascular tumors: evaluation with CT. Radiology 1986; 159:181–185
5. Mafee MF, Lachenauer CS, Kumar A, Arnold PM, Buckingham RA, Valvassori GE. CT and MR imaging of intralabyrinthine schwannoma: report of two cases and review of the literature. Radiology 1990; 174:395–400
6. May M. The facial nerve. New York: Thieme; 1986
7. Pulec JL. Facial nerve tumors. Ann Otol Rhinol Laryngol 1969; 78:962–982
8. Swartz JD, Harnsberger HR. The facial nerve. In: Swartz JD, Harnsberger HR (eds), Imaging of the temporal bone. New York: Thieme; 1992:268–297

*Notes*

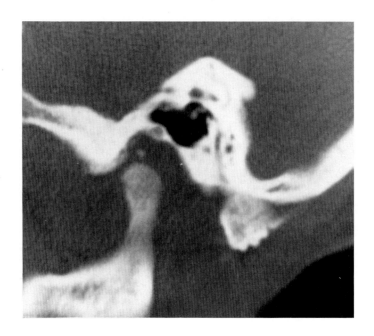

*Figure 15-1*

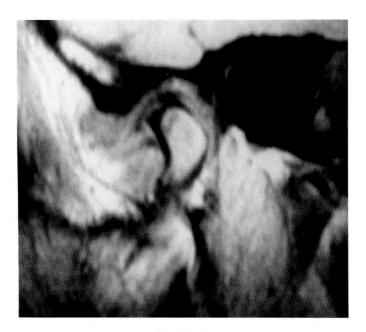

SE 800/20

*Figure 15-2*
*Figures 15-1 through 15-4.* This 53-year-old woman presented with pain referable to her left temporomandibular joint. You are shown a sagittal CT scan (Figure 15-1), a sagittal T1-weighted MR image (Figure 15-2), several coronal T1-weighted MR images (Figure 15-3), and a coronal T2-weighted MR image (Figure 15-4) of the left temporomandibular joint.

# Case 15: Temporomandibular Joint Synovial Chondromatosis

## Question 66

Which *one* of the following is the MOST likely diagnosis?

(A) Meniscal dislocation
(B) Synovial chondromatosis
(C) Septic arthritis
(D) Post-traumatic joint hemorrhage
(E) Rheumatoid arthritis

The direct sagittal CT scan (Figures 15-1 and 15-5) of the left temporomandibular joint (TMJ) shows widening of the joint, apparently by a soft tissue mass or joint effusion. Also apparent are an irregular cortical outline of the mandibular condyle, irregular calcifications along the inferior margin of the articular eminence, and calcifications within the joint space. There is erosion of the posterior aspect of the glenoid fossa. The sagittal T1-weighted MR scan (Figures 15-2 and 15-6) of the left TMJ shows moderate widening of the joint space (Figure 15-4). The articular disk is irregular, but its position is normal. There is an intra-articular hypointense area within the anterior joint space. This is due to the intra-articular calcification (loose body) seen in Figure 15-1. The coronal T1-weighted MR scans (Figures 15-3 and 15-7) of the left TMJ shows marked expansion of the joint capsule and a few hypointense areas in the superior joint space, consistent with intra-articular calcifications. The articular disk is seen as a hypointense curvilinear band. The coronal T2-weighted MR scan (Figures 15-4 and 15-8) of the left TMJ shows hyperintense fluid within the joint space and hypointense loose bodies. There is also expansion of the joint capsule as a result of a joint effusion.

The CT findings of calcifications within the joint space and along the inferior margin of the articular eminence are features suggestive of, but

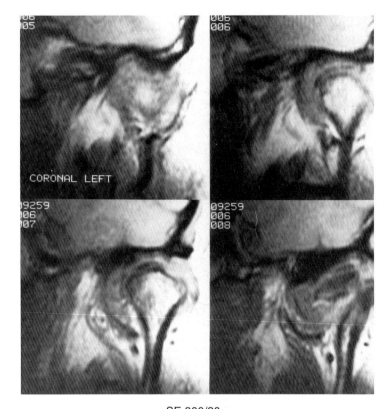

SE 800/20

*Figure 15-3*

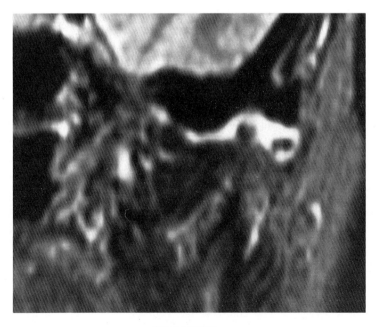

SE 2,000/80

*Figure 15-4*

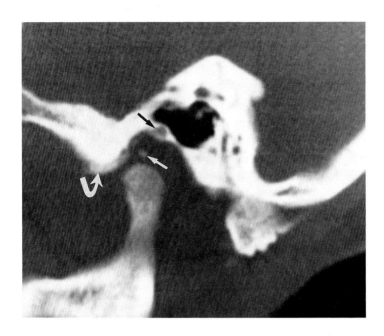

*Figure 15-5* (Same as Figure 15-1). This direct sagittal CT scan of the left TMJ, obtained with the mouth closed, shows widening of the TMJ. Note the lack of a sharp cortical outline of the mandibular condyle, irregular calcifications along the inferior margin of the articular eminence (curved arrow), and calcifications within the joint space (straight white arrow). There is erosion of the posterior aspect of the glenoid fossa (black arrow).

not specific for, synovial chondromatosis. The striking expansion of the TMJ capsule seen on the MR scans is known to be a common finding at surgery in patients with synovial chondromatosis. The loose cartilaginous or calcified bodies within the joint space, seen as hypointense areas on the MR scans, are consistently present within the joint in patients with synovial chondromatosis. Thus these CT and MR findings show the characteristic features of synovial chondromatosis **(Option (B) is correct).** The articular disk is shown to be irregular but in a normal position; this eliminates the possibility of meniscal dislocation (Option (A)). The irregularity of the disk is also consistent with the diagnosis of synovial chondromatosis.

Infectious (septic) arthritis (Option (C)) of the TMJ can arise as a hematogenous infection or by direct extension from an adjacent infection arising in the parotid gland or the ear. Expansion of the joint is related to accumulation of pus or inflammatory exudate. In the later stages of

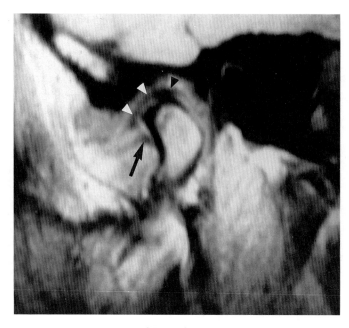

SE 800/20

*Figure 15-6* (Same as Figure 15-2). This sagittal T1-weighted MR scan of the left TMJ, obtained with the mouth closed, shows moderate widening of the joint. The articular disk (arrowheads) is irregular, but its position is normal. Note the intra-articular hypointense area (arrow) within the anterior joint space.

infection, dystrophic calcifications and fibrous or bony ankylosis may develop, leading to marked degenerative narrowing of the TMJ, with associated reactive sclerosis of the condyle and glenoid fossa. Depending on the severity of the infection, various degrees of disk destruction and osteomyelitis of the condyle may be present. Except for the intra-articular fluid collection and the expansion of the joint capsule, the CT and MR findings in the test patient are incompatible with septic arthritis.

Post-traumatic joint hemorrhage (Option (D)) represents the immediate intra-articular TMJ response to injury. The most common finding is an increase in the intra-articular space, which is seen as expansion of the joint capsule. In some instances an intracapsular or extracapsular fracture is present. The T2-weighted MR image (Figure 15-4) shows hyperintense joint fluid consistent with either exudate or subacute or old hemorrhage; however, the signal intensity of the joint fluid on the T1-weighted MR images (Figures 15-2 and 15-3) is inconsistent with subacute or chronic hemorrhage (methemoglobin).

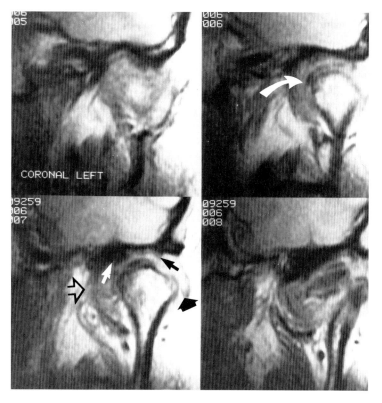

SE 800/20

*Figure 15-7* (Same as Figure 15-3). This series of coronal T1-weighted MR scans of the left TMJ, obtained with the mouth closed, shows marked expansion of the joint capsule (open arrow and wide black arrow) and a few areas of hypointensity in the superior joint space (small arrows). The articular disk is seen as a hypointense curvilinear band (curved arrow in the top right panel).

Rheumatoid arthritis (RA) (Option (E)) presents as a chronic inflammatory disease of the synovial tissues of the joints, including the TMJ. Initially there may not be any osseous changes; however, bone erosion of the condyle and glenoid fossa occurs later. The irregularity of the condyle and the bone erosion of the glenoid fossa in the test case are not inconsistent with chronic RA. However, joint exudate is less common than fibrosis in the late stages of RA. The clinical presentation, the lack of history of any other joint problems, and the CT and MR findings (Figures 15-1 through 15-4), along with the fact that about 50 to 80% of

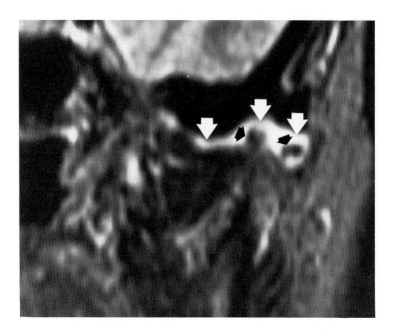

SE 2,000/80

*Figure 15-8* (Same as Figure 15-4). This coronal T2-weighted MR scan of the left TMJ, obtained with the mouth closed, shows hyperintense fluid within the joint space (white arrows) and hypointense loose bodies (black arrows). Note the expansion of the joint capsule as a result of joint effusion.

patients with RA show bilateral evidence of TMJ disease, make the diagnosis of RA unlikely.

The chief symptom in the test patient was progressively increasing pain in her left TMJ, which was exacerbated by function. This was associated with preauricular swelling. These symptoms are consistent with synovial chondromatosis.

## Discussion

The TMJ is subject to involvement by types of osteoarthritis similar to those that occur in other joints in the body. These include infectious arthritis, RA, degenerative arthritis, psoriatic arthritis, metabolic arthritis (gout and pseudogout), and traumatic arthritis. Synovial chondromatosis of the TMJ is a benign condition of unknown origin that can present

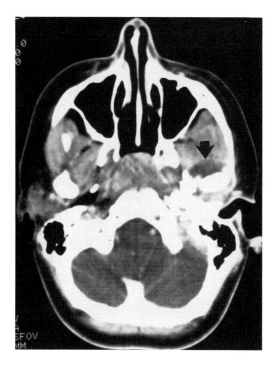

*Figure 15-9.* Acute septic (gonococcal) arthritis of the left TMJ. Axial CT scan shows fluid collection (pus) in the left TMJ (arrow).

with symptoms and signs similar to those of acute or chronic TMJ arthritis.

*Infectious arthritis.* The TMJ may be involved as part of a systemic infection such as staphylococcal or streptococcal septicemia, gonorrhea, tuberculosis, syphilis, or one of the mycoses. A more common cause of TMJ infection is direct extension from an adjacent infection, e.g., of parotid, otic, or dental origin. Infection may also arise consequent to penetrating injury of the TMJ and as a complication of arthroscopy or other surgical procedures of the TMJ (e.g., infection of a prosthetic TMJ). The onset of septic arthritis is usually accompanied by chills, fever, and sweating. This is followed by redness, swelling, and tenderness in the region of the joint, leading to accumulation of pus and inflammatory exudate within the joint capsule (Figures 15-9 and 15-10) and to limitation of movement. Later, depending on the severity of the infection, various degrees of destruction, ranging from partial to complete damage of the articular disk to osteomyelitis of the condyle and glenoid fossa, may develop. In the late stages of infection, fibrosis and dystrophic

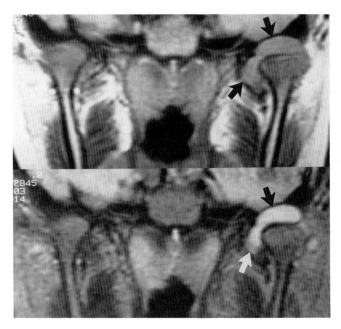

SE 2,000/80

*Figure 15-10.* Same patient as in Figure 15-9. Acute septic (gonococcal) arthritis of the left TMJ. Proton-density (top) and T2-weighted (bottom) MR scans show expansion of the superior and medial portion of the left TMJ (arrows) owing to fluid collection (pus and inflammatory exudate).

calcifications occur, leading to fibrous or bony ankylosis. In children, the disease may affect the growth potential of the condyle, which in turn may lead to facial asymmetry and malocclusion. The rapid development of TMJ ankylosis (Figure 15-11) requires that treatment begin as soon as the first signs of acute infectious arthritis appear.

The findings on conventional radiographs in the early stage (days 7 through 10) of septic arthritis are ordinarily insignificant owing to a lack of osseous involvement. However, the intra-articular collection of pus or inflammatory exudate can be easily seen by CT and, especially, MRI (Figures 15-9 and 15-10). In the later stages, when bone rarefaction and erosion occur, CT may be superior to MRI in delineating changes within the soft and hard tissues of the joint. Both CT and MRI are extremely useful in delineating any adjacent infection of the ear, parotid gland, masticatory space, or parapharyngeal space. Necrotizing external otitis is a condition predominantly of elderly, poorly controlled diabetic patients and is usually caused by *Pseudomonas aeruginosa*. The infection may

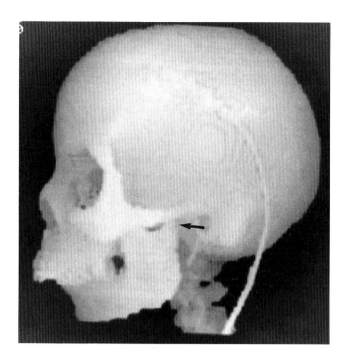

*Figure 15-11.* TMJ ankylosis following neonatal meningitis and presumed TMJ infection. Three-dimensional CT image shows deformity of the left mandibular condyle (arrow) and absence of the normal condyle-fossa relationship as a result of ankylosis. The patient has a ventriculo-peritoneal shunt.

spread along several routes: directly via bony erosion into the adjacent mastoid air cells and middle ear; anteriorly into the parotid gland, masticatory space, and TMJ; and inferiorly into the soft tissues of the parapharyngeal space and the infratemporal fossa. In this condition, involvement of the TMJ and adjacent soft tissue structures is best evaluated by MRI. On the other hand, bone erosions and sequestra due to osteomyelitis are best evaluated by high-resolution CT.

*Degenerative arthritis (osteoarthritis).* Degenerative arthritis of the TMJ may be primary or secondary in origin. Primary degenerative osteoarthritis is caused by the normal joint wear and tear associated with aging, and it usually begins in the fifth decade. Secondary degenerative arthritis of the TMJ is often seen in 20- to 40-year-old patients and is frequently caused by acute trauma. However, it can also be a sequela of chronic myofascial pain dysfunction (MPD) syndrome. This MPD syndrome, the most common disorder of the TMJ, is characterized by facial

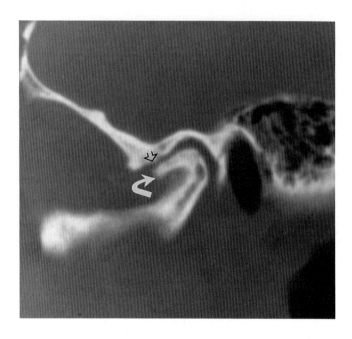

*Figure 15-12.* Degenerative arthritis of the TMJ. Direct sagittal CT scan shows flattening of the mandibular condyle, anterior lipping (curved arrow), and deformity, as well as flattening of the articular eminence (open arrow).

pain and mandibular dysfunction. The pain is often localized in the ear or jaw, and the mandibular dysfunction is manifested by limitation of movement. It is thought that such patients have increased musculature tension and hyperexcitable reflexes related to emotional tension. There is also associated pain and tenderness in some of the muscles of mastication and occasionally in the muscles of the neck and shoulder.

Facial pain and limited ability to open the jaw without evidence of TMJ disease may also be associated with infections, such as Lyme disease, and with malignant tumors. CT is the modality of choice to delineate features of degenerative arthritis of the TMJ. The earliest CT finding is subchondral sclerosis of the condyle or glenoid fossa or both. If the condition progresses, condylar flattening and marginal lipping may be noted (Figure 15-12). In the later stages, there may be erosion of the cortical plate or osteophyte formation (Figure 15-13). There may also be formation of degenerative subcortical bone cysts (Figure 15-13) and internal derangement of the articular disk. Narrowing of the joint space usually indicates degenerative changes in the articular disk. MRI is the

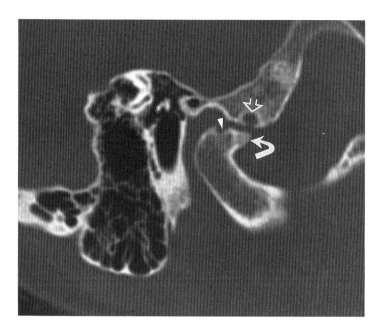

*Figure 15-13.* Degenerative arthritis of the TMJ. Direct sagittal CT scan shows subcortical erosion of the mandibular condyle (arrowhead), marginal osteophyte (curved arrow), and subcortical cyst formation (open arrow) involving the anterior articular eminence.

modality of choice to show various degrees of internal derangement of the articular disk (Figures 15-14 through 15-16).

*Traumatic arthritis.* Traumatic arthritis represents the intra-articular response to injury of the TMJ. The resultant inflammation and occasional hemarthrosis result in pain, joint tenderness, and limitation of jaw movement. At this stage CT is the modality of choice to evaluate the TMJ, since there may be an intracapsular fracture present. A hemarthrosis of the TMJ is seen on CT as an increased size of the joint space. The density of the blood may not be higher than the density of the periarticular soft tissues or the density of the adjacent muscles. MRI is more specific in detecting hemarthrosis (acute or chronic). In patients with severe TMJ trauma, degenerative arthritis may eventually occur. The CT findings of degenerative arthritis vary with the severity of the process. The common findings include narrowing of the joint and subchondral sclerosis of the condyle and glenoid fossa, and there may be fibrous or bony ankylosis of the TMJ (Figure 15-17).

*Rheumatoid arthritis.* RA is a chronic systemic disease of unknown etiology, manifested primarily by inflammatory arthritis of the periph-

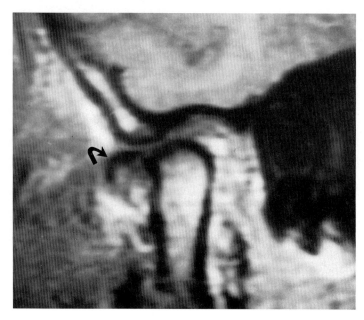

SE 600/20

*Figure 15-14.* Internal derangement and nonreduced disk dislocation. Sagittal T1-weighted MR scan, obtained with the mouth open, shows a deformed, anteriorly displaced meniscus (arrow).

eral joints. The serum and joint fluid of the majority of patients with RA contain antibodies specific for immunoglobulin G (IgG; rheumatoid factor). As many as 50 to 80% of patients with RA show some involvement of the TMJ. TMJ involvement may interfere with mastication, and in children the disease may lead to malocclusion. The TMJs are swollen and painful, and the pain may be referred to the middle ear and throat. Juvenile RA differs from the disease in adults by the more frequent occurrence of systemic manifestations, by more frequent monoarticular joint involvement, and by the infrequent occurrence of typical rheumatoid factor and rheumatoid nodules. Generalized lymphadenopathy, splenomegaly, and hepatomegaly are often present. The name "Still's disease" is sometimes used for juvenile RA when the arthritis is polyarticular and occurs in combination with adenopathy, splenomegaly, and hepatomegaly. Involvement of TMJs may produce micrognathia because of destruction of the condyle, leading to impaired mandibular growth. Fibrous or bony ankylosis is a sequela at all ages. Radiographic findings of TMJ involvement in patients with RA depend on the stage of the

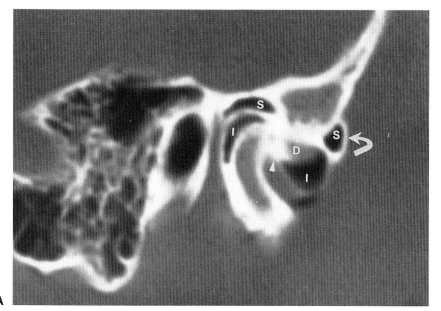

A

B

SE 1,000/75

*Figure 15-15.* Anterior dislocation of the left TMJ disk. (A) Double-contrast CT arthrogram, obtained with the mouth closed, shows anteriorly displaced disk (D). Air is present in the superior (S) and inferior (I) joint spaces. Note the presence of iodinated contrast (arrowhead) in the inferior joint space and along the anterior joint capsule (curved arrow). (B) Sagittal T1-weighted MR scan, obtained with the mouth closed, shows anterior displacement of the disk (arrows).

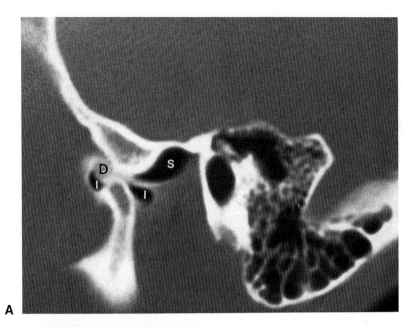

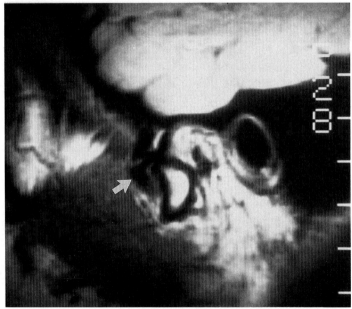

SE 1,500/25

*Figure 15-16.* Anterior displacement of the right TMJ disk without reduction. (A) Double-contrast CT arthrogram, obtained with the mouth
open, shows anteriorly displaced disk (D). Air is present in the superior
(S) and inferior (I) joint spaces. (B) Sagittal proton-density MR scan, obtained with the mouth open, shows a deformed, anteriorly displaced disk
(arrow).

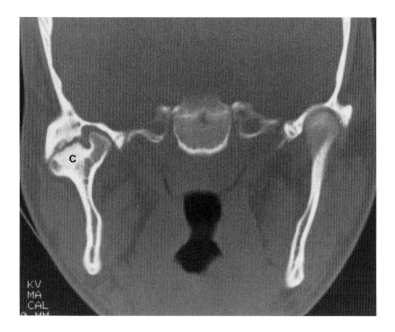

*Figure 15-17.* Post-traumatic ankylosis of the right TMJ. Coronal CT scan shows deformity of the right condyle (c) and glenoid fossa, as well as pseudoarthrosis. There is marked subchondral sclerosis involving the mandibular condyle and temporal bone of the glenoid fossa.

disease. Initially, there may not be any osseous changes to be detected by standard radiographs or CT scans. As the process progresses, however, there is bilateral evidence of loss of bone density (demineralization), condylar irregularity and flattening, and erosion. Erosion of the glenoid fossa may also be present. Intra-articular calcification is infrequent.

*Synovial chondromatosis.* Synovial chondromatosis is a rare, benign joint disorder characterized by metaplasia of the synovium with the formation of numerous foci of cellular hyaline cartilage. These foci may detach from the synovium and become loose bodies within the joint space, and they may also calcify. The disease is usually monoarticular, is of unknown origin, and occurs most often in larger joints such as the knee, shoulder, and hip. Synovial chondromatosis of the TMJ was first described by Axhausen in 1933, and it has been reported to occur in individuals ranging from age 18 to 75 years, with a mean age of 46 years. There is a predilection for women. It is a benign disease, although chondrosarcoma has been reported to develop in association with synovial chondromatosis. Such cases probably represent a primary tumor. None

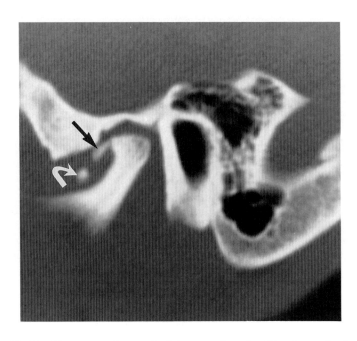

*Figure 15-18.* Degenerative arthritis associated with a loose body. Direct sagittal CT scan shows flattening of the mandibular condyle and glenoid fossa, anterior marginal osteophyte (black arrow), and an intra-articular calcification (loose body) (white arrow).

of these cases involved the TMJ. The clinical findings of synovial chondromatosis of the TMJ include pain, restriction of mandibular movement, and, often, preauricular swelling. Radiographic findings of synovial chondromatosis of the TMJ include widening of the joint space, the presence of calcified loose bodies, and erosive and sclerotic changes in the condyle and condylar fossa (Figure 15-5). These findings are not specific for synovial chondromatosis; all or some of them may be seen in patients with degenerative arthritis (Figure 15-18). Radioopaque loose bodies in the TMJ are not pathognomonic for synovial chondromatosis and can be found in patients with other disorders, such as degenerative arthritis (Figure 15-18), osteochondritis dissecans, condylar fracture, tuberculous arthritis, RA, and neuropathic arthropathy. CT has been helpful in the diagnosis of synovial chondromatosis, because it identifies intra-articular as well as extra-articular calcifications that are not seen on conventional radiography (Figure 15-5). Erosion and sclerosis of the condyle and glenoid fossa can best be evaluated on direct sagittal CT scans. Expansion of the joint capsule and the presence of a large volume of fluid within the joint cavity are common findings in patients with synovial chondromatosis, and these findings are better delineated by MRI than by CT (Figures 15-7 and 15-8). The presence of fluid within the joint space can be confirmed by gradient-echo images (Figure 15-19). In a patient with unilateral TMJ pain associated with preauricular swelling, the CT and MR findings of loose bodies, expansion of the joint capsule, erosion of the condyle and glenoid fossa, and the presence of intra-articular effusion are highly suggestive of synovial chondromatosis.

Craniofacial disorders may cause various and seemingly unrelated clinical manifestations that mimic TMJ disorders, leading to misdiagnosis and ineffective treatment planning. It is thus imperative for the clinician to obtain a thorough history and to perform the most appropriate diagnostic tests, including imaging studies. CT and MRI can provide exceedingly valuable information in evaluating TMJ diseases and other craniofacial disorders that may present as TMJ pain and dysfunction. For example, negative CT and MR studies of the TMJ in a patient who presented with intractable facial pain or what appears to be a case of TMJ MPD syndrome that does not respond to therapy should raise the question of Lyme disease. The patient should be tested for Lyme borreliosis even though not all patients with active Lyme disease produce antibodies.

*Mahmood F. Mafee, M.D.*

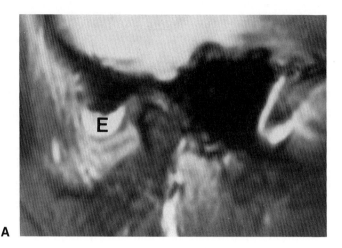

GRE 27/14/60°

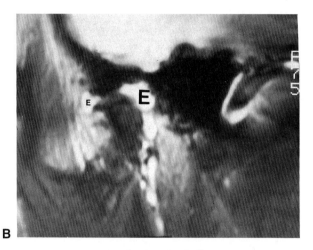

GRE 27/14/60°

*Figure 15-19.* Synovial chondromatosis of the left TMJ. (A) Gradient-echo sagittal MR scan of the left TMJ, obtained with the mouth closed, shows hyperintense effusion (E) in the anterior joint space. (B) Gradient-echo sagittal MR scan of the left TMJ, obtained with the mouth open, shows hyperintense effusion (E) in the anterior and posterior joint spaces. (C) Gradient-echo sagittal MR scan of the right TMJ shows a normal right TMJ with no evidence of effusion in the right joint.

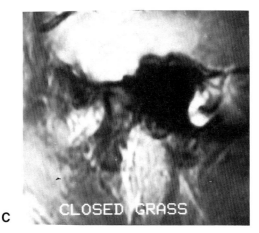

C

GRE 27/14/60°

*SUGGESTED READINGS*

SYNOVIAL CHONDROMATOSIS

1. Blenkinsopp PT. Loose bodies of the temporo-mandibular joint, synovial chondromatosis or osteoarthritis. Br J Oral Surg 1978; 16:12–20
2. Hamilton A, Davis RI, Hayes D, Mollan RA. Chondrosarcoma developing in synovial chondromatosis. A case report. J Bone Joint Surg (Br) 1987; 69:137–140
3. Herzog S, Mafee M. Synovial chondromatosis of the TMJ: MR and CT finding. AJNR 1990; 11:742–745
4. Nokes SR, King PS, Garcia R Jr, Silbiger ML. Jones JD III, Castellano ND. Temporomandibular joint chondromatosis with intracranial extension: MR and CT contributions. AJR 1987; 148:1173–1174

SEPTIC ARTHRITIS

5. Bounds GA, Hopkins R, Sugar A. Septic arthritis of the temporo-mandibular joint—a problematic diagnosis. Br J Oral Maxillofac Surg 1987; 25:61–67
6. Wurman LH, Flannery JV Jr, Sack JG. Osteomyelitis of the mandibular condyle secondary to dental extractions. Otolaryngol Head Neck Surg 1979; 87:190–198

OTHER TMJ DISORDERS

7. Larheim TA, Kolbenstvedt A. Osseous temporomandibular joint abnormalities in rheumatic disease. Computed tomography versus hypocycloidal tomography. Acta Radiol 1990; 31:383–387
8. Laskin DM. Diagnosis of pathology of the temporomandibular joint: clinical and imaging perspectives. Radiol Clin North Am 1993 (in press)

9. Cohen SG, Quinn PD. Facial trismus and myofascial pain associated with infections and malignant disease. Report of five cases. Oral Surg Oral Med Oral Pathol 1988; 65:538–544

10. Lader E. Lyme disease misdiagnosed as a temporomandibular joint disorder. J Prosthet Dent 1990; 63:82–85

*Notes*

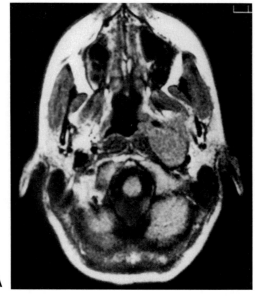

SE 700/25

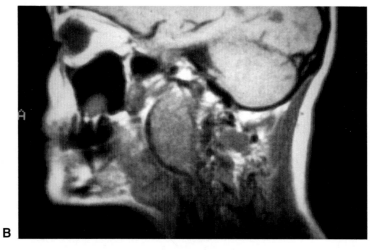

SE 550/20

*Figure 16-1.* This 56-year-old man presented with dysphagia. You are shown T1-weighted axial (A) and sagittal (B) MR images.

# Case 16: Parapharyngeal Space Schwannoma

## Question 67

Which *one* of the following is the MOST likely diagnosis?

(A) Glomus vagale tumor
(B) Schwannoma
(C) Minor salivary gland tumor
(D) Deep-lobe parotid tumor
(E) Carotid aneurysm

The T1-weighted axial (Figure 16-1A) and sagittal (Figure 16-1B) MR images show an ovoid mass (ca. 4 by 3 cm) of fairly homogeneous low to intermediate signal intensity. Overall, the mass is fairly clearly delineated from the adjacent soft tissues, and thus the lesion should not be considered infiltrative.

In the axial plane, a zone of high-intensity fat separates the posterolateral margin of the mass from the parotid gland (Figure 16-2A, small arrow) and the internal carotid artery is seen as an ovoid signal void along the anterior margin of the lesion. This artery is also seen draped anteriorly over the mass on the sagittal scan. This constellation of findings makes schwannoma the most likely diagnosis **(Option (B) is correct)**.

The vast majority of the schwannomas that arise in the parapharyngeal space develop in the vagus nerve. Since the vagus nerve lies posterior to the internal carotid artery, these schwannomas tend to displace this artery anteriorly (Figure 16-2A, white arrow; Figure 16-2B, open arrow). The schwannomas are ovoid masses that usually have low to intermediate signal intensity on T1-weighted images and slightly higher signal intensity on T2-weighted images. Areas of necrosis and hemorrhage can occur within these tumors. The sites of necrosis have low signal intensity on T1-weighted images and high signal intensity on T2-weighted images. Areas of hemorrhage usually have high signal intensity on both T1- and

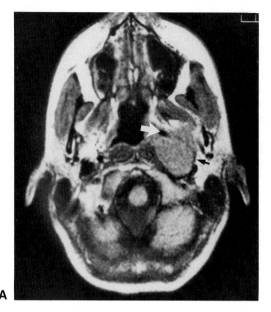

SE 700/25

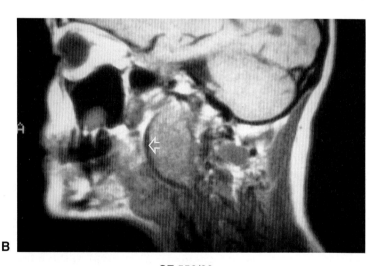

SE 550/20

*Figure 16-2* (Same as Figure 16-1). Parapharyngeal space schwannoma.
(A) Axial T1-weighted MR scan showing an ovoid mass in the left parapharyngeal space. The mass has a fairly homogeneous low to intermediate signal intensity and is fairly well delineated from the adjacent soft
tissues. There is anterior displacement of the left internal carotid artery
(white arrow) and a thin zone of fat (small arrow) separating the mass
from the parotid gland. (B) Sagittal T1-weighted MR scan showing the
same left parapharyngeal space mass. The anterior displacement of the
internal carotid artery is clearly seen (open arrow).

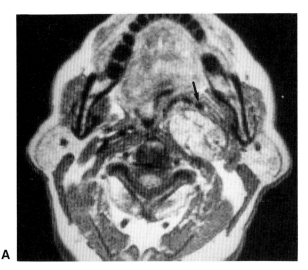

A

SE 1,800/30

*Figure 16-3.* Glomus vagale tumor. Axial proton-density (A) and T2-weighted (B) MR scans showing an ovoid left parapharyngeal space mass that is separate from the parotid gland and well delineated from the adjacent soft tissues. The carotid arteries are anteriorly displaced (arrow in panel A), and there are serpiginous flow voids within the mass. On the T2-weighted image, the lesion has a "salt-and-pepper" appearance.

T2-weighted images owing to the presence of methemoglobin. Such areas, if present, give a heterogeneous MR appearance to these schwannomas. The tumors are separated from the deep portion of the parotid gland by a zone of parapharyngeal space fat.

Glomus vagale tumors (Option (A)) arise from paraganglionic cells around the nodose (lower) ganglion of the vagus nerve. As a result of this, they develop posterior to the internal carotid artery and thus also tend to displace this artery anteriorly. They are ovoid masses with sharply defined margins and are separated from the deep portion of the parotid gland by a zone of parapharyngeal space fat. However, once these tumors are larger than 1 to 1.5 cm in greatest diameter, their tumor vessels are large enough to be seen on MR images as areas of circular, ovoid, or serpiginous regions of signal void. In addition, these tumors have a salt-and-pepper appearance on T2-weighted images as a result of flow voids and areas of slowly flowing blood (Figure 16-3). No such signal voids are seen in the fairly sizable mass in the test images.

Minor salivary gland tumors in the parapharyngeal space (Option (C)) arise from salivary rest cells in the fat of the parapharyngeal space. This

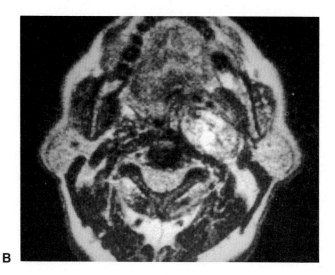

B

fat lies anterior to the carotid sheath structures; thus, these tumors tend to displace the internal carotid artery posteriorly, unlike the anterior displacement in the test images. These tumors are ovoid masses with low to intermediate signal intensity on T1-weighted images and higher signal intensity on T2-weighted images. They also have clearly defined borders and are separated from the deep portion of the parotid gland by a zone of parapharyngeal space fat (Figure 16-4).

Deep-lobe parotid tumors (Option (D)) arise from the parotid gland, and thus no zone of parapharyngeal space fat (as is seen in the test images) is seen between the mass and the parotid gland. In addition, the deep portion of the parotid gland lies in the stylomandibular tunnel, which is delimited anteriorly by the back of the ramus of the mandible, superiorly by the undersurface of the skull base, and posteriorly by the styloid process and the stylomandibular ligament. The carotid sheath structures are posterior to the styloid process, and as a result, the deep portion of the parotid gland lies anterior to the internal carotid artery. Therefore, tumors of the deep portion of the parotid gland tend to displace the internal carotid artery posteriorly, unlike the situation in the test images. The tumors have clearly defined margins with the parapharyngeal space and its surrounding structures. The MR signal intensities are similar to those of schwannomas (Figure 16-5).

Since the carotid artery is clearly seen as a separate structure along the anterior margin of the mass in the test images, it is unlikely that a carotid aneurysm (Option (E)) is present. An aneurysm usually shows

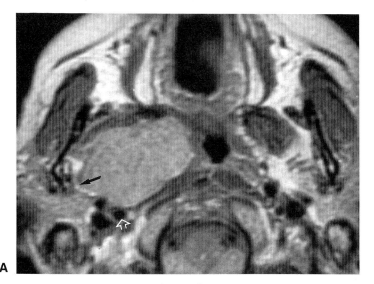

SE 716/20

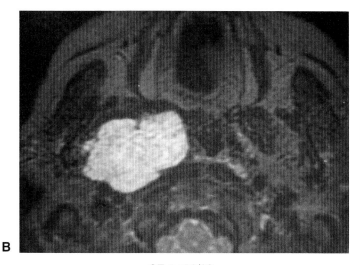

SE 2,500/80

*Figure 16-4.* Extraparotid pleomorphic adenoma. Axial T1-weighted (A) and T2-weighted (B) MR scans showing a well-delineated right parapharyngeal space mass that has a low to intermediate signal intensity on T1-weighted images and a high signal intensity on T2-weighted images. The mass is anterior to the internal carotid artery (open arrow), and there is a fat plane (black arrow) between the lesion and the parotid gland. The slightly scalloped contour in this large tumor is a fairly characteristic finding.

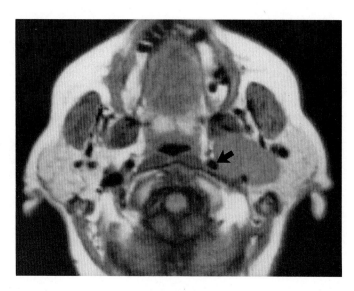

SE 500/20

*Figure 16-5.* Parotid pleomorphic adenoma. Axial T1-weighted MR scan showing an ovoid mass in the deep portion of the left parotid gland. There is no fat plane between the mass and the parotid gland, and the lesion is anterior to the internal carotid artery (arrow). The parapharyngeal space fat is clearly identified along the medial margin of the mass.

evidence of continuity with the internal carotid artery at either the cranial or caudal margin of the aneurysm. No such relationship is seen in the test images. Areas of signal void (Figure 16-6) or variably higher signal intensity are seen on T1-weighted images, reflecting the variable flow or presence of thrombus within the aneurysm. This is not consistent with the MR appearance of the mass in the test images.

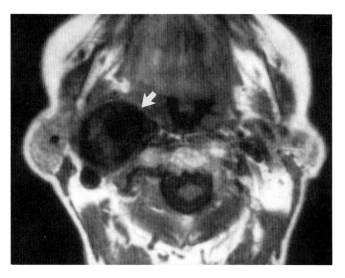

SE 600/27

*Figure 16-6.* Carotid aneurysm. Axial T1-weighted MR scan showing an ovoid mass in the right parapharyngeal space region (arrow). The mass has low, heterogeneous signal intensity, and the internal carotid artery cannot be identified.

## Question 68

Concerning schwannomas of the parapharyngeal space,

(A) they usually arise in the third division of the trigeminal nerve
(B) they usually displace the internal carotid artery posteriorly
(C) they are hypovascular lesions
(D) they usually develop in the prestyloid compartment
(E) they often contain scattered calcification

Most schwannomas that arise in the parapharyngeal space develop from the vagus nerve **(Option (A) is false).** The next most common nerve of origin is the superior sympathetic plexus. In theory, such schwannomas could arise from any minor nerve branch; however, the vagus and superior sympathetic plexus are the nerves of origin for virtually all such reported cases. The mandibular nerve or third division of the trigeminal nerve actually lies in the masticator space and not in the parapharyngeal space.

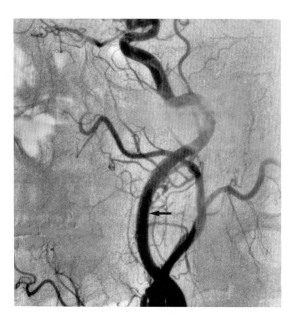

*Figure 16-7.* Schwannoma. Right lateral subtraction angiogram showing anterior displacement of the internal carotid artery (arrow) by a hypovascular mass. This is the typical angiographic appearance of a schwannoma.

Because the vagus nerve and the superior sympathetic plexus both lie posterior to the internal carotid artery, tumors that arise in these nerves tend to displace this artery anteriorly, if at all **(Option (B) is false).**

Schwannomas are hypovascular lesions, as demonstrated on angiography (Figure 16-7), and no vascular flow voids are seen on MR studies **(Option (C) is true).** These tumors can, however, enhance on postcontrast CT scans (Figure 16-8) and on contrast MR examinations. The reason appears to be that the contrast agent leaks into the tumor matrix through the few (but abnormal) tumor vessels. Since schwannomas are hypovascular lesions, there is no good venous system to remove any contrast material that has leaked into the tumor. As a result, the relative contrast agent concentration can transiently increase in these lesions, and they can appear as enhancing "vascular" masses on sectional imaging. However, dynamic scanning and angiography will demonstrate the hypovascular nature of these lesions and the slow buildup and slow elimination of the contrast agent within the tumor. By comparison, a vascular tumor shows rapid accumulation and rapid elimination of contrast material on both dynamic scans and angiography (Figure 16-9).

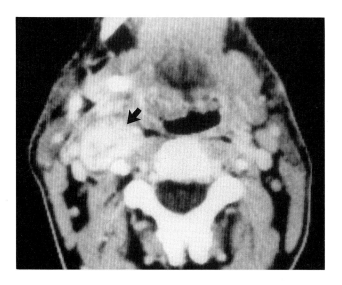

*Figure 16-8.* Schwannoma. Axial postcontrast CT scan showing an enhancing right parapharyngeal space mass (arrow). On the basis of this CT scan, one might conclude that this mass should be vascular in origin. However, this is a hypovascular schwannoma that demonstrates extravascular accumulation of contrast agent within the tumor.

These schwannomas, as mentioned above, arise almost exclusively from the vagus nerve or branches of the superior sympathetic trunk, both of which are directly related to the carotid sheath. The vagus nerve lies within this sheath, posterior to the internal carotid artery and the internal jugular vein. The superior sympathetic trunk lies along the medial margin of the carotid sheath. The primary anatomic divisions of the parapharyngeal space are the prestyloid and retrostyloid compartments. The retrostyloid compartment is essentially the carotid sheath and its related nerves and vessels. The prestyloid compartment is filled with fat and is the area into which the deep portion of the parotid gland extends. Thus, schwannomas usually develop in the retrostyloid compartment and not the prestyloid compartment **(Option (D) is false).**

Dystrophic calcifications usually do not occur within schwannomas **(Option (E) is false),** although in rare cases one or two calcifications are seen on CT scans.

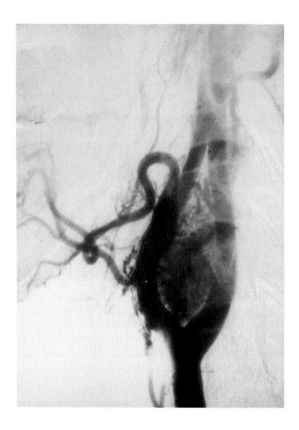

*Figure 16-9.* Vascular carotid body tumor. Right lateral subtraction angiogram showing a vascular mass in the carotid bifurcation. This carotid body tumor also enhances intensely on CT, so that a contrast CT scan would appear similar to Figure 16-8, although this angiogram is quite different from Figure 16-7.

## Question 69

Concerning extraparotid salivary gland tumors of the parapharyngeal space,

    (A) they usually arise in salivary rest tissue
    (B) they usually develop in the prestyloid compartment
    (C) they usually are benign mixed tumors
    (D) MRI usually shows a fat plane separating the tumor from the parotid gland

    Extraparotid salivary gland tumors of the parapharyngeal space have been shown to arise in salivary rest tissue within the fat that fills the parapharyngeal space **(Option (A) is true).** These salivary rests lie along the embryologic course of the ascent of the parotid gland and are completely separate from the parotid gland.

The salivary rest tissue lies in the anterior or prestyloid compartment of the parapharyngeal space. The retrostyloid compartment of the parapharyngeal space is essentially the carotid sheath structures. Tumors that arise in these salivary rests also lie in the prestyloid compartment **(Option (B) is true)** and are anterior to the carotid sheath and the internal carotid artery.

Almost all of the extraparotid salivary gland tumors that arise in the parapharyngeal space are benign mixed tumors (pleomorphic adenomas) **(Option (C) is true).** Malignant tumors in such extraparotid lesions are rare. The very high relative incidence of benign tumors is similar to that in the parotid gland; considering the embryologic origin of these salivary rests, this is not surprising.

On sectional imaging the characteristic finding that differentiates a deep-lobe parotid tumor from an extraparotid salivary gland tumor of the parapharyngeal space is the presence in the latter case of a zone of parapharyngeal space fat between the posterolateral margin of the tumor and the parotid gland **(Option (D) is true).** If this plane of fat is identified on all scans through the tumor, the lesion cannot arise in the parotid gland and therefore must be extraparotid in origin. If the fat plane is not seen on all scans through the mass, the lesion must be considered to arise from the parotid deep lobe (Figure 16-10). Although this fat can be seen on CT scans, it is much more clearly identified on T1-weighted and proton density MR scans.

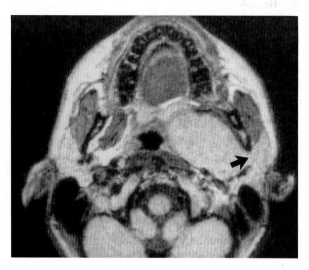

SE 2,500/27

*Figure 16-10.* Deep-lobe parotid pleomorphic adenoma. Axial proton-density MR scan showing a large left parapharyngeal space mass that is attached to the parotid gland by a narrow isthmus of tissue (arrow). This connection was not seen on CT and emphasizes why MRI is the modality of choice in such cases.

## Question 70

Concerning deep-lobe parotid tumors,

    (A)  they frequently extend into the prestyloid compartment
    (B)  they usually are malignant mixed tumors
    (C)  if dumbbell shaped, they extend through the stylomandibular tunnel
    (D)  they often have calcifications along their periphery

    Classically, the deep lobe refers to the portion of the parotid gland that lies deep (medial) to the plane of the facial nerve. However, from a practical point of view, the deep lobe refers to the portion of the parotid gland that is behind and deep to the ramus of the mandible. This small portion of the parotid gland represents about 20% of the volume of the gland and extends behind the mandibular ramus through the stylomandibular tunnel. This triangular space is defined anteriorly by the posterior edge of the ramus of the mandible, superiorly by the undersurface of the skull, and posteriorly by the styloid process and the stylomandibular ligament.

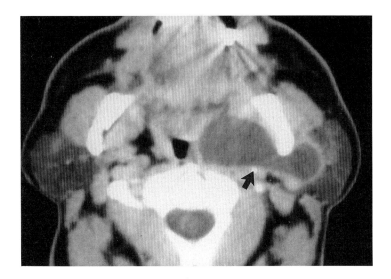

*Figure 16-11.* Deep-lobe parotid branchial cleft cyst. Axial CT scan showing a cystic mass in the left parapharyngeal space and parotid deep lobe. The mass extends through the stylomandibular tunnel. The styloid process is clearly seen (arrow). The dumbbell shape of this branchial cleft cyst also occurs with solid tumors that extend through and are constricted by the stylomandibular tunnel.

The stylomandibular tunnel anatomically brings the parotid deep lobe into the anterior or prestyloid compartment of the parapharyngeal space, and therefore tumors arising in the parotid deep lobe extend into the prestyloid compartment of the parapharyngeal space **(Option (A) is true).** Accordingly, these tumors lie anterior to the carotid sheath structures. Thus, both parotid deep-lobe tumors and extraparotid parapharyngeal space salivary gland tumors usually displace the internal carotid artery posteriorly.

Most parotid tumors are benign, and although there is a slight increase in the ratio of malignant to benign tumors when lesions in the deep portion of the parotid gland are compared with those arising in the superficial portion of the gland, the vast majority (ca. 80%) of these lesions are benign **(Option (B) is false).**

The stylomandibular tunnel is a rigid ring that resists expansion or remodeling by tumors. As a result, a parotid neoplasm that extends through the tunnel tends to be constricted at the level of the stylomandibular tunnel and hence has a dumbbell shape **(Option (C) is true),** with expanded areas of the tumor lying external (lateral) and internal (medial) to the plane of the tunnel (Figure 16-11).

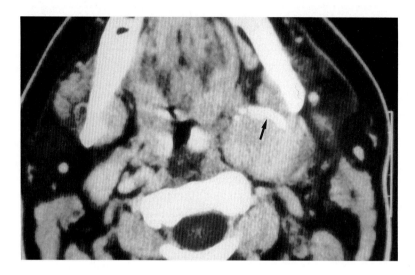

*Figure 16-12.* Axial CT scan showing a left parapharyngeal space mass with a curvilinear peripheral calcification (arrow). This appearance is highly suggestive of an aneurysm.

Calcifications in salivary gland tumors are uncommon **(Option (D) is false).** When they do occur, they are usually dystrophic and are small and scattered throughout the lesion. Peripheral-rim calcifications are highly suggestive of an aneurysm and should not be interpreted as indicating a parotid lesion (Figure 16-12). In fact, such rim calcifications are an important finding and should prompt further workup to evaluate the possible presence of an aneurysm.

## Question 71

Concerning the parapharyngeal space,

(A) it is immediately posteromedial to the masticator space
(B) its boundaries run from the skull base to the level of the hard palate
(C) mycotic aneurysm is a potential complication of an abscess within it
(D) the surgical approach to a mass within it is determined by the intraparotid or extraparotid origin of the mass

Parapharyngeal spaces are present on each side of the pharynx in the upper neck, under the middle cranial fossa. These spaces have also been referred to as the lateral pharyngeal, peripharyngeal, pharyngomaxillary, pterygopharyngeal, pterygomandibular, and pharyngomasticatory spaces. The boundaries of this space are somewhat controversial in the anatomic literature. However, there is general agreement about the overall contours of this space. Medially, the fascia over the nasopharynx and superior pharyngeal constrictor muscle forms the boundary. Laterally and extending anteriorly to posteriorly, the fascia over the medial portion of the masticator space and the deep aspect of the parotid gland is the boundary **(Option (A) is true).** The masticator space fascia extends primarily from the medial pterygoid muscle up to the skull base, attaching to the skull base along a line that runs from the medial pterygoid plate to the medial margin of the foramen ovale. This means that the mandibular nerve, which extends through the foramen ovale, lies within the masticator space and not the parapharyngeal space. Posteriorly, the boundary is the posterior fascia about the carotid sheath structures.

The parapharyngeal space extends from the skull base caudally to the hyoid bone. However, because there is fusion of the various adjacent fascial planes, from a functional point of view the parapharyngeal space extends down to the level of the styloglossus muscle, near the level of the angle of the mandible. In either case, it extends caudad to the palate **(Option (B) is false).**

The parapharyngeal space is often thought of as a "highway" that connects a number of adjacent spaces. These include the pharynx, masticator space, retropharyngeal space, parotid gland and submandibular gland spaces, and submaxillary space. An infection in any one of these adjacent areas can enter the parapharyngeal space and extend to other spaces. Once infection enters the parapharyngeal space, the resulting cellulitis can develop into an abscess. Such a parapharyngeal space abscess can cause a mycotic aneurysm in the adjacent internal carotid artery within 10 days **(Option (C) is true).** Thus, if an abscess is seen on sectional imaging, surgery should be performed immediately.

Traditionally, the only surgical approach to a parapharyngeal space mass was via the parotid gland. In this approach, the facial nerve must be lifted out of the way so that the mass can be extirpated. However, in the past 10 to 15 years, an alternative surgical approach has become popular for removing extraparotid parapharyngeal space masses. This approach is through the neck and does not require any manipulation of the facial nerve. Since even in the most expert surgical hands there is some associated facial nerve morbidity when the nerve must be moved, an approach that avoids this nerve is desirable as long as there is adequate access to the tumor. As a result, the findings on preoperative sectional imaging of a patient with a parapharyngeal space mass will influence the selection of the surgical approach **(Option (D) is true).** If no fat plane can be demonstrated between the posterolateral margin of the parapharyngeal space mass and the parotid gland, the lesion must be considered to have a parotid origin and a transparotid surgical approach is necessary. If a fat plane is demonstrated between the mass and the deep portion of the parotid gland on all scans through the lesion, a transcervical approach is used.

*Peter M. Som, M.D.*

## SUGGESTED READINGS

1. Kumar AJ, Kuhajda FP, Martinez CR, Fishman EK, Jezic DV, Siegelman SS. Computed tomography of extracranial nerve sheath tumors with pathological correlation. J Comput Assist Tomogr 1983; 7:857–865
2. Lloyd GA, Phelps PD. Demonstration of tumours of the parapharyngeal space by magnetic resonance imaging. Br J Radiol 1986; 59:675–683
3. Mancuso AA, Hanafee WN. Computed tomography and magnetic resonance imaging of the head and neck, 2nd ed. Baltimore: Williams & Wilkins; 1985:428–497
4. Olsen WL, Dillon WP, Kelly WM, Norman D, Brant-Zawadzki M, Newton TH. MR imaging of paragangliomas. AJR 1987; 148:201–204
5. Som PM. Parapharyngeal space. In: Som PM, Bergeron RT (eds), Head and neck imaging, 2nd ed. St. Louis: Mosby-Year Book; 1991:467–496
6. Som PM, Lanzieri CF, Sacher M, Lawson W, Biller HF. Extracranial tumor vascularity: determination by dynamic CT scanning. Part I. Concepts and signature curves. Radiology 1985; 154:401–405
7. Som PM, Lanzieri CF, Sacher M, Lawson W, Biller HF. Extracranial tumor vascularity: determination by dynamic CT scanning. Part II. The unit approach. Radiology 1985; 154:407–412

*Notes*

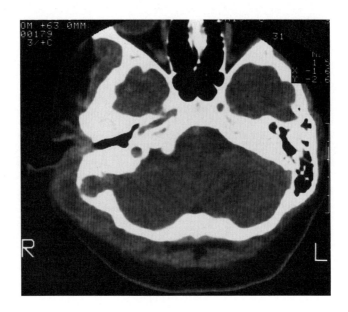

*Figure 17-1*

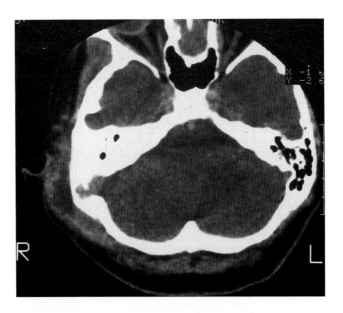

*Figure 17-2*
*Figures 17-1 through 17-4.* This 17-year-old girl has a history of recent mastoiditis. You are shown two axial postcontrast CT scans (Figures 17-1 and 17-2), as well as axial (Figure 17-3) and coronal (Figure 17-4) high-resolution CT scans.

# Case 17: Coalescent Mastoiditis

## Question 72

The images demonstrate:

- (A) serous otitis media
- (B) subperiosteal mastoid abscess
- (C) perisinus abscess
- (D) coalescent mastoiditis
- (E) cerebellar abscess

The middle ear cleft (eustachian tube, tympanum [middle ear], mastoid antrum, and mastoid air cells) constitutes an extension of the upper respiratory tract and is subject to bacterial invasion by way of the eustachian tube. Clinical manifestations of infection depend upon bacterial virulence, host response, and effectiveness of treatment. Acute otitis media responds to antibiotic treatment and is more common in children than in adults. Acute otomastoiditis can be a complication of preexisting serous otitis media (SOM) or other chronic diseases of the middle ear, including cholesteatoma. Before the advent of antibiotics it was a common and widespread condition, associated in some instances with serious complications. The mucosa of the tympanic cavity and its extensions into the mastoid share with the rest of the respiratory mucosa an inherent ability to overcome acute infection. As a result, acute otitis media and mastoiditis may be self-limiting infections. However, severe suppurative and necrotizing infections of the middle ear can be associated with systemic signs and symptoms of infection and can lead to dangerous complications, such as brain abscess. Imaging examinations are indicated in patients with acute otitis media when there is clinical suggestion of coalescent mastoiditis, because coalescence signifies the transition from mucoperiosteal disease to bone disease and eventually to intracranial, extracranial, and other systemic complications.

The middle ear cleft is a unified anatomic structure and must be considered in its entirety when it is affected by an inflammatory process. The clinical course of acute otitis media is usually short, and the process

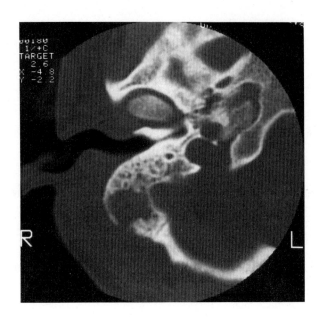

*Figure 17-3*

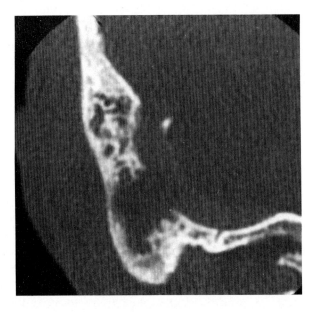

*Figure 17-4*

usually terminates as a result of three factors: the infection-resistant properties of the mucosal lining, the immune system of the host, and the susceptibility of the primary causative bacteria (beta-hemolytic strepto-

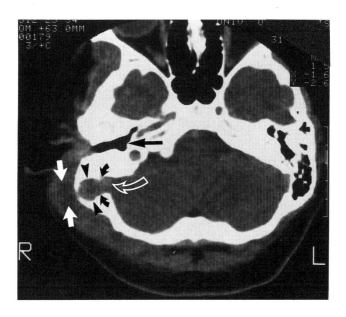

*Figure 17-5* (Same as Figure 17-1).   This postcontrast axial CT scan
shows soft tissue swelling of low density over the right mastoid (white
arrows), which is compatible with a subperiosteal abscess. There is irregular enhancement (abscess) within the mastoid cavity (arrowheads)
and along the sinodural angle and sigmoid sinus plate (small curved black
arrows) secondary to perisinus abscess and granulation tissue formation.
The mastoid abscess, indicative of coalescent mastoiditis, is more clearly
seen in Figure 17-7. There is medially displaced enhanced dura (open
curved arrow), indicating that the abscess is not within the cerebellum.
The middle ear and eustachian tube (large black arrow) are well aerated.
If SOM were present, there would be fluid (secretions) within the middle
ear, and this would appear as an opacified middle ear on the CT scan.

cocci or *Streptococcus pneumoniae*) to antibiotics. However, a small pro-
portion (1 to 5%) of untreated or inadequately treated patients may
experience complications.

The sources of acute otomastoiditis vary. This condition can be a complication of preexisting SOM or other chronic diseases. SOM is common
in children and is known to resolve spontaneously. Eustachian tube
obstruction has been documented as a cause of SOM in experimental
animals; a similar mechanism has been reported to explain the high
incidence of SOM in patients with upper respiratory tract infection.
Allergy as a factor in the pathogenesis of SOM has been a subject of
controversy; some researchers argue that all chronic middle ear disease
in adults is the result of secondary SOM experienced in childhood.

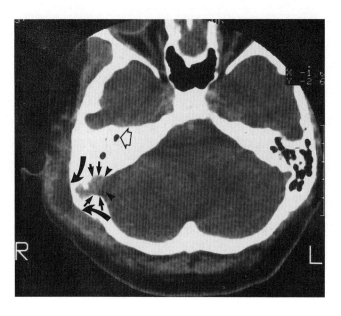

*Figure 17-6* (Same as Figure 17-2). This postcontrast axial CT scan shows low-density soft tissue swelling over the right mastoid (curved black arrows) compatible with a subperiosteal abscess. Note the irregular enhancement along the sinodural angle and sigmoid sinus plate (small arrows) as a result of a perisinus abscess and granulation tissue formation. There is also an enhancing, medially displaced dura (arrowheads), and the epitympanic recess is aerated (open arrow).

CT scans have contributed greatly to an understanding of the pathologic processes by which otomastoiditis and its complications develop. The test images (Figures 17-1 through 17-4) are CT scans of a patient with recent mastoiditis (see legends to Figures 17-5 through 17-8 for a detailed description of the findings). In patients with acute otomastoiditis, the lumen of the mastoid cells is seen as being filled because of the swollen mucosal lining and the presence of mucus or mucopurulent secretions (Figure 17-9). As the mucoperiosteum thickens, free drainage of these secretions is obstructed. With effective therapy, the inflammatory process can be arrested and the appearance of the mastoid cells returns to normal. If the process continues, the normally sharply delineated trabeculae of the mastoid become less well defined and appear decalcified. This is the result of mechanical compression of the spongy bone by the retained secretions, together with the effects of inflammatory hyperemia and associated localized acidosis. If the infection progresses, the trabeculae are absorbed, the separate air cells begin to coalesce into an irregular

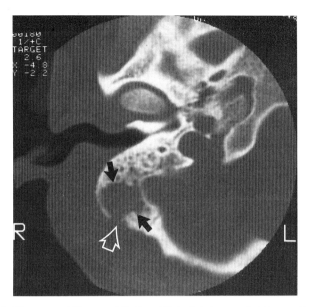

*Figure 17-7* (Same as Figure 17-3). This high-resolution axial CT scan shows a large mastoid cavity (black arrows) filled with material of soft tissue density, compatible with a mastoid abscess and granulation tissue formation. There is erosion of the outer cortex of the mastoid (open arrow), which provided a pathway for the formation of a subperiosteal abscess (better seen in Figures 17-5 and 17-6) over the outer cortex of the mastoid. Formation of a cavity in the mastoid following simple acute mastoiditis indicates development of an acute coalescent mastoiditis.

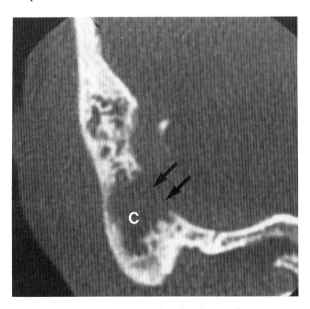

*Figure 17-8* (Same as Figure 17-4). This high-resolution coronal CT scan shows a large mastoid cavity (C) due to a mastoid abscess. There is erosion of the cortex of the inner table of the right mastoid along the sigmoid sinus plate (arrows), which provided a pathway for the formation of a perisinus abscess (more clearly seen in Figures 17-5 and 17-6) over the inner cortex of the mastoid.

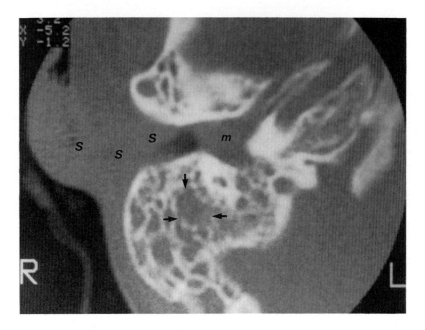

*Figure 17-9.* Acute otomastoiditis. This axial CT scan shows soft tissue opacification of the middle ear (*m*), eustachian tube, and mastoid air cells. There is soft tissue swelling (*S*) in the external auditory canal and periauricular region and slight lack of sharpness and partial demineralization of some of the trabeculae (arrows). The remaining trabeculae are intact, indicating simple acute mastoiditis and therefore not an acute frank coalescent mastoiditis. The early rarefaction of some of the trabeculae should be carefully studied by follow-up CT scans to rule out an incipient coalescent mastoiditis.

cavity (coalescent mastoiditis), and empyema develops. Therefore, coalescent mastoiditis best explains all of the findings in the test images **(Option (D) is true)**. By comparison, in patients with SOM, the middle ear cavity and mastoid air cells are opacified and the mastoid air cells are not destroyed **(Option (A) is false)**. As the inflammatory process continues, the pus retained in the closed mastoid perforates the mastoid cortex and migrates beneath the periosteum (subperiosteal abscess, a common complication of coalescent mastoiditis) **(Option (B) is true)**. In rare instances this abscess invades the external auditory canal or advances into the zygomatic roots of the zygomatic process of the temporal bone and is seen both clinically and on the CT or MR scans as an abscess anterior to the auricle. The osteoclastic resorption of bone proceeds in all directions. The subperiosteal abscess may break through the tip of the mastoid into the neck (Bezold's abscess) or the inner table, forming a perisinus (sigmoid) abscess **(Option (C) is true)** or other abscess, such as an epidural abscess (see Figure 17-10). No cerebellar lesion is present in the test images **(Option (E) is false).**

## Question 73

Complications of acute otomastoiditis include:

(A) thrombosis of lateral and sigmoid sinuses
(B) thrombosis of petrosal and cavernous sinuses
(C) facial nerve palsy
(D) leptomeningitis
(E) labyrinthitis
(F) Gradenigo syndrome

Complications of fulminating, persistent acute otitis media and otomastoiditis include thrombosis of the lateral and sigmoid sinuses, thrombosis of the petrosal and cavernous sinuses, facial nerve palsy, leptomeningitis, suppurative labyrinthitis, apex petrositis (with or without the full Gradenigo syndrome), and brain abscess **(Options (A) through (F) are all true).** The pathologic process by which a complication develops depends upon the stage of infection. Early in the course of infection there may be a progressive thrombophlebitis of venules in the tympanum and mastoid mucoperiosteum. Later this infection can extend even through an intact bone to the sigmoid sinus, meninges, brain, labyrinth, or facial nerve. The beta-hemolytic streptococci and type III *S. pneumoniae* are particularly capable of producing thrombophlebitic complications. Later in the course of acute otomastoiditis, complications are the result of the progressive bone erosion of coalescent mastoiditis, as in the test case (Figures 17-1 through 17-8). Any patient with acute otitis media or acute coalescent mastoiditis, particularly if there is the slightest clinical evidence of cerebellar or meningeal abnormality, should undergo contrast-enhanced CT or MR scanning of the head to search for otitic intracranial complications such as abscess, meningitis, or thrombosis.

Extradural (epidural) abscess can occur when pus collects between the dura mater and the bones of the middle or posterior cranial fossae (Figure 17-10). The dura may become thickened and covered with granulation tissue. This thickening is seen on a CT scan as an area of contrast enhancement (Figure 17-10) and can easily be overlooked if the abscess

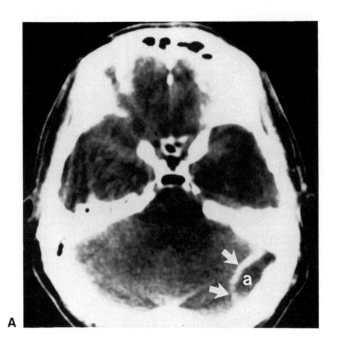

A

*Figure 17-10.* Otogenic epidural abscess. (A) This axial postcontrast CT scan shows an epidural abscess (a) in the posterior cranial fossa. There is marked enhancement of the thickened dura (arrows). (B) This axial postcontrast CT scan shows extension of the posterior fossa epidural abscess (a) over the high-convexity parietal region. Again, there is marked enhancement of the thickened dura (arrows).

is small (Figure 17-11). When infection penetrates the dura, it may cause subdural abscess, meningitis, and brain abscess. Subdural abscess is more common with chronic otomastoiditis than with acute otomastoiditis and consists of a collection of purulent material between the dura mater and the brain. Meningitis is a serious complication of otomastoiditis (Figure 17-12). The microorganisms can reach the meninges by way of soft tissue pathways, areas of bone erosion, extradural pathways, an infected labyrinth, or infected venous sinuses. Enhancement of the leptomeninges on contrast-enhanced CT or MR scans is characteristic of meningitis (Figure 17-12).

Otogenic meningitis may at times be due to an anomaly of the inner ear. The inner ear anomaly may not be known to the clinicians. In general, when there is recurrent meningitis in a child, a cerebrospinal fluid (CSF) leak should be considered. The suspected sites of CSF leakage should include the middle ear cleft. If congenital deafness is associated

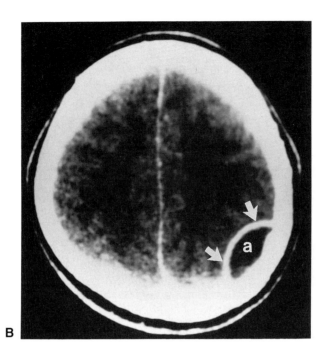

with recurrent meningitis, a developmental anomaly of the inner ear must be considered. The Mondini-type anomaly has been the most frequent inner ear anomaly associated with CSF otorrhea. The Mondini-type anomaly is caused by the incomplete formation of the bony and membranous labyrinth. The cochlea, vestibule, and semicircular canals may be dilated. The cochlea and vestibule may have a cyst-like appearance. Many patients also have an anatomic defect in the stapes footplate. Patients with Mondini dysplasia are predisposed to developing a CSF leak and, therefore, repeated episodes of otogenic meningitis.

Lateral and sigmoid sinus thrombophlebitis are known to result from extradural abscess in more than half of all cases. The epidural abscess may lead to thrombosis of the superior and inferior petrosal sinuses and eventually to thrombosis of the cavernous sinus. Depending on the degree of mastoid pneumatization, the bone surrounding the sigmoid sinus can be relatively thin. It can be easily eroded by granulation tissue or cholesteatoma, and a perisinus inflammation can eventually lead to a localized phlebitis and mural thrombosis. The thrombus may become infected and release septic emboli. Characteristic clinical features of otogenic dural sinus thrombophlebitis and thrombosis include otalgia, headache, irritability, lethargy, and signs of increased intracranial

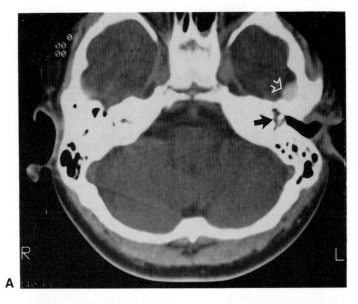

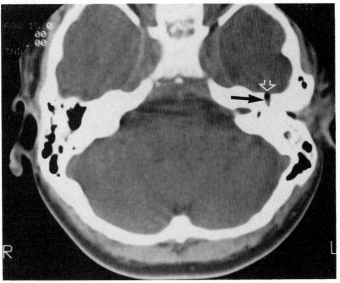

*Figure 17-11.* Acute otitis media with middle cranial fossa epidural abscess. (A) This axial postcontrast CT scan shows soft tissues in the middle ear (solid arrow) and an enhancing epidural abscess (open arrow). (B) This axial postcontrast CT scan, obtained 5 mm above the level seen in panel A, shows an air-fluid level in the anterior epitympanic recess (solid arrow). There is bone dehiscence along the anterior epitympanic recess (open arrow). This is most probably the cause of the epidural abscess seen in panel A.

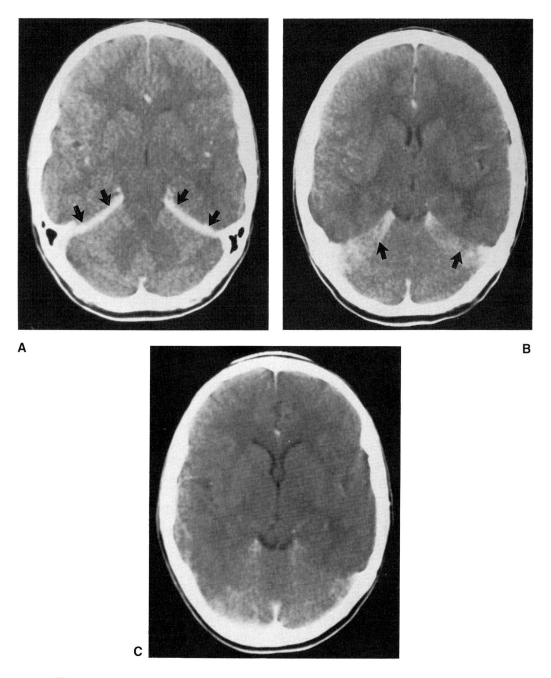

*Figure 17-12.* Acute otitis media with associated meningitis. (A) Axial postcontrast CT scan shows prominent tentorial enhancement and thickening (arrows). This is indicative of meningeal inflammation. (B) Postcontrast CT scan, obtained 5 mm above the level seen in panel A, shows prominent increased enhancement of the tentorium and leptomeninges (arrows). (C) This postcontrast CT scan, obtained 4 days later than and at the same level as the scan in panel B, shows decreased tentorial enhancement following antibiotic treatment.

pressure. Thrombosis tends to be more difficult to diagnose than other intracranial complications of acute otomastoiditis, such as epidural abscess or meningitis. Traditionally, cerebral angiography was required to confirm such a diagnosis. CT has proved effective in detecting many instances of deep vein and dural venous sinus thrombosis. CT signs that point toward the diagnosis of venous sinus thrombosis include the following: (1) increased density as a result of congealed blood in and along the course of the venous sinuses on noncontrast CT; (2) filling defects within the sinuses on contrast-enhanced CT; (3) intense inflammatory enhancement of sinus walls and adjacent dura; and (4) failure of a sinus to opacify. Other suggestive but nonspecific findings associated with sinus thrombosis include cerebral or cerebellar edema, intense tentorial enhancement from collateral venous flow, multifocal bilateral parasagittal hemorrhages, and gyral cerebral or cerebellar enhancement. Some of the aforementioned CT features are readily depicted on the series of pre-and postcontrast MR scans in Figures 17-13 through 17-19.

Venous sinus thrombophlebitis is an uncommon but serious complication of otomastoiditis. Early effective antibiotic therapy is usually sufficient to control it. Although antibiotics have altered its characteristic clinical and imaging features, such complications still occur. Figures 17-13 through 17-19 exemplify the MR features of the disease as seen today. The abnormalities associated with this lateral (transverse) and sigmoid sinus thrombophlebitis range from perisinus granulations and pus formation to mural thrombus formation, occlusive thrombophlebitis, intrasinus empyema, and, finally, organization of the thrombus. Propagation of sinus thrombosis proximally is believed to be the cause of otitic hydrocephalus. Showering of the circulation with septic emboli may lead to lung abscesses, peritonitis, or septic arthritis. The septic form of venous thrombophlebitis often requires both medical and surgical therapy. There is general agreement that an appropriate form of mastoidectomy should be performed, that the middle fossa tegmen and posterior fossa petrous bone plate should be skeletonized, and that the sigmoid sinus plate should be removed. Removal of granulations and pus from the surface of the sinus and adjacent dura and needling the sinus to rule out the presence of pus suffice in most cases. In the patient in Figures 17-13 through 17-19, a satisfactory outcome was achieved with medical treatment because of early diagnosis by MRI.

Today contrast-enhanced MRI is the imaging modality of choice for demonstrating deep venous sinus thrombophlebitis, epidural abscess, intradural abscess, and brain abscess. Contrast-enhanced MRI is also excellent for demonstrating facial nerve involvement (Figure 17-20) and

SE 2,600/30

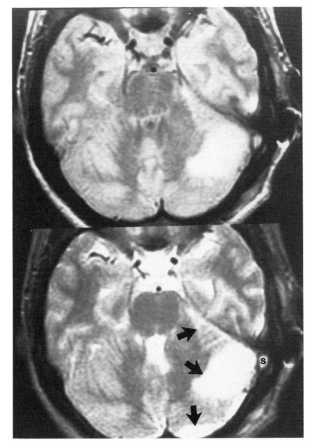

SE 2,600/80

*Figure 17-13.* Focal encephalitis and clinically presumed sigmoid sinus thrombophlebitis. Following a radical mastoidectomy for an infected cholesteatoma, this 31-year-old woman developed fever, headache, and cerebellar symptoms and signs. These axial proton-density (top) and T2-weighted (bottom) MR scans show increased signal intensity in the left sigmoid sinus (s) and marked edema in the left cerebellar hemisphere (arrows), resulting in deformity of the fourth ventricle. The increased signal intensity in the left sigmoid sinus is due either to slow blood flow or to thrombosis.

labyrinthitis, two serious complications of otomastoiditis. It is assumed that in patients with facial nerve paralysis secondary to acute otomastoiditis, the pathophysiologic changes reflect venous congestion, tissue edema, neural toxicity, or direct invasion. The site of involvement is often

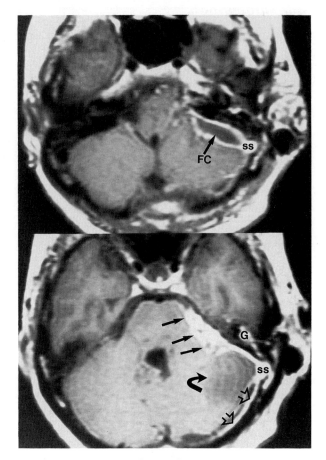

*Figure 17-14.* Same patient as in Figure 17-13. These axial postcontrast T1-weighted MR scans show increased enhancement of the left sigmoid sinus (ss) and lateral sinus (open arrows). There is a normal flow pattern in the right sigmoid sinus. There is evidence of focal cerebritis (curved arrow) and a focal intradural fluid collection (FC), and there is marked enhancement of the anterolateral dura (straight arrows), which most probably represents inflammation of the dura and granulation tissue. The enhancement of the active inflammatory process and granulation tissue (G) in the left middle ear should also be noted.

the tympanic segment of the facial nerve, where the canal is dehiscent in more than 40% of cases (Figure 17-21).

Labyrinthitis can be serous or suppurative. In many cases, serous labyrinthitis is a diagnosis of exclusion, whereas suppurative labyrinthi-

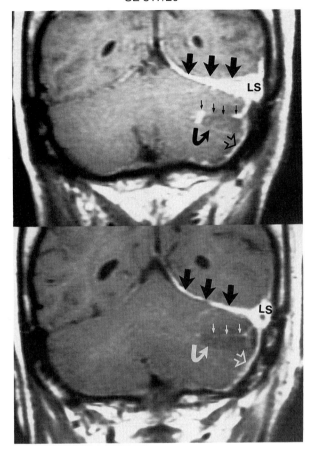

SE 817/20

*Figure 17-15.* Same patient as in Figures 17-13 and 17-14. These coronal postcontrast T1-weighted MR scans show marked thickening as well as increased enhancement of the left tentorial leaf (large black arrows). There is increased enhancement of the left lateral (transverse) sinus (LS), related to either slow blood flow or thrombophlebitis. The flow pattern of the right lateral sinus is normal. There is also increased linear enhancement (small arrows), leading toward the lateral sinus. This was believed to represent phlebitis of a deep vein. There is focal cerebritis (curved arrow) adjacent to this presumed phlebitis and increased enhancement of the left posterior fossa dura (open arrow).

tis frequently occurs after a purulent process, such as otitis media and mastoiditis, that may spread to the labyrinth through preformed pathways such as the round and oval windows. Before the advent of MRI, only the chronic or sclerotic type of labyrinthitis could be demonstrated

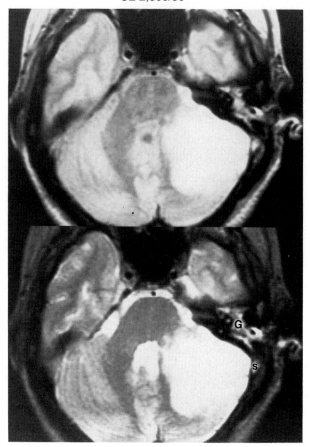

*Figure 17-16.* Same patient as in Figures 17-13 through 17-15. Focal encephalitis and clinically presumed sigmoid sinus and lateral sinus thrombophlebitis. These axial proton-density (top) and T2-weighted (bottom) MR scans, taken 7 days after the scans seen in Figure 17-13, show progression of the left cerebellar edema. The signal from the left sigmoid sinus (s) remains hyperintense, and the granulation tissue (G) persists in the left ear.

by either complex-motion tomography or CT scanning, appearing as obliteration of the lumen of the labyrinth ("ossifying or obliterative labyrinthitis"). Today, with the use of paramagnetic contrast material, serous or suppurative labyrinthitis is easily seen on MRI as enhancement of the labyrinth (Figure 17-22).

Otitic brain abscess is seen most often in the temporal lobe (Figure 17-23) or in the anterior portion of the lateral lobe of the cerebellum

SE 850/20

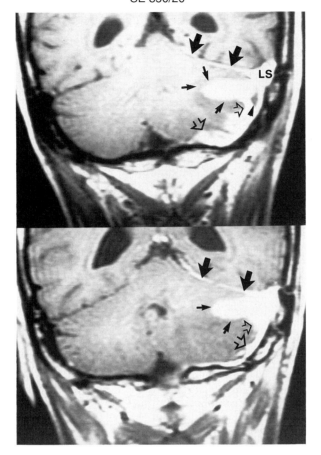

SE 850/20

*Figure 17-17.* Same patient as in Figures 17-13 through 17-16. These coronal postcontrast T1-weighted MR scans, obtained 7 days after the scans seen in Figure 17-13, show marked contrast enhancement (small arrows) in the region of the focal cerebritis. There is less enhancement of the tentorium (large arrows). However, there is increased enhancement along the left sigmoid sinus and adjacent dura (open arrows) of the left cerebellar hemisphere. There is a suggestion of a filling defect (arrowhead) in the left sigmoid sinus. The signal intensity of the right lateral and sigmoid sinuses is normal.

(Figure 17-24) but is occasionally found in other areas of the brain if the infection is transported through the blood or by thrombophlebitis. Focal otogenic encephalitis that precedes abscess formation (Figures 17-13 and 17-14) resembles brain abscess clinically but consists of a focal area of brain edema and inflammation without intracranial suppuration. The

SE 2,800/30

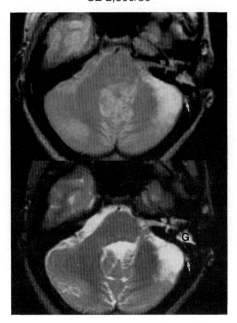

SE 2,800/80

*Figure 17-18.* Same patient as in Figures 17-13 through 17-17. Resolving focal encephalitis. These proton-density (top) and T2-weighted (bottom) MR scans, obtained 3 months after the scans seen in Figure 17-13, show marked resolution of the left cerebellar edema following medical treatment. The granulation tissue (G) persists in the left mastoid antrum. The signal from the left sigmoid sinus (arrows) remains somewhat hyperintense.

focal encephalitis is frequently associated with either thrombophlebitis of the dural veins or an extradural abscess. Adequate antibiotic treatment and timely surgical intervention are necessary to control infection in the temporal bone and adjacent (epidural) area. Focal cerebritis can be diagnosed with a high degree of certainty by using CT and MRI, eliminating the need for intracranial tests through burr holes.

SE 1,000/30

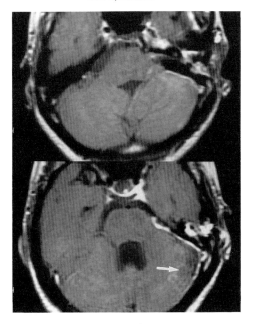

SE 1,000/30

*Figure 17-19.* Same patient as in Figures 17-13 through 17-18. Focal encephalitis and resolving clinically presumed thrombophlebitis of the sigmoid sinus. These postcontrast T1-weighted MR scans, obtained 13 weeks after the scans seen in Figure 17-14, show marked resolution of the dural as well as the sigmoid sinus enhancement following medical treatment. There is residual edema or gliosis (arrow) in the left cerebellar hemisphere.

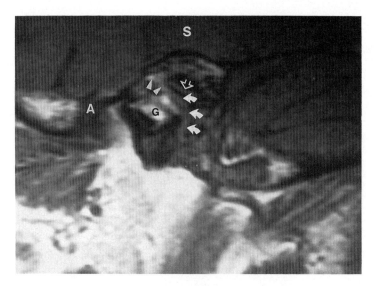

SE 800/20

*Figure 17-20.* Otogenic facial nerve palsy. This postcontrast sagittal T1-weighted MR scan shows granulation tissue (G) within the middle ear. Note increased enhancement at the geniculate portion and proximal tympanic portion (arrowheads) of the facial nerve. At surgery, active granulation tissue was found in the middle ear and around the geniculate and proximal tympanic portion of the facial nerve. The tympanic and mastoid segments of the facial nerve (curved arrows) and lateral semicircular canal (open arrow) can also be identified. A = anterior; S = superior.

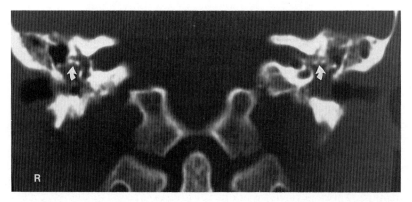

*Figure 17-21.* Otogenic right facial nerve palsy. This coronal CT scan shows opacification of both middle ear cavities as a result of acute otitis media. Note the tympanic segment of the facial nerve canal (arrows). Both facial nerve canals appear to be dehiscent, with the right side possibly more so than the left side. The patient developed facial paralysis on the right side as a result of a dehiscent facial nerve canal. Facial paralysis resolved after the otitis media had been cured.

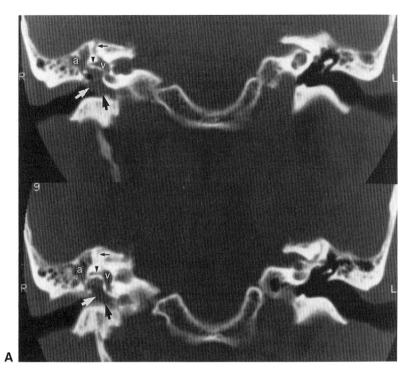

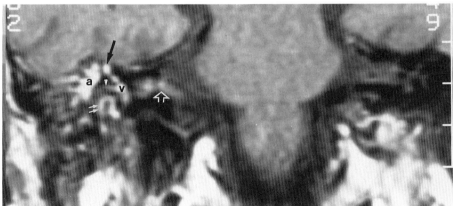

SE 700/20

*Figure 17-22.* Granulomatous labyrinthitis following otomastoiditis. (A) These coronal CT scans show opacification of the right mastoid air cells, including the mastoid antrum (a), with a soft tissue mass (large arrows) in the middle ear. At surgery the mass was found to be due to active granuloma. The vestibule (v) and horizontal (arrowhead) and superior (small arrow) semicircular canals appear unremarkable. (B) This coronal postcontrast T1-weighted MR scan shows marked contrast enhancement in the mastoid antrum (a), superior semicircular canal (large black arrow), lateral semicircular canal (arrowhead), vestibule (v), and middle ear (small white arrows) and within the internal auditory canal (open arrow). The labyrinthine involvement and neuronal involvement of the internal auditory canal were not detected by the contrast CT scan (panel A). There is normal nonenhancing labyrinth on the left side.

403

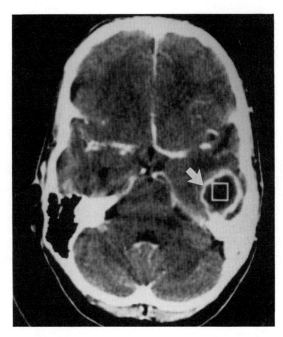

*Figure 17-23.* Otogenic temporal lobe abscess. This axial postcontrast CT scan shows a mass (abscess) with ring enhancement (arrow) involving the left inferior temporal lobe.

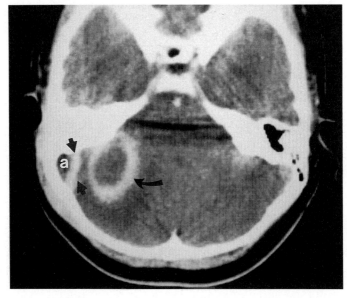

*Figure 17-24.* Otogenic cerebellar abscess. This axial postcontrast CT scan shows enhancing thickened dura (straight arrows) with associated epidural abscess (a) and a right cerebellar hemispheric abscess (curved arrow), as well as opacification of the right mastoid air cells.

404 / *Head and Neck Disorders IV*

# Question 74

Features of Gradenigo syndrome include:

    (A) apex petrositis
    (B) abducens nerve paresis
    (C) gasserian ganglionitis
    (D) facial paralysis

CT is the radiographic modality of choice for evaluating infralabyrinthine and petrous apex air cells (present in 30% of cases). Apex petrositis (petrous apicitis) is now uncommon because antibiotic treatment limits the course of otomastoiditis. However, apex petrositis should be suspected whenever an acute or chronic suppurative ear infection is associated with deep ipsilateral pain or whenever purulent otorrhea and deep-seated pain persist after what seems to have been an adequate simple mastoidectomy for acute coalescent mastoiditis. When the diagnosis of apex petrositis is made, aggressive radical surgical drainage is indicated. Ramedier and Lempert first described the now classic approach to the petrous apex by a radical exposure of the carotid canal through the glenoid fossa. In 1907, Gradenigo described a condition consisting of abducens nerve paresis or paralysis **(Option (B) is true),** deep pain along the trigeminal nerve, and discharge of purulent matter from the ear as a result of apex petrositis **(Option (A) is true).** The deep facial pain associated with Gradenigo syndrome is due to involvement of the dura over the petrous apex (focal meningitis) or direct irritation of the gasserian ganglion (gasserian ganglionitis) in Meckel's cave **(Option (C) is true)** (Figures 17-25 and 17-26). The abducens nerve is involved as it courses through Dorello's canal under the petroclinoid ligament. The classic triad (otomastoiditis, abducens nerve paralysis, and deep facial pain) of Gradenigo syndrome may not be present in every patient with apex petrositis. Patients with Gradenigo syndrome may have facial paralysis related to other complications of otomastoiditis; however, facial paralysis or paresis is not part of the triad of Gradenigo syndrome **(Option (D) is false).** With dramatic advances in antimicrobial therapy, imaging techniques, and early surgical treatment of otitis media and mastoiditis, the incidence of complications has fallen precipitously. Nevertheless, despite these advantages, the morbidity from suppurative ear disease persists.

*Mahmood F. Mafee, M.D.*

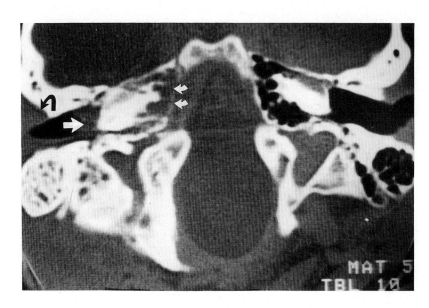

*Figure 17-25.*   Gradenigo syndrome. This 16-year-old girl presented with right sixth nerve palsy a few days after a right external auditory canal abscess was drained following an episode of otomastoiditis. This axial CT scan, imaged for bone details, shows opacification of the right mastoid air cells. There is also opacification of the right petrous apex air cells, associated with bone resorption (curved white arrows). In addition, the soft tissue (granulation tissue) in the right middle ear (straight white arrow), as well as soft tissue swelling of the right external canal (black arrow), can be seen.

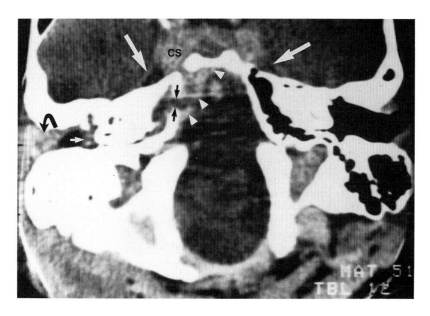

*Figure 17-26.* Same patient as in Figure 17-25. Gradenigo syndrome. This axial postcontrast CT scan imaged for soft tissue details shows increased dural enhancement at the right petrous apex (arrowheads), indicative of focal apical meningitis. This apical petrous meningitis was responsible for a sixth cranial nerve palsy. The cistern of each gasserian ganglion (large white arrows) is seen along the posterior aspect of the cavernous sinus (CS). Involvement of the leptomeninges around this ganglion (focal meningitis) is responsible for the deep pain (trigeminal ganglionitis) of Gradenigo syndrome. There is focal erosion of the medial cortex of the petrous apex (small black arrows) and there is granulation tissue in the right middle ear (small white arrow) and in the right external auditory canal (curved black arrow).

## SUGGESTED READINGS

1. Hara HJ. Otitic meningitis in the antibiotic ear: observations on 28 adult patients treated in Los Angeles County Hospital, 1950–1957. Ann Otol Rhinol Laryngol 1959; 82:305–314

2. Lederer FL, Torok N. Otogenic meningitis. In: Maloney WH (ed), Otolaryngology, vol 2. New York: Harper & Row; 1966:1–25

3. Lempert J. Complete apicectomy (mastoidotympanoapicectomy). New technique for complete apical exenteration of apical carotid of petrous pyramid. Arch Otolaryngol 1937; 25:144–177

4. Mafee MF, Singleton EL, Valvassori GE, Espinosa GA, Kumar A, Aimi K. Acute otomastoiditis and its complications: role of CT. Radiology 1985; 155:391–397

5. Mafee MF, Valvassori GE, Kumar A, Levin BC, Siedentop KH, Raju S. Otogenic intracranial inflammations: role of CT. Otolaryngol Clin North Am 1988; 21:245–263

6. Neely JG. Complications of temporal bone infection. In: Cummings GW, Harker LA (eds), Otolaryngology—head and neck surgery. St. Louis: CV Mosby; 1986:2988–3015

7. Shambaugh GE Jr, Quie PG. Acute otitis media and mastoiditis. In: Paparella M, Shumrick D (eds), Otolaryngology, vol 2. The ear. Philadelphia: WB Saunders; 1973:113–120

8. Venezio FR, Naidich TP, Shulman ST. Complications of mastoiditis with special emphasis on venous sinus thrombosis. J Pediatr 1982; 101:509–513

9. Zizmor J, Noyek AM. Inflammatory diseases of the temporal bone. Radiol Clin North Am 1974; 12:491–504

*Notes*

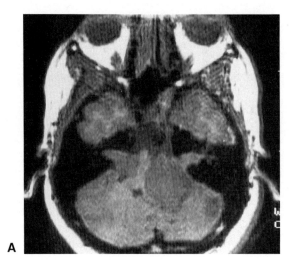

SE 500/20

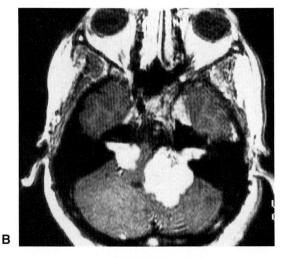

SE 500/20

*Figure 18-1.* This 26-year-old woman has had decreased hearing on the left side for several years and on the right side for the past 7 to 8 months. You are shown a series of MR scans, including T1-weighted images without enhancement (A) and with gadolinium DTPA enhancement (B and C) and T2-weighted images (D through F).

# Case 18: Neurofibromatosis 2

## Question 75

Which *one* of the following is the MOST likely diagnosis?

(A) Neurofibromatosis 2
(B) Multiple leptomeningeal metastases
(C) Ruptured dermoid cyst
(D) Meningiomatosis
(E) Lymphoma

The T1-weighted precontrast axial test image (Figure 18-1A) shows slightly hypointense masses in both cerebellopontine angles (CPAs) and in the left Meckel's cave (see Figure 18-2). The fourth ventricle is compressed and displaced superiorly and to the right by the large left CPA mass. On the postcontrast T1-weighted axial images (Figures 18-1B and C), the two masses in the CPAs show heterogeneous enhancement and each mass extends into and is centered about an expanded internal auditory canal. These masses represent bilateral acoustic nerve tumors. The mass in the left Meckel's cave shows dense enhancement and extends forward into the left cavernous sinus (Figure 18-1C) along the course of the left trigeminal nerve. There is another small enhancing nodule in the right Meckel's cave, suggesting a contralateral right trigeminal ganglion tumor.

The postcontrast T1-weighted images also show multiple small enhancing nodules adjacent to the dura. These nodules are attached to the left anterior clinoid process, to the left side of the tentorium, and along the dura near the uncus of the right temporal lobe. These represent multiple small meningiomas.

Patchy, nonconfluent white matter lesions are seen bilaterally in the periventricular central white matter on the T2-weighted axial image (Figure 18-1D). The etiology of these lesions is unclear. They may represent hamartomas or early neoplasms. There is also an intramedullary tumor with high T2-weighted signal intensity in the medulla and upper cervical cord (Figure 18-1E). This intramedullary tumor is most likely a

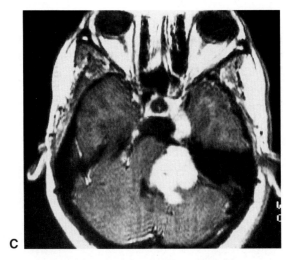

C

SE 500/20

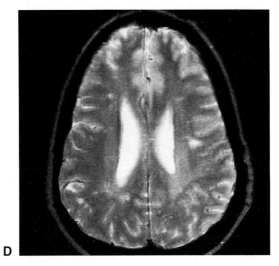

D

SE 2,500/90

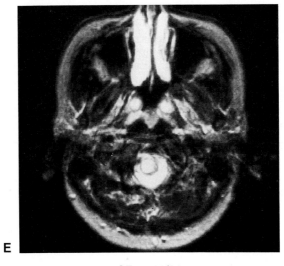

E

SE 2,500/90

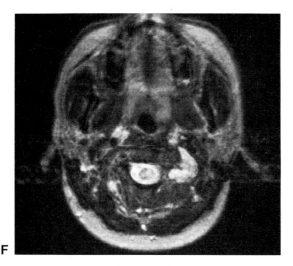

SE 2,500/90

cystic ependymoma. Such a spinal cord neoplasm may be seen without clinical symptomatology. A separate mass is noted in the left side of the neck adjacent to the spinal canal at the level of the C3 neural foramen (Figure 18-1F). This approximately 2- by 3-cm lesion has high T2-weighted signal intensity and represents a schwannoma or neurofibroma of C3. The findings in this patient of multiple central nervous system tumors, and specifically bilateral acoustic schwannomas, are characteristic of neurofibromatosis 2 **(Option (A) is correct).**

Multiple leptomeningeal metastases (Option (B)) may involve the cranial nerves but rarely expand to the size of the lesions seen in both CPAs in the test images. Typically, there are additional small nodules scattered throughout the cisternal spaces (Figure 18-3), unlike the focal meningiomas depicted in the test images. Furthermore, leptomeningeal metastases usually do not show patchy periventricular lesions with high T2-weighted signal intensity without any associated parenchymal tumors. Finally, the clinical course of leptomeningeal metastatic disease would be very unlikely to extend over several years as did the symptoms in the test patient.

Rupture of a dermoid cyst (Option (C)) usually leads to dissemination of the cyst contents throughout the subarachnoid spaces. These deposits are detected by MRI, provided that they demonstrate sufficient T1 shortening to make them appear brighter than cerebrospinal fluid (CSF) on T1-weighted images. Such deposits are seen on the noncontrast

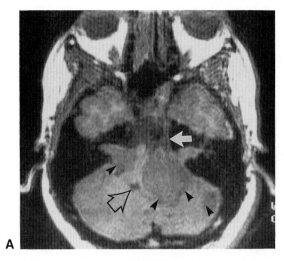

SE 500/20

*Figure 18-2* (Same as Figure 18-1). Neurofibromatosis 2. (A) Axial MR image. There are bilateral slightly hypointense masses in the cerebellopontine angles (CPAs) (arrowheads) and in the left Meckel's cave (solid arrow). The fourth ventricle (open arrow) is compressed and displaced laterally to the right by the larger left CPA mass. (B and C) Postcontrast axial MR images. The two masses (m) in the CPAs show heterogeneous enhancement extending well into the internal auditory canals bilaterally; these represent acoustic nerve tumors. The mass in the left Meckel's cave (open arrow, panel C) shows dense enhancement and extends forward into the left side of the cavernous sinus. There is another small enhancing nodule in the right Meckel's cave region (solid arrow, panel C). These represent trigeminal ganglion tumors. (D through F) Axial MR images. Multiple patchy and confluent white matter lesions (arrows, panel D) are noted in the periventricular and central white matter bilaterally. These are believed to represent foci of Schwann cell heterotopia or melanin deposition. There is a long-T2 lesion in the upper portion of the cervical cord (arrows, panel E). There is a mass in the left side of the neck extending from the neural foramen. This lesion demonstrates T2 lengthening involving the left C3 nerve root (arrows, panel F). These abnormalities are due to schwannomas of the cervical nerves.

T1-weighted images as areas of high signal intensity scattered throughout the CSF pathways (Figure 18-4); by comparison, the lesions in the test patient were slightly hypointense on the T1-weighted images. Moreover, the subarachnoid deposits of a ruptured dermoid cyst do not enhance, unlike the multiple lesions in the test images.

Meningiomatosis (Option (D)) represents another hereditary form of multiple neoplasms. It is a less common disorder than neurofibromatosis

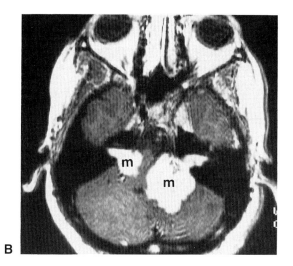

B

SE 500/20

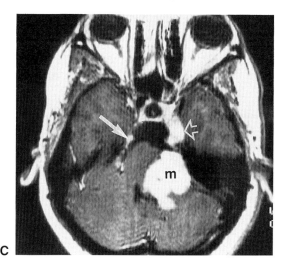

C

SE 500/20

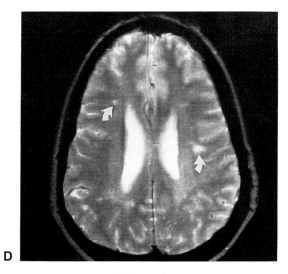

D

SE 2,500/90

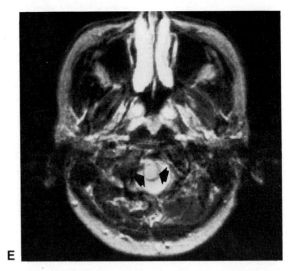

E

SE 2,500/90

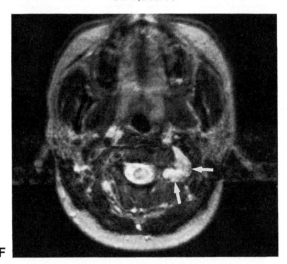

F

SE 2,500/90

2. Patients with meningiomatosis have multiple enhancing meningiomas, all of which are attached to a dural surface within the central nervous system (Figure 18-5). The bilateral CPA tumors and the left Meckel's cave mass in the test patient could represent meningiomas. There is no known association, however, of meningiomatosis with intramedullary spinal cord tumors or with periventricular areas of T2 lengthening without associated parenchymal masses, unlike the situation shown in the test images.

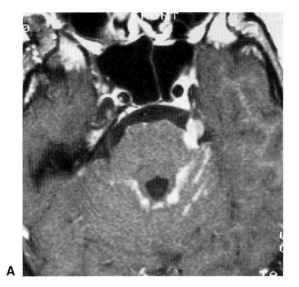

SE 460/15

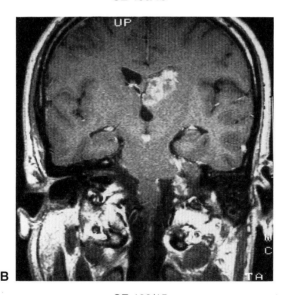

SE 460/15

*Figure 18-3.* Metastatic brain tumor with subarachnoid seeding (primary adenocarcinoma). (A) Postcontrast axial MR image. There are several enhanced nodules along the surface of the brain, including a 1.5-cm-diameter nodule along the left trigeminal nerve. Other, smaller nodules are present in the superior cerebellar folia. (B) Postcontrast coronal MR image. A large heterogeneously enhancing mass is located partially in the left lateral ventricle. Smaller nodules are located in the third ventricle, beneath the left margin of the tentorium, and adjacent to the left flocculus of the cerebellum. Additional smaller nodules are scattered in the cerebral sulci and upper cervical spinal canal.

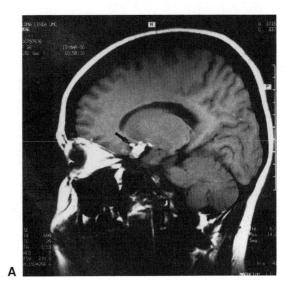

SE 600/20

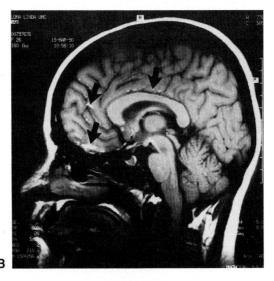

SE 600/20

*Figure 18-4.* Ruptured dermoid cyst with subarachnoid seeding. (A) Sagittal MR image. This unenhanced T1-weighted image documents a high-intensity lobulated mass in the left parasellar region extending into the transverse fissure (arrow). The signal is characteristic of fat. (B) Sagittal MR image. Multiple high-intensity nodules are scattered throughout the interhemispheric fissure region, in the subfrontal subarachnoid space, and in the pericallosal cistern (arrows).

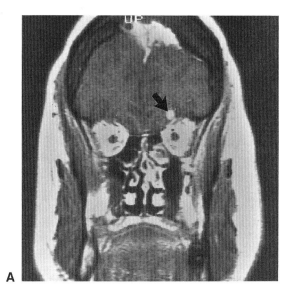

SE 600/17

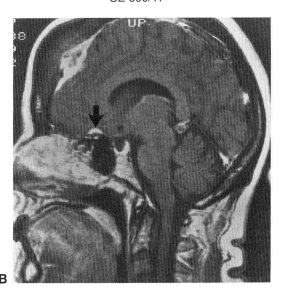

SE 600/17

*Figure 18-5.* Meningiomatosis with multiple en plaque meningiomas. Postcontrast coronal (A) and sagittal (B) MR images. There are multiple enhancing extra-axial tumors. A large lesion, approximately 2 by 4 cm with associated irregularity and blistering of the overlying frontal bone, is straddling the frontal falx. Smaller enhancing lesions are noted near the left orbital roof and along the planum sphenoidale (arrow).

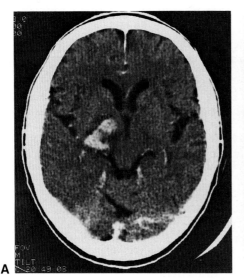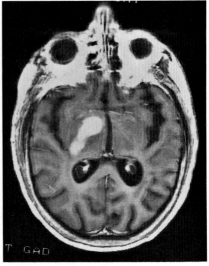

A                                                                                          B

SE 500/20

*Figure 18-6.* Primary thalamic lymphoma. (A) Axial postcontrast CT
scan. There is an enhanced tumor involving the right internal capsule
and thalamus. The lesion is surrounded by a slightly low-density area,
reflecting edema, and shows a slight mass effect causing deformity of the
third ventricle. (B and C) Postcontrast axial MR images. There is a somewhat lobulated, intensely enhancing lesion involving the right internal
capsule, thalamus, and uppermost portion of the midbrain.

The central nervous system may be affected by both primary and
metastatic lymphoma (Option (E)). Primary malignant lymphoma may
be multicentric and often extends contiguously in a structure such as the
brain stem. Such parenchymal lymphomas typically involve the deep
brain structure, including the white matter, and these tumors usually
show enhancement after administration of contrast material (Figure
18-6). Metastatic lymphoma can involve the leptomeninges and the
parenchymal structures of the brain. Like multiple leptomeningeal
metastases discussed above, these metastatic lymphomatous foci rarely
grow to the size of the lesions seen in both CPAs in the test images and
would not be likely to be associated with symptoms extending over
several years. Furthermore, leptomeningeal lymphomas do not typically
expand into the internal auditory canals, unlike the situation in the test
images.

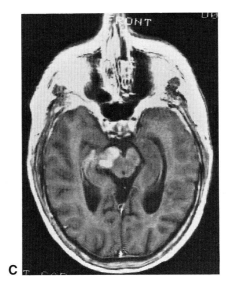

SE 500/20

## Question 76

Typical features of neurofibromatosis 2 include:

(A) a genetic locus on chromosome 22
(B) plexiform neurofibromas
(C) white matter lesions
(D) bilateral acoustic schwannomas
(E) multiple meningiomas
(F) optic nerve glioma

Neurofibromatosis is the most common disorder among the spectrum of phakomatoses (neurocutaneous disorders). It was originally studied by von Recklinghausen in 1882 and was further defined by Henneberg and Koch in 1903; two basic forms, neurofibromatosis types 1 and 2 (NF-1 and NF-2), are currently recognized. Both forms are inherited in an autosomal dominant fashion with variable penetrance. NF-1 (von Recklinghausen's disease) designates the peripheral form of neurofibromatosis and is caused by an abnormality within a gene locus near the centromere on the long arm of chromosome 17. This disorder affects approximately 1 of every 3,000 to 5,000 people and is characterized clinically by multiple

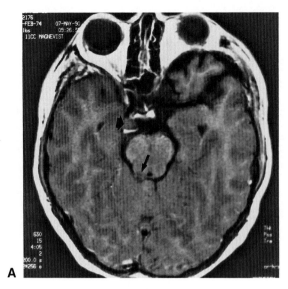

SE 630/15

*Figure 18-7.* Neurofibromatosis 1. (A) Postcontrast axial MR image. There is an isointense lesion without enhancement in the right peri-mesencephalic cistern along the course of the third cranial nerve (short arrow). A slightly hypointense lesion is noted in the right tectal plate (long arrow). There is a defect in the greater wing of the left sphenoid bone, with dysplasia of the left anterior temporal lobe. (B and C) Axial MR images. A hyperintense area, representing the site of a low-grade tectal neoplasm, is noted in the right tectal plate. The defect in the greater wing of the left sphenoid bone with bulging forward of the contents of the left middle cranial fossa is evident. An arachnoid cyst that deforms the dysplastic left anterior temporal lobe is present in the left temporal pole. There is associated proptosis of the left globe as well as bulging of the anterior chamber (arrow, panel C). The expanded globe is caused by congenital glaucoma or buphthalmos.

café-au-lait spots, Lisch nodules, peripheral neurofibromas, and, in only 5 to 10% of patients, central nervous system tumors. NF-1 accounts for more than 90% of all cases of neurofibromatosis. The diagnostic criteria for this disease are described as two or more of the following: (1) six or more café-au-lait macules over 5 mm in greatest diameter (over 15 mm in greatest diameter in postpubertal individuals); (2) two or more neurofibromas of any type or one plexiform neurofibroma; (3) freckling in the axillary or inguinal areas; (4) optic glioma; (5) two or more Lisch nodules (iris hamartomas); (6) a distinctive osseous lesion, such as sphenoid dysplasia or thinning of a long bone cortex, with or without

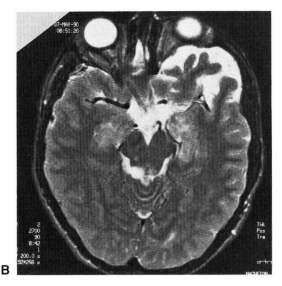

B

SE 2,700/90

pseudoarthrosis; and (7) a first-degree relative (parent, sibling, or offspring) with NF-1 also established by these criteria.

Patients with NF-1 may manifest certain structural intracranial abnormalities such as aqueductal stenosis. They may also have dysplasias of the cerebral vasculature. A common structural anomaly with NF-1 is very severe congenital glaucoma, which is typically unilateral. This anomaly is referred to as buphthalmos and may be associated with a large orbital plexiform neurofibroma or with dysplasia of the sphenoid wing leading to secondary pulsatile proptosis (Figure 18-7).

NF-2 represents the central form of NF and probably stems from an abnormality within a gene locus near the center of the long arm of chromosome 22 **(Option (A) is true).** Although much less common than NF-1, NF-2 demonstrates a near-100% penetrance.

Patients with NF-2 may present early in life with mental retardation and seizure disorders or, more typically, may display initial symptoms in their teens or early twenties. Neurologic symptoms are related to the specific locations of the patient's tumors, and the most common symptoms include hearing loss, facial weakness, sensory and visual changes, and headaches. Characteristically, meningiomas, tumors of various cranial nerves, and bilateral acoustic schwannomas are seen, with the bilateral acoustic schwannomas representing the most frequent intracranial manifestation of NF-2 (Figures 18-1 and 18-2) **(Options (D) and (E) are true).** Multiple glial neoplasms, hamartomas, meningoangiomatosis, and

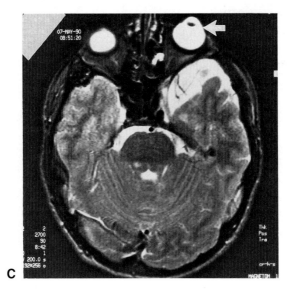

C

SE 2,700/90

areas of heterotopic tissue are also associated with NF-2. Unlike patients with NF-1 (Figure 18-8), patients with NF-2 almost never have optic nerve or chiasmal gliomas **(Option (F) is false)**. Intraspinal manifestations of NF-2 include intradural extramedullary neurofibromas or meningiomas, intramedullary ependymomas (Figure 18-1E), astrocytomas, and syringohydromyelia (Figure 18-9). Plexiform neurofibromas are extremely rare in patients with NF-2 **(Option (B) is false)**. The diagnostic criteria for NF-2 consist of either one of the following: (1) bilateral eighth-nerve masses seen with CT or MRI or (2) NF-2 in a first-degree relative and either a unilateral eighth-nerve mass or two of the following: neurofibroma, meningioma, glioma, schwannoma, or juvenile posterior subcapsular lenticular opacity.

Despite the propensity toward multiplicity, pathologically the tumors in patients with NF-2 are the same as those that occur sporadically in other patients. However, the hamartomatosis process of meningoangiomatosis demonstrates an infiltration of meningothelial cells and small blood vessels into the brain cortex. Areas of heterotopic tissues include clusters of atypical glial cells, subependymal glial nodules, ependymal ectopias, and intramedullary schwannosis. Heterotopias are found most frequently in the cerebral cortex and less often in the basal ganglia, hypothalamus, cerebral peduncles, and spinal cord. Recent investigators have demonstrated a proximal direct and possibly a causal relationship between heterotopias and neoplastic lesions.

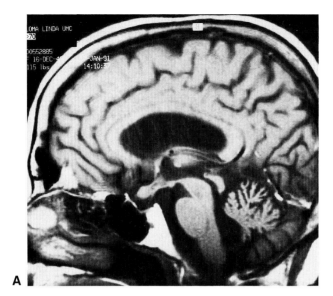

SE 600/15

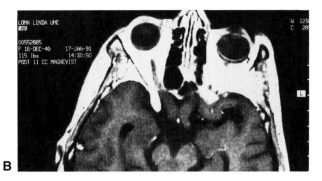

SE 600/15

*Figure 18-8.* Neurofibromatosis 1. (A) Sagittal MR image. There is marked thickening of the optic chiasm with deformity of the prechiasmatic sulcus. There are high-intensity lesions along the margin of the medial tentorium that are caused by ossifications with associated marrow formation. (B) Postcontrast axial MR image. The expanded cranial portions of the optic nerves and optic chiasm are clearly visible. There is no evidence of enhancement. The findings are characteristic of a low-grade neoplasm of the optic nerves and chiasm.

Certain structural anomalies are also seen in association with NF-2 but are not obligatory components of the disorder. These anomalies include meningocele, aqueductal stenosis, arachnoid cysts, hydrocephalus, macrocranium, and cerebrovascular occlusions.

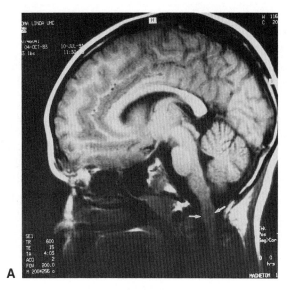

SE 600/15

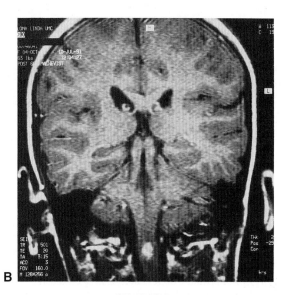

SE 600/15

*Figure 8-9.* Neurofibromatosis 2. The patient from whom these images were obtained was the daughter of the test patient. (A) Sagittal MR image. There is focal expansion of the upper cervical cord, with a hypointense central portion (arrows). (B) Postcontrast coronal MR image. A homogeneously enhancing nodule is present in the upper cervical cord. This intramedullary neoplasm was demonstrated on a routine screening MR image and was not associated with clinical findings.

In addition to multiple tumors, certain nontumoral radiologic manifestations of NF-2 have been described. Calcifications are well known to occur with many tumors, particularly meningiomas. However, cerebellar, subependymal, and abnormal choroid plexus calcifications are now being recognized as early, perhaps even prodromic, features of NF-2. Abnormal, extensive calcification of the choroid plexus of the lateral ventricles involves the entire choroid plexus from the foramen of Monro to the temporal horn of one or both lateral ventricles. Third ventricular choroid plexus calcifications also occur. Calcifications involving the cerebellum are nodular and occasionally almost confluent, favoring a location peripherally in the folia of the cerebellar hemispheres. These calcifications may be related to foci of meningoangiomatosis. Subependymal calcifications similar to those seen in tuberous sclerosis have also been associated with NF-2.

Cranial MR scans of patients with NF-1 or NF-2 have demonstrated relatively well-defined areas of hyperintensity on T2-weighted images within the basal ganglia, internal capsule, midbrain, cerebellum, or subcortical white matter **(Option (C) is true)** (Figure 18-1D). More recently, attention to T1-weighted images has revealed areas that are also hyperintense with respect to cerebral white matter and that involve the globus pallidus and occasionally the posterior lateral portion of the thalamus. These areas are always bilateral and are usually symmetrical. Frequently there is communication across the anterior commissure, resulting in a dumbbell configuration. These areas of T1 shortening correspond to the above-mentioned areas of T2 lengthening, although the former findings are usually more extensive. It has been speculated that these areas of abnormal signal intensity are related to Schwann cell heterotopias or melanin deposits. In no case has associated edema, enhancement with gadolinium chelates, or neoplasia been found.

High-resolution imaging is important for diagnosis and follow-up in patients with NF-1 and NF-2. MRI has superseded CT as the method of choice, because of its increased sensitivity for small asymptomatic lesions and its better visualization of the posterior fossa. Additionally, changes within the basal ganglia have been reliably identified only with MRI. For the same reasons, MRI is the method of choice for screening asymptomatic first-degree relatives of patients.

Current treatment options for NF-2 are limited and are directed toward symptomatic, potentially symptomatic, and progressive lesions. Specifically, the high frequency of bilateral acoustic schwannomas and the potential for deafness require regular screening and early intervention.

No therapy to retard either the appearance or the growth rate of the multiple associated tumors is currently available.

## Question 77

Concerning multiple leptomeningeal metastases,

(A) most patients have hydrocephalus
(B) they typically result from further dissemination of an intraventricular metastasis
(C) involvement of the cranial nerves is best evaluated by T2-weighted MRI
(D) in adults they are most commonly seen with adenocarcinoma
(E) they are usually asymptomatic

Both metastatic neoplasms and primary malignant tumors of the central nervous system can disseminate via the subarachnoid cisternal pathways to locations distant from the initial tumor nidus. This type of metastatic spread may be manifested as either a diffuse spread along the leptomeningeal surfaces of the brain or loculated deposits of tumor nodules at distant sites within the subarachnoid spaces or ventricular system (Figure 18-3). The most common dissemination in children is from primitive neuroectodermal tumors (including the subtypes of medulloblastoma and ependymoblastoma) and ependymomas. Since both ependymomas and primitive neuroectodermal tumors are rare in adults, such seeding in this age group is presumably from a glioblastoma multiforme or a distant tumor. The incidence of leptomeningeal seeding from a glioblastoma is less than 5% in all age groups. The tumors that most commonly seed to the leptomeninges are sarcomas, carcinomas, and particularly adenocarcinomas (of the breast, colon, stomach, or kidneys) **(Option (D) is true).** Leptomeningeal metastases from various lymphoproliferative tumors are also common in both children and adults.

A large metastatic focus that involves the ependyma of the ventricular system may in turn seed throughout the CSF spaces. This type of tumor is rare **(Option (B) is false).** Both primary and metastatic intraventricular tumors shed tumor cells into the ventricular system, causing seeding inside as well as outside the ventricles. These tumor cells may be deposited adjacent to the cranial nerves along their course through the posterior and middle cranial fossae.

Patients with leptomeningeal metastases most often present with a variety of symptoms, which are usually multifocal. Headache, change of mental status, cranial nerve deficits, and gait disturbances are the most common **(Option (E) is false).**

The most common change observed on contrast-enhanced CT or MRI is abnormal enhancement along the margins of the tentorium, Sylvian fissures and basal cisterns, cortical subarachnoid spaces, and ventricular walls. Metastatic deposits are visualized best on T1-weighted postcontrast images as areas of either nodular or linear enhancement following the contours of the known meningeal surfaces (Figure 18-3A). The enhancement of these tumor deposits is seen clearly on T1-weighted images against the low-intensity CSF. The T2-weighted images are less sensitive because of the surrounding high signal intensity of the CSF. Only very large nodular metastases are seen clearly on T2-weighted images **(Option (C) is false).** In most cases, hydrocephalus is not present. It is primarily in those few patients who live long enough to develop extensive disease that communicating hydrocephalus may be found. Thus in most patients, hydrocephalus is not a feature of multiple leptomeningeal metastases **(Option (A) is false).**

Intracranial leptomeningeal metastases tend to be diffuse throughout the subarachnoid spaces. Microscopically, the tumor cells infiltrate the leptomeninges as a single layer or as thicker, multilayered aggregates. The earliest infiltration is along cortical vessels and is limited to the perivascular Virchow–Robin spaces. There is no transgression of the pia. Whenever the tumor cells form larger aggregates, they may appear as "sugar coating" on the surface of the brain, in the cisterns and fissures, along the tentorium, or on the ependymal lining of the ventricles.

## Question 78

Concerning meningiomatosis,

    (A) it is usually a manifestation of dissemination from a single neoplasm
    (B) it is usually a familial disease
    (C) it is a specific form of phakomatosis
    (D) it is a common component of neurofibromatosis 1

Meningiomatosis is a distinct clinical syndrome characterized by multicentric meningiomas, usually of the en plaque variety, although more-nodular masses may also be present. These multiple meningiomas show an extensive diffuse distribution that involves the leptomeninges without the accompaniment of large circumscribed masses (Figure 18-5). These neoplasms infiltrate the brain from multiple sites and do not represent dissemination of a single tumor **(Option (A) is false).** Microscopically, the subarachnoid tumor infiltrate frequently dips into the sulci and spreads along the Virchow–Robin spaces. These concentric perivascular cellular perforations are indistinguishable from the cells of an endotheliomatous meningioma.

It is now well established that patients with multiple meningiomas or meningiomatosis have only one of the chromosome 22 pair. The loss of heterozygosity at the level of chromosome 22 is an important step in all meningioma tumorigenesis. This disease is thought to be familial since several kindred with multiple meningiomas have been identified, many of whom reveal a loss of one chromosome 22 **(Option (B) is true).**

The meningiomatosis syndrome appears to represent a specific form of phakomatosis **(Option (C) is true),** separate from NF-1 or NF-2 **(Option (D) is false).** It is similar to NF-1 and NF-2 in that there is a chromosomal basis for the disease. It is even close in its cytogenetics to NF-2, with the loss of one chromosome 22. As mentioned above, NF-2 has a likely gene locus abnormality on the center of the long arm of chromosome 22.

*Anton N. Hasso, M.D.*
*Monika L. Kief-Garcia, M.D.*

## SUGGESTED READINGS

### NEUROFIBROMATOSIS AND MENINGIOMATOSIS

1. Aoki S, Barkovich AJ, Nishimura K, et al. Neurofibromatosis types 1 and 2: cranial MR findings. Radiology 1989; 172:527–534
2. Bognanno JR, Edwards MK, Lee TA, Dunn DW, Roos KL, Klatte EC. Cranial MR imaging in neurofibromatosis. AJR 1988; 151:381–388
3. Mayfrank L, Mohadjer M, Wullich B. Intracranial calcified deposits in neurofibromatosis type 2. A CT study of 11 cases. Neuroradiology 1990; 32:33–37
4. Mirowitz SA, Sartor K, Gado M. High-intensity basal ganglia lesions on T1-weighted MR images in neurofibromatosis. AJR 1990; 154:369–373
5. Neurofibromatosis. Conference statement. National Institutes of Health Consensus Development Conference. Arch Neurol 1988; 45:575–578
6. Wertelecki W, Rouleau GA, Superneau DW, et al. Neurofibromatosis 2: clinical and DNA linkage studies of a large kindred. N Engl J Med 1988; 319:278–283

## LEPTOMENINGEAL METASTASES

7. Bentson JR, Steckel RJ, Kagan AR. Diagnostic imaging in clinical cancer management: brain metastases. Invest Radiol 1988; 23:335–341
8. Krol G, Sze G, Malkin M, Walker R. MR of cranial and spinal meningeal carcinomatosis: comparison with CT and myelography. AJR 1988; 151:583–588
9. Lee YY, Tien RD, Bruner JM, DePena CA, VanTassel P. Loculated intracranial leptomeningeal metastases: CT and MR characteristics. AJR 1990; 154:351–359
10. Russell DS, Rubinstein LJ. Pathology of tumours of the nervous system, 5th ed. Baltimore: Williams & Wilkins; 1989:825–841

## RUPTURED DERMOID CYSTS

11. Smith AS, Benson JE, Blaser SI, Mizushima A, Tarr RW, Bellon EM. Diagnosis of ruptured intracranial dermoid cyst: value of MR over CT. AJNR 1991; 12:175–180

## LYMPHOMA

12. Jack CR Jr, O'Neill BP, Banks PM, Reese DF. Central nervous system lymphoma: histologic types and CT appearance. Radiology 1988; 167:211–215
13. Schwaighofer BW, Hesselink JR, Press GA, Wolf RL, Healy ME, Berthoty DP. Primary intracranial CNS lymphoma: MR manifestations. AJNR 1989; 10:725–729

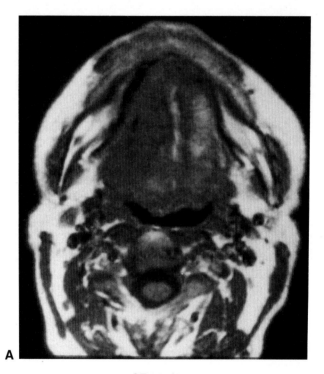

A

SE 800/20

*Figure 19-1.* This 50-year-old man has a newly diagnosed carcinoma of the tongue. You are shown T1- and T2-weighted axial MR scans (A and B), as well as axial and coronal T1-weighted scans obtained after intravenous administration of gadolinium DTPA (C and D).

# Case 19: Carcinoma of the Tongue

## Question 79

The tumor involves the:

    (A) free margin of the tongue
    (B) contralateral tongue
    (C) mandible
    (D) floor of the mouth
    (E) pterygoid plate

The tongue can be divided into two general regions: the anterior (or mobile) portion and the posterior (or pharyngeal) portion, which is also known as the base of the tongue. The tongue is readily accessible to direct examination, and so most tumors, especially those of the anterior tongue, are readily detected clinically. Usually the radiologist's role in imaging is to determine the depth of the lesion.

As an example, the tumor presented in the test case (Figure 19-1) would be easily visible on clinical examination of the patient's mouth. The images show this superficial involvement of the lateral margin of the tongue **(Option (A) is true)** but also show the deeper extension of the tumor. The lesion, though large and infiltrating, does not violate the midline **(Option (B) is false)** (Figure 19-2). The midline is an important landmark when a surgeon is deciding how much of the tongue must be removed. Also, the closer a lesion is to the midline, the more likely it is to spread to contralateral cervical lymph nodes. Because of the extensive lymphatic network, however, contralateral nodes can be involved even if the tumor does not cross midline.

On the coronal postcontrast scan (Figure 19-1D), the abnormality can be followed inferiorly along the lateral border of the geniohyoid/genioglossus muscle complex and then across the floor of the mouth **(Option (D) is true).** The tumor does seem to "climb" slightly along the tonsillar pillar or fossa, but at this point there is no deep invasion and the mandible is not involved. The signal void of the cortex of the mandible is

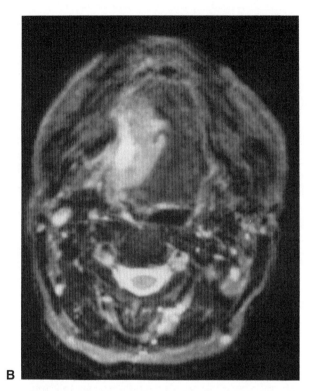

B

SE 2,727/80

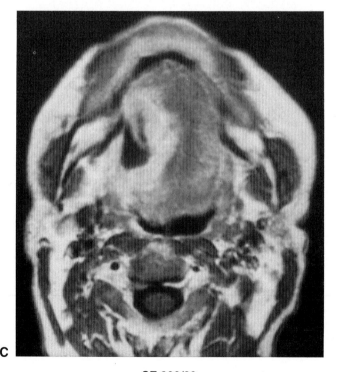

C

SE 800/20

*Figure 19-1 (Continued)*

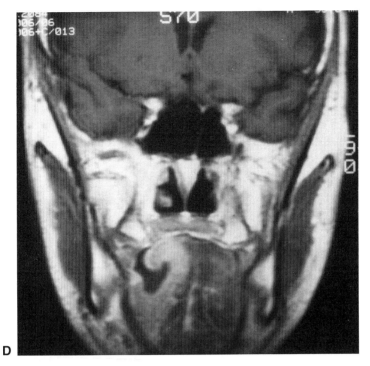

SE 2,727/80

intact, and the bright signal of the mandibular marrow fat is not obliterated **(Option (C) is false).** The pterygoid plates are seen superiorly and are easily separated from the abnormality **(Option (E) is false).**

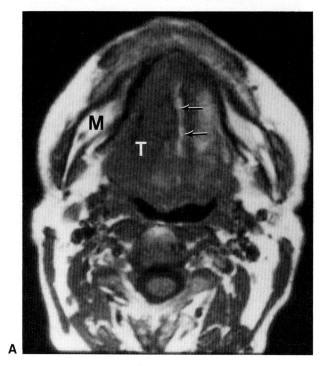

SE 800/20

*Figure 19-2* (Same as Figure 19-1). Carcinoma of the tongue extending across the floor of the mouth to the tonsillar pillar. (A) Axial T1-weighted image. The tumor (T) is difficult to differentiate from the musculature of the tongue. There is no evidence of transgression by tumor of the high signal intensity of fat (arrows) in the midline raphe. The high signal intensity of fat in the marrow of the mandible (M) is also normal. (B) T2-weighted axial image shows the higher signal of the tumor (T) compared with the uninvolved tongue musculature. (C) Gadolinium-enhanced axial image more clearly defines the edges of the lesion (arrowheads). There is extension into the region (solid arrow) of the tonsillar pillar. The tumor (open arrow) does appear to touch the lingual side of the mandible, but this actually represents the free margin of the tongue, which is separated from the mandible by the lateral oral cavity. The tumor was readily visible clinically, and its free edge was separate from the mandible. (D) Gadolinium-enhanced coronal image. The tumor (T) is seen replacing the lateral free margin of the tongue. The extension (arrowheads) across the floor of the mouth and toward the tonsillar pillar is more clearly seen in this coronal image. The pterygoid plates (P) are not involved by the tumor. The mylohyoid muscle (open arrow) is intact, and the mandible (M) is uninvolved. Again, note the high signal intensity of the fat in the midline of the tongue.

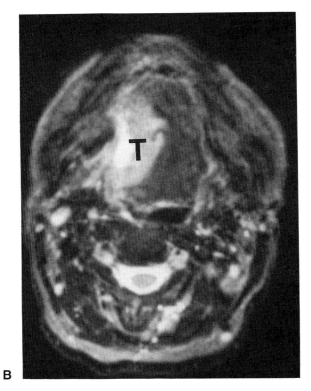

B

SE 2,727/80

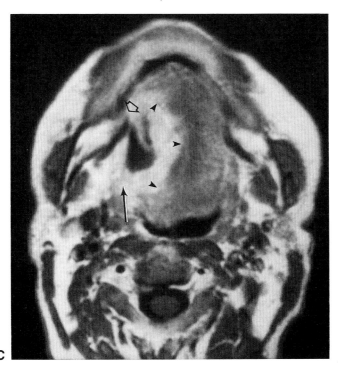

C

SE 800/20

437

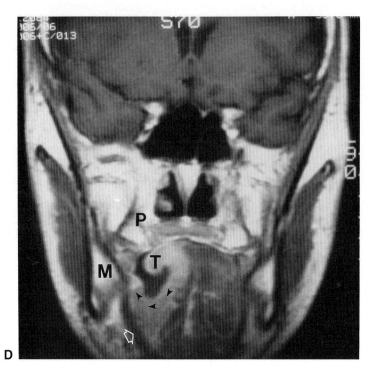

SE 2,727/80

## Question 80

Which *one* of the following is LEAST likely in a patient with carcinoma of the tongue base?

(A) Metastasis to a jugulodigastric node
(B) Involvement of the supraglottic larynx
(C) Perineural spread to the pterygopalatine fossa
(D) Simultaneous carcinoma of the esophagus
(E) Involvement of the mandible

Local extension within the tongue will determine how much of the tongue must be removed at surgery. However, extension beyond the limits of the tongue will often greatly increase the amount of surgery necessary and may have a more profound effect upon survival. The most important methods of extension away from the primary lesion are direct extension or encroachment, perineural spread, and lymphatic metastasis. Hematogenous metastasis is rare in lesions of the tongue.

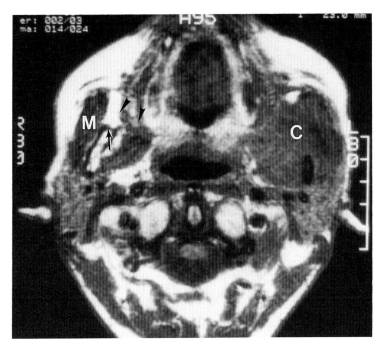

SE 500/20

*Figure 19-3.* Carcinoma of the retromolar trigone extending into the mandible. Axial T1-weighted MR image. Carcinoma (C) involves the retromolar trigone and extends into the masticator muscles. The cortex of the mandible has been destroyed, and the remaining fat of the marrow has been obliterated. Compare with the normal side. The retromolar trigone (arrowheads), masseter muscles (M), and cortex of the mandible (arrow) are indicated. Note the fat in the medullary cavity of the mandible on the normal side.

By direct extension, the tumor can spread across the floor of the mouth onto the gingival surface of the mandible. Lateral extension from the more posterior portion of the tongue brings the tumor to the region of the tonsillar pillars and fossa. The tonsillar region is in turn bordered anteriorly by the retromolar trigone, which is the mucosa-covered area along the anterior border of the mandibular ramus. Thus, although tumors localized in the tongue do not involve the mandible, several routes of extension away from the tongue bring tumor into the proximity of the bone (Figure 19-3). Involvement of the mandible (Option (E)) is one of the most significant considerations in determining the surgical procedure most appropriate for a given tumor in this region.

If a clear separation is shown between the lesion and the bone, the bone need not be resected. An osteotomy of the mandible may still be

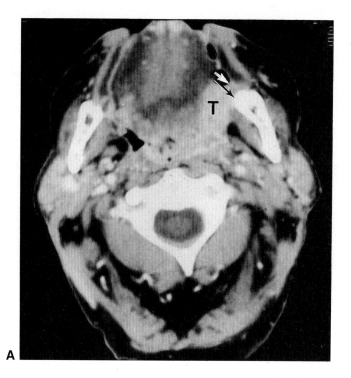

*Figure 19-4.* Tumor of the tonsillar pillar tunneling up into the soft palate and down into the tongue. (A) Axial CT scan shows obvious tumor (T) in the region of the tonsillar pillar. The lesion abuts the mandible (black arrow) but does not cause bone erosion. The retromolar trigone (white arrow) is anterior and lateral to the lesion. Compare with the opposite side. (B) Axial CT scan slightly higher than that in panel A. The tumor (T) is infiltrating into the soft palate and extending across the midline. (C) Axial CT scan, more caudal than that in panel A, shows the inferior extent of the tumor (T) as the lesion extends from the tonsillar pillar into the tongue itself.

necessary to gain access to the tumor, but this will be repaired during surgical closure. If the tumor abuts the bone but does not erode it extensively, then a marginal mandibulectomy is often sufficient. In this procedure, the cortex of the mandible is removed where it is contiguous to the tumor. However, enough of the mandible remains that this important bone is structurally intact. For significant erosion, especially when the medullary cavity of the mandible has been reached, a more extensive resection is required. A segmental resection removes a section of the body of the mandible; this is much more debilitating. Often the surgeon will re-establish the integrity of the mandible with metal plates or with bone grafts.

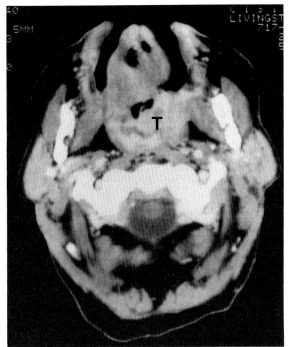

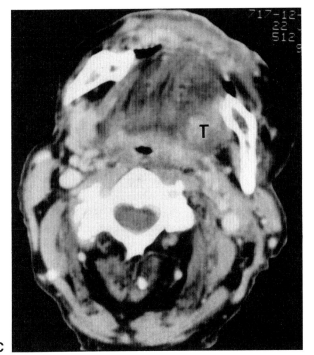

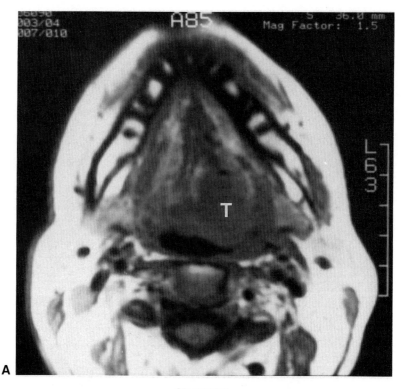

SE 500/20

*Figure 19-5.* Tumor of the base of the tongue. (A) Axial T1-weighted MR image shows the tumor (T) bulging in the lateral pharyngeal portion of the base of the tongue. (Reprinted with permission from Strong and Spiro [5].) (B) Sagittal T1-weighted MR image shows that the tumor (T) in the base of the tongue extends across the floor of the vallecula onto the epiglottis (arrowheads). Note that the lesion has not extended into the pre-epiglottic fat (arrow) of the larynx.

A tumor of the tongue that reaches the tonsillar area can extend submucosally along the pillar to reach the soft palate or even the level of the nasopharynx. This submucosal tumor spread can be undetectable clinically, and so evaluation at the time of imaging is very important (Figure 19-4). If such submucosal tumor spread is detected, this area can be included in the primary resection. Failure to identify this type of tumor extent may require the surgeon to change the surgical plan intraoperatively or, worse, may result in tumor being left at the margin of the resection.

Posteriorly, the base of the tongue borders the supraglottic larynx (Figure 19-5). Posterior and inferior extension from the tongue base

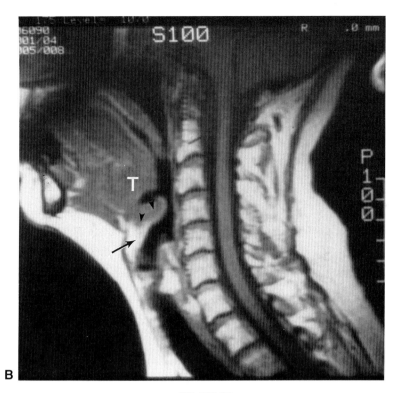

B

SE 400/20

brings the tumor to the valleculae. With further inferior extension, there is involvement of the epiglottis or the pre-epiglottic space of the supraglottic larynx (Option (B)). If there is significant involvement, a supraglottic laryngectomy or even a total laryngectomy may be required. Combining a supraglottic laryngectomy with a tongue base resection requires careful patient selection because the patient will have to learn to swallow without aspirating. This can be very difficult once a significant portion of the tongue has been resected.

The tumor can also follow the nerves out of the tongue. This phenomenon, called perineural extension, is most common with adenoid cystic carcinoma arising in the minor salivary glands, but it occasionally occurs with squamous cell carcinoma. The nerves that traverse the region of the base of the tongue are the lingual, glossopharyngeal, and hypoglossal nerves. The lingual nerve is a branch of the third division of the trigeminal nerve (V3), which passes through the foramen ovale. The glossopharyngeal and hypoglossal nerves extend posteriorly toward the inter-

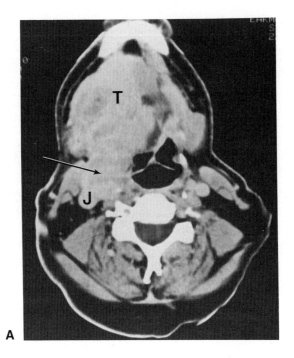

**A**

*Figure 19-6.* Adenoid cystic carcinoma of the tongue with perineural extension along the hypoglossal nerve. (A) The tumor (T) infiltrates along the floor of the mouth where there is posterolateral extension (arrow) toward the carotid artery and jugular vein (J). This would be approximately the course of the hypoglossal nerve close to the hyoid bone. (B) Slightly higher slice through the upper tongue shows the inhomogeneity of the tumor (arrows). Note the mass (arrowhead) in the post-styloid region representing gross enlargement of the hypoglossal nerve. S = tip of the styloid process. (C) Higher slice shows soft tissue mass (short arrow) between the carotid artery (arrowhead) and the jugular vein (long arrow). The soft tissue between the carotid artery and jugular vein again represents the enlargement of the nerve. MP = medial pterygoid muscle. (D) Photograph taken at surgery. The grossly enlarged hypoglossal nerve (arrows) is seen crossing the external (E) and internal (C) carotid arteries. This nerve normally should be closer to the size of the vagus nerve (arrowhead).

nal carotid artery and then through the skull base via the jugular foramen and the hypoglossal canal, respectively (Figure 19-6). Perineural extension to the pterygopalatine fossa should not occur in a tumor of the base of the tongue because the second division of the trigeminal nerve (V2), which is the nerve passing through the pterygopalatine fossa, does not have a direct connection to the tongue **(Option (C) is correct).**

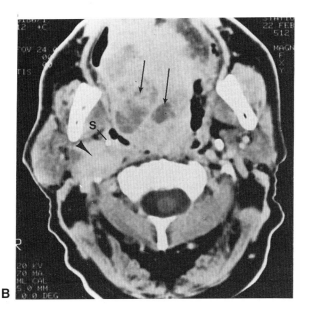

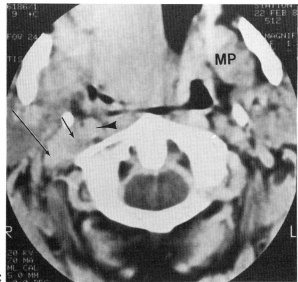

Tumors of the tongue have a very high frequency of lymphatic spread. Approximately one-third of patients with squamous cell carcinoma of the tongue will have clinically evident nodal metastases when initially seen by the clinician. The larger and more infiltrating a lesion is, the more likely it is to spread to the lymph nodes of the neck. Several nodal groups

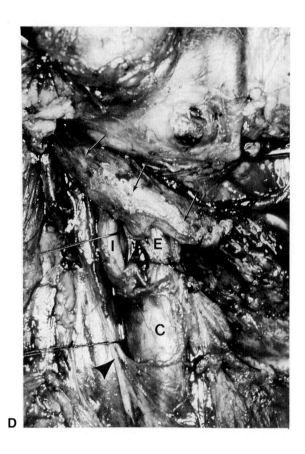

can be affected. Tumors arising in the anterior tongue and floor of the mouth often drain to the area beneath the mylohyoid muscle to either the submental nodes in the midline or the submandibular nodes more laterally. These nodes in turn drain to the jugulodigastric region, which is at the angle of the mandible just posterior to the submandibular gland. Tumors of the posterior tongue can drain to the retropharyngeal nodes or directly to the jugulodigastric nodes. In either case involvement of the jugulodigastric node (Option (A)) is very likely to occur. Bilateral nodal involvement is not unusual, especially in tumors that are large and infiltrating. The radiologist attempts to identify nodal metastasis but must realize that even nodes that are negative by imaging criteria may still harbor microscopic foci of tumor. Several studies have shown that the false-negative rate for the clinical evaluation is at least 25%, whereas the false-negative rate for imaging is closer to 10%. Many patients are treated by either neck dissection or radiation therapy of the neck even in the face of negative clinical and radiologic evaluations because delayed nodal recurrences occur in a significant percentage of these cases.

A patient with a squamous cell carcinoma of the upper aerodigestive tract has a substantial risk (10 to 20%) of developing a second, completely separate primary carcinoma. The second cancer may be present at the time of the initial diagnosis or may develop later. The second lesion is predicted to be in another site of the upper aerodigestive tract or in the esophagus (Option (D)). To exclude such a second lesion, endoscopy or a barium swallow is generally done as part of the preoperative workup.

*Hugh D. Curtin, M.D.*

*SUGGESTED READINGS*

CARCINOMA OF THE TONGUE

1. Curtin HD, Tabor EK. Radiologic evaluation. In: Myers EN, Suen JY (eds), Cancer of the head and neck, 2nd ed. New York: Churchill Livingstone; 1988:39–74
2. Dillon WP. The pharynx and oral cavity. In: Som PM, Bergeron RT (eds), Head and neck imaging, 2nd ed. Chicago: Mosby-Year Book; 1991:407–466
3. Mancuso AA, Hanafee WN. Elusive head and neck cancer beneath intact mucosa. Laryngoscope 1983; 93:133–139
4. Mancuso AA, Hanafee WN. Oral cavity and oropharynx including tongue base, floor of mouth and mandible. In: Mancuso AA, Hanafee WN (eds), Computed tomography and magnetic resonance imaging of the head and neck, 2nd ed. Baltimore: Williams & Wilkins; 1985:358–427
5. Strong EW, Spiro R. Cancer of the oral cavity. In: Myers EN, Suen JY (eds), Cancer of the head and neck, 2nd ed. New York: Churchill Livingstone; 1988:417–464

LYMPH NODES

6. Friedman M, Mafee MF, Pacella BL Jr, Strorigl TL, Dew LL, Toriumi DM. Rationale for elective neck dissection in 1990. Laryngoscope 1990; 100:54–59
7. Johnson JT. A surgeon looks at cervical lymph nodes. Radiology 1990; 175:607–610
8. Som PM. Lymph nodes of the neck. Radiology 1987; 165:593-600

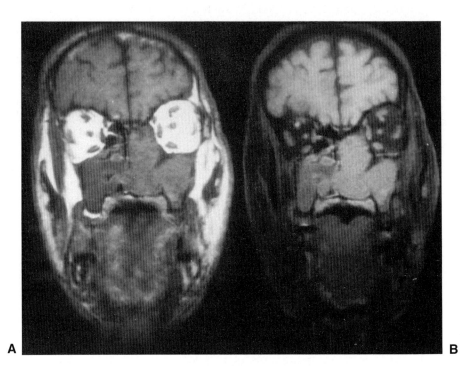

SE 600/15

*Figure 20-1*

*Figures 20-1 through 20-3.*    This 55-year-old man presented with chronic nasal stuffiness and pain. You are shown coronal T1-weighted MR images through the nasal vault without (A) and with (B) fat saturation (Figure 20-1), a coronal postcontrast T1-weighted MR image (Figure 20-2), and an axial noncontrast CT scan through the maxillary sinuses and nasal vault (Figure 20-3).

# Case 20: Squamous Cell Carcinoma of the Nasal Cavity

## Question 81

Which *one* of the following is the MOST likely diagnosis?

(A) Concha bullosa
(B) Inverted papilloma
(C) Squamous cell carcinoma
(D) Hemangioma of the nasal turbinate
(E) Nasopharyngeal angiofibroma

The test images include coronal MR scans (Figures 20-1 and 20-2) and an axial CT scan (Figure 20-3). The MR scans demonstrate a slightly enhancing mass involving the left nasal vault and maxillary sinus. The coronal T1-weighted MR scans without and with fat saturation demonstrate a fairly homogeneous mass (solid arrows, Figure 20-4) with slightly higher signal intensity than the adjacent obstructed sinus secretions (open arrows, Figure 20-4). Erosion of the lateral nasal wall is apparent. On the fat-saturated sequence, the signal intensity of the mass apparently increases. However, the absolute signal intensity is actually unchanged. The mass appears brighter simply because of the suppression of higher-intensity fat. After contrast agent administration, the mass (open arrows, Figure 20-5) enhances to a lesser degree than the adjacent mucosa (solid arrows, Figure 20-5). The axial CT scan demonstrates that the mass erodes the medial and posterior walls of the left maxillary sinus (arrows, Figure 20-6), an indication of malignant behavior. The appearance of an aggressive mass in the nasal vault with associated bone erosion is most consistent with a squamous cell carcinoma **(Option (C) is correct)**.

Aeration of the middle turbinate, termed concha bullosa (Option (A)), is a common normal variant present in 34% of individuals evaluated by coronal CT of the sinus. A concha bullosa is easily recognized on coronal

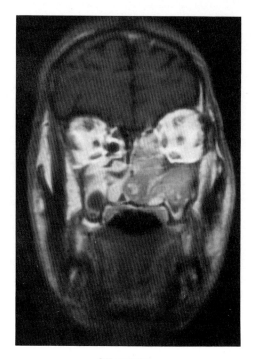

SE 600/15

*Figure 20-2*

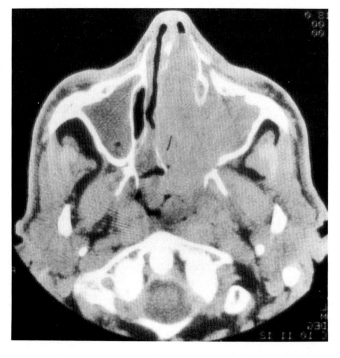

*Figure 20-3*

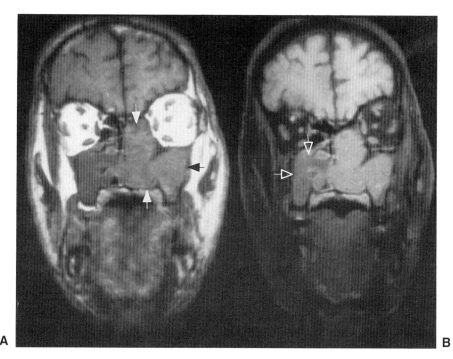

A

B

SE 600/15

*Figure 20-4* (Same as Figure 20-1).   Squamous cell carcinoma of the nasal vault and left maxillary sinus. Coronal T1-weighted MR scans without (A) and with (B) fat saturation show a homogeneous mass filling the lumen of the left maxillary sinus and nasal vault (solid arrows). The mass is slightly higher in signal intensity than the obstructed secretions within the right maxillary sinus (open arrows). In addition, there is bone erosion of the left lateral nasal wall. The tumor does not extend through the cribriform plate or into the orbit.

CT scans, appearing as an air-filled lumen of variable size (usually within the middle turbinate). The lumen of the turbinate is usually largest at its inferior margin and tapers superiorly near the junction of the turbinate with the cribriform plate (Figure 20-7). Occasionally this normal variant is large enough to obstruct the ostium of the maxillary sinus. However, its association with sinusitis is controversial. Zinreich et al. reviewed the coronal CT scans of 320 patients with symptomatic sinusitis and found no difference in the frequency of inflammatory disease in the osteomeatal complex between patients with and those without concha bullosa. However, they cited several instances in which apparent obstruction of the osteomeatal complex occurred as a result of an enlarged middle turbinate. Lloyd, on the other hand, found that concha bullosa was the

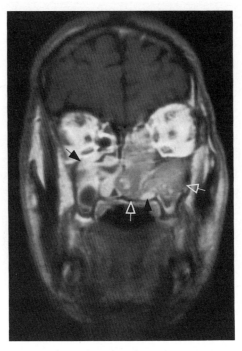

SE 600/15

*Figure 20-5* (Same as Figure 20-2). Squamous cell carcinoma of the nasal vault and left maxillary sinus. Postcontrast coronal T1-weighted MR scan through the same level as Figure 20-4. The mass inhomogeneously enhances (open arrows) but to a lesser degree than surrounding inflammatory mucosa (solid arrows).

only anatomic variant of the paranasal sinuses that was associated with an increased likelihood of sinus infection (85%). Yousem reviewed 100 consecutive coronal CT scans performed to evaluate patients with sinusitis and found that obstruction of the lumen of a concha bullosa was rare and could lead to mucocele formation of the concha (Figure 20-8). The test images do not have the appearance expected of a concha bullosa, because the middle turbinate is not aerated and a concha bullosa is not associated with destruction of the maxillary sinus walls.

Inverted papilloma (Option (B)) is one of the more common benign lesions of the nasal vault and sinuses, accounting for about 4% of all nasal neoplasms. The name is derived from its histologic appearance of papillary fronds that palisade inward toward the center of the tumor and down the stalk of the lesion, usually extending under the nasal mucosa at the base of the mass. Inverted papilloma usually arises from the lateral

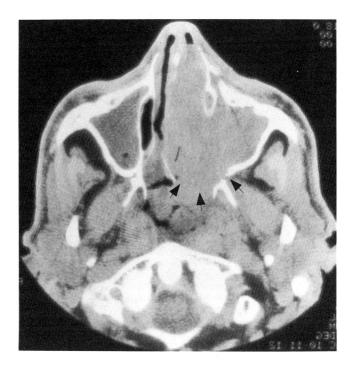

*Figure 20-6* (Same as Figure 2-3). Squamous cell carcinoma of the nasal vault and left maxillary sinus. Axial noncontrast CT scan demonstrates erosion of the medial and posterior walls of the left maxillary sinus (arrows) and deviation with possible erosion of the nasal septum. Such aggressive bone destruction favors a malignant process.

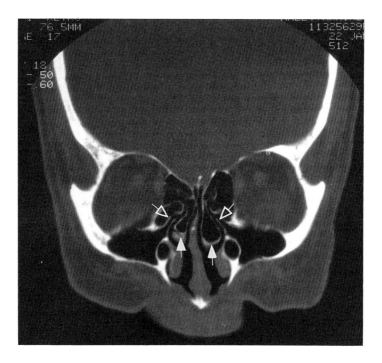

*Figure 20-7.* Concha bullosa. Coronal 3-mm CT scan through the level of the osteomeatal unit (open arrows) demonstrates bilateral conchae bullosae (solid arrows). The conchae bullosae are wider inferiorly and taper superiorly, near their attachment at the cribriform plate.

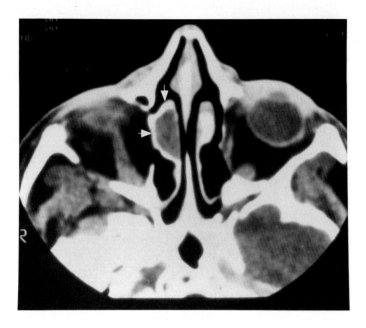

*Figure 20-8.* Mucocele of a concha bullosa. Axial CT scan through the nasal vault demonstrates an opacified expanded lumen of the right middle turbinate (arrows). A mucocele of a concha bullosa is generally surrounded by a thin rim of bone (the turbinate) and is located in a typical position. These features assist in differentiation of the mucocele from a neoplastic process.

nasal wall, and as it grows, it often results in bone remodeling of the medial wall of the sinus and nasal septum. Rarely, there is even more aggressive bone erosion of the nasal vault. The test images demonstrate a mass with aggressive destruction of the posterior and medial walls of the maxillary sinus; therefore, it is unlikely to be a benign inverted papilloma.

Hemangioma (Option (D)) is considered by most authors to be a benign tumor, although in some cases it acts like a vascular malformation. It occurs primarily in the soft tissues of the head and neck; however, a capillary hemangioma occasionally arises from the mucosa of the lateral nasal vault (Figure 20-9). In these instances, the clinical presentation usually involves a young adult with epistaxis or chronic nasal stuffiness. Unlike osseous hemangiomas, bone destruction is not a typical feature of mucosal hemangiomas. The MR features of nasal hemangioma are nonspecific. The presence of fresh or older blood products within or near the lesion on MR images may suggest the presence of a vascular lesion.

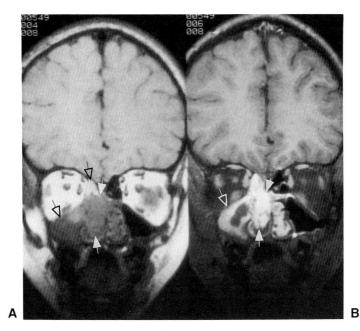

SE 600/15

*Figure 20-9.* Nasal hemangioma. Coronal T1-weighted MR images without contrast enhancement or fat saturation (A) and with fat saturation and post-gadolinium DTPA administration (B) show that before contrast administration, the right nasal mass (solid arrows) appears slightly lower in signal intensity than gray matter. Obstructed sinonasal secretions are either lower or higher in signal intensity than the mass (open black arrows, panel A). After contrast medium administration, the mass enhances (solid arrows, panel B) to an intensity equal to that of the surrounding mucosa (open white arrow) and nasal turbinates. (C) Axial T1-weighted MR image following contrast administration and with fat saturation shows intense enhancement of the right nasal mass (solid arrows). Note also the enhancement of the inflamed right maxillary sinus mucosa (open arrow).

Intense enhancement of the lesion is also the rule. In this setting, angiography is usually normal and is therefore of limited value. The test images do not show enhancement to the degree that would be expected with a hemangioma. The history also does not support the diagnosis of a vascular lesion. In addition, the presence of aggressive bone erosion of the sinus walls, as in the test patient, is not typical of a mucosal hemangioma.

Juvenile angiofibroma (Option (E)) is a benign vascular tumor that generally affects young adolescent males. Patients typically present with

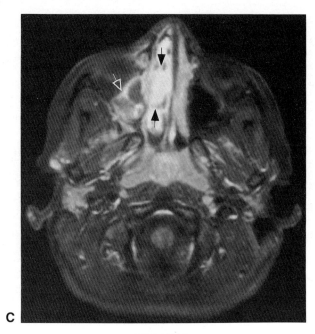

C

SE 600/15

either epistaxis or nasal congestion. The mass arises near the spheno-palatine foramen, which is located in the upper posterior nasal cavity wall. Bone destruction, when present, is centered at the pterygoid fossa, and there may be anterior bowing or remodeling of the posterior wall of the maxillary sinus. On CT or MRI, the juvenile angiofibroma intensely enhances following contrast administration (Figure 20-10). The tumor is usually slow growing and often results in bone remodeling rather than aggressive bone destruction. On angiography the tumor has a typical hypervascular blush fed by the branches of the internal maxillary artery. The age of the test patient (55 years) is not typical for juvenile angio-fibroma, the mass is not centered at the sphenopalatine foramen, and there is associated obstruction of the medial maxillary sinus wall; all of these make juvenile angiofibroma an unlikely diagnosis.

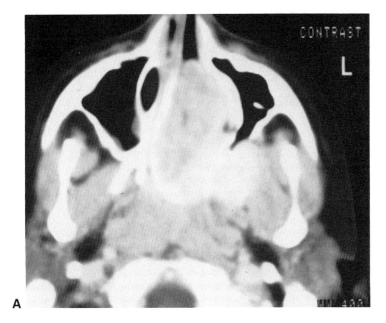

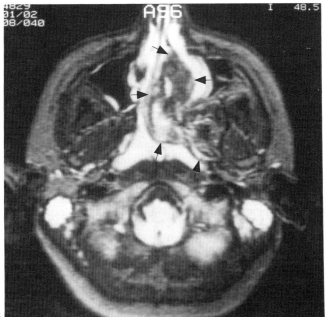

SE 2,800/80

*Figure 20-10.* Juvenile nasopharyngeal angiofibroma in a 16-year-old boy with epistaxis and nasal stuffiness. (A) Axial CT scan obtained after intravenous contrast administration demonstrates a large, smoothly marginated, intensely enhancing mass that has eroded the left pterygoid plate and remodeled the medial wall of the left maxillary sinus. (B) Axial T2-weighted MR scan shows that the mass has an intermediate to low signal intensity (arrows) relative to muscle, probably reflecting fibrous constituents within the tumor. The low signal intensity is easily distinguished from the surrounding higher signal intensity of the mucosa and lymphoid tissue.

# Question 82

Concerning inverted papilloma,

   (A) the most common site is within the ethmoid sinuses
   (B) it is associated with the development of squamous cell carcinoma
   (C) it is often confused clinically with a benign nasal polyp
   (D) bone invasion is common
   (E) it recurs after surgical resection in about 50% of cases

Inverted papilloma is a benign tumor with an overall frequency of about 4% of all primary nasal tumors. It usually arises on the lateral wall of the nasal vault near the ostium of the maxillary sinus (Figure 20-11). This tumor rarely arises within the ethmoid sinuses **(Option (A) is false).** The incidence of inverted papilloma is highest in the fifth to seventh decades. The name "inverted papilloma" is derived from its histologic appearance, which consists of centrally directed papillary fronds within the papilloma and its stalk. Squamous cell carcinoma develops from or in association with inverted papilloma in 10 to 24% of cases **(Option (B) is true).** In one study, patients with squamous cell carcinoma were older, were more likely to have epistaxis, and had less time between the onset of symptoms and clinical presentation than those without carcinoma. Nests of carcinoma may be found within or adjacent to an inverted papilloma, and it is unclear whether this represents malignant degeneration or synchronous occurrence of tumors of different histologic types. The clinical presentation and radiographic appearance of inverted papillomas are similar to those of a nasal polyp **(Option (C) is true).** If the tumor extends through the ostium of the maxillary sinus, it may be confused on imaging with an antrochoanal polyp. On CT, inverted papilloma often appears as a well-circumscribed soft tissue mass usually centered near the ostium of the maxillary sinus. Bone remodeling of the lateral nasal vault wall and nasal septum is common (Figure 20-11). Aggressive bone invasion or destruction is rare, and its presence should alert the physician to the possibility of a malignant transformation or coexistent cancer (Figure 20-12) **(Option (D) is false).** Surgical resection is required for cure. There is a high frequency of tumor recurrence if the base of the lesion is not resected. However, a complete wide surgical resection is rarely associated with recurrence **(Option (E) is false).**

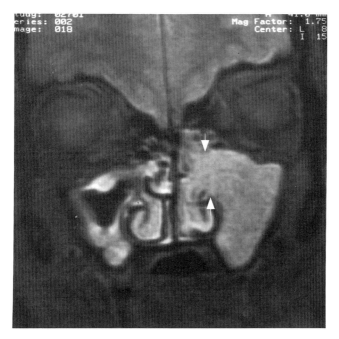

SE 2,800/80

*Figure 20-11.* Inverted papilloma. A coronal T2-weighted MR scan through the maxillary sinuses reveals a homogeneous mass with increased signal intensity extending from the left lateral nares into the left maxillary sinus (compare with the signal intensity of the inflamed mucosa in the right maxillary sinus). The ostium of the maxillary sinus is enlarged (arrows). At biopsy this proved to be an inverted papilloma. The differential diagnosis includes antrochoanal polyp and carcinoma; however, the lack of aggressive bone destruction favors a benign process.

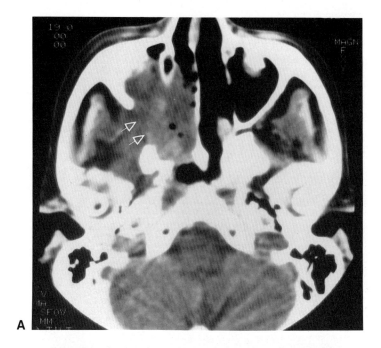

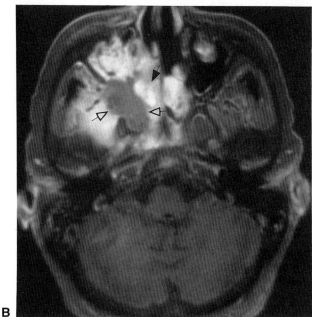

SE 600/15

*Figure 20-12.* Inverted papilloma with synchronous squamous cell carcinoma of the maxillary sinus. (A) Axial CT scan through the right maxillary sinus and nasal vault demonstrates a soft tissue mass that has eroded the posterior wall of the maxillary sinus (arrows). (B) Axial contrast-enhanced, fat-suppressed, T1-weighted MR scan through the same level as panel A demonstrates a lower-intensity mass in the region of the destroyed maxillary sinus wall and pterygoid plate (open arrows). Medially, intensely enhancing tissue (solid arrow) is evident within the nasal vault. At biopsy the nasal mass proved to be an inverted papilloma and the low-intensity mass destroying the bone proved to be a squamous carcinoma.

# Question 83

Concerning carcinoma of the nasal cavity and paranasal sinuses,

(A) adenocarcinoma is the most frequent histologic type
(B) extension into the tonsillar pillar is typical
(C) the lesions usually have a higher signal intensity than mucous secretions on T2-weighted MR sequences
(D) it cannot be reliably differentiated from lymphoma by CT

Carcinoma of the nasal vault and paranasal sinuses represents 15% of head and neck neoplasms of the upper respiratory tract. Approximately 80% of cancers of the paranasal sinuses arise in the antrum. Nearly 95% of patients are over 40 years old, and the majority are men. Squamous cell carcinoma is the most common histologic type (80 to 90%) of nasal vault and paranasal sinus cancer, with minor salivary gland carcinomas (such as adenoid cystic carcinoma, adenocarcinoma, and mucoepidermoid carcinoma) being much less common **(Option (A) is false).** Chronic sinusitis, nasal polyposis, and inverted papilloma are all associated with squamous cell carcinoma of the nasal cavity and paranasal sinuses. Patients present with a variety of symptoms that are directly related to the extent of disease. Early symptoms of nasal stuffiness or recurrent sinusitis are nonspecific complaints that often result in a delay of diagnosis of 6 to 8 months. Cancer is usually not suspected until the tumor is large and has invaded surrounding structures. Symptoms of advanced tumor growth depend on the structures involved. Extension into the orbit results in proptosis, whereas involvement of the fifth cranial nerve may lead to pain or hypesthesia. Carcinoma of the maxillary sinus rarely involves the mucosal airway, tonsils, or pharynx **(Option (B) is false).** Medial, anterior, and inferior extension produces the classic symptoms of facial swelling, visible tumor in the nasal cavity, and a tumor bulge palpable or visible (in 40 to 60% of cases) in the oral cavity. Lymphatic metastases are unusual, occurring in only 15% of patients.

MRI is useful in the evaluation of tumors of the sinonasal region for several reasons. First, it easily distinguishes obstructed sinonasal secretions from tumor. Neoplasms usually have a lower signal intensity than inflammatory secretions on T2-weighted sequences **(Option (C) is false).** Coronal and sagittal images are optimal for determining the superior extent of sinonasal tumors. Detection of tumor spread to the anterior skull base is critical for proper planning of surgical and radiation therapy. MRI may also assist in differentiating benign inflammatory disease from malignant tumor. Som et al. have demonstrated that aggressive benign diseases, such as nasal polyps, that invade the skull base can be differentiated from malignant tumors on the basis of MR signal intensity and the contour of the lesion. The presence of permeative bone destruction is more typical of malignant disease. A homogeneous mass with a low signal intensity on T2-weighted sequences is more typical of malignant disease, a feature that can be used to distinguish tumor from obstructed sinonasal secretions.

Imaging with CT or MRI cannot reliably differentiate malignant from benign disease in all cases. However, the presence of extensive osseous erosion is more typical of aggressive infectious or malignant disease than of benign neoplasms. Squamous cell carcinoma tends to be more aggressive in its appearance than other cancers such as lymphoma, but in an individual instance, CT or MR cannot reliably differentiate among the various cancers **(Option (D) is true).**

## Question 84

Concerning fat suppression in MRI,

(A) it results in high signal intensity of fat on T1-weighted sequences
(B) it improves contrast between enhancing lesions and fat on gadolinium-enhanced MR images
(C) it has a lower frequency of susceptibility artifacts than does conventional spin-echo imaging
(D) it can be used to verify a diagnosis of lipoma

Most authors agree that MRI is superior to CT in the evaluation of the nasopharynx, upper oropharynx, internal auditory canal, and skull base. However, it has some disadvantages, which must be overcome for it to reach its full potential in evaluating other regions of the head and neck. For instance, contrast-enhanced CT is still the best method for evaluating cervical adenopathy. Although MRI clearly differentiates lymph nodes from vascular structures, it is not yet as specific as contrast-enhanced CT for elucidating the internal architecture of nodes. Specifically, some researchers believe that capsular nodal enhancement and central nodal necrosis are better imaged by CT than by MRI.

Lesion enhancement on T1-weighted MR images is often poorly seen or obscured by the high signal intensity of adjacent fat. Thus, despite "contrast" administration, a loss of contrast between fat and the enhancing lesion actually results. This problem also severely limits the use of contrast-enhanced MRI in the evaluation of lesions of the orbit and optic nerve, which are also surrounded by fat.

Recently, pulse sequences that allow the high signal intensity of fat to be suppressed while maintaining the signal intensity of enhancing structures have been developed. These "fat suppression" techniques result in lower signal intensity of fat on T1-weighted images **(Option (A) is false).** Currently several pulse sequences are available for fat saturation, including STIR (short-tau inversion-recovery) imaging, frequency-selective presaturation (Chemsat), and the Dixon-Chopper two-part and three-part techniques.

STIR is an inversion-recovery pulse sequence that yields both T1 and T2 information. The inversion-recovery sequence uses a 180° radiofrequency (RF) pulse to invert the longitudinal magnetization vector. After the RF pulse, the magnetization vector begins its return to equilibrium. As it does this, it crosses over from the negative (inverted plane) into the positive plane. This is referred to as the nullpoint, since no longitudinal magnetization vector is available for a signal to be generated. One can null the signal for various tissues by varying the time (TI) between the initial 180° pulse and the subsequent 90° pulse. The nullpoint for fat is about 160 msec, depending on the TR and field strength of the magnet. Thus, if an interval of 160 msec is allowed to elapse after the initial 180° pulse before the 90° pulse is initiated, fat will not be able to participate in signal generation. Disadvantages of STIR include a relatively long imaging time, the potential to null signal from enhanced tissues, and the dependence of T1 and T2 relaxation parameters on signal generation.

Chemsat employs an RF pulse placed in the frequency axis overlying the resonant frequency of fat. Before each TR, hydrogen protons in fat are preferentially excited by the RF pulse. This signal is then spoiled by a "spoiler" gradient pulse just before the imaging sequence (Figures 20-13 and 20-14). This technique is therefore a T1-weighted spin-echo sequence with suppression of the high-intensity signal of fat. This has two important effects. First, the contrast among the remaining structures is improved, because as the signal of fat is suppressed, the gray scale dynamic range is spread over a more narrow range of signal intensities, thereby resulting in improved soft tissue contrast. Second, after contrast administration, any enhancing regions now assume the highest signal intensity in the dynamic range, resulting in improved detection of these regions of enhancement **(Option (B) is true).** The areas of the head and neck that benefit most from Chemsat imaging include the orbit, skull base, and neck (Figure 20-15).

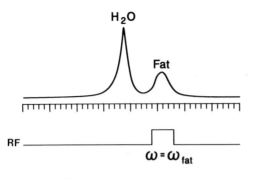

H₂O

Fat

RF

$\omega = \omega_{fat}$

**Frequency selective pulse**

*Figure 20-13.* Diagram of the chemical-shift technique of fat saturation. The spectrum shown is typical of that seen in tissues examined at 1.5 T. Protons of fat and water precess at slightly different frequencies, depending on the field strength. At 1.5 T, this separation is approximately 3 ppm. This allows separation of these two groups of protons based on their "chemical shift" (upper spectrum). A radiofrequency (RF) pulse at the specific frequency ($\omega$) of fat protons is placed prior to the slice-selective 90° RF pulse. Note that this RF pulse ideally avoids the frequency of water protons. After placement of this frequency-selective RF pulse, a "spoiler" gradient (not shown) is applied to dephase those excited fat protons. This is then followed by the routine spin-echo pulse sequence, typically a T1-weighted sequence. However, the fat protons have been previously dephased and will not contribute any signal, thus appearing "suppressed" or saturated on the image.

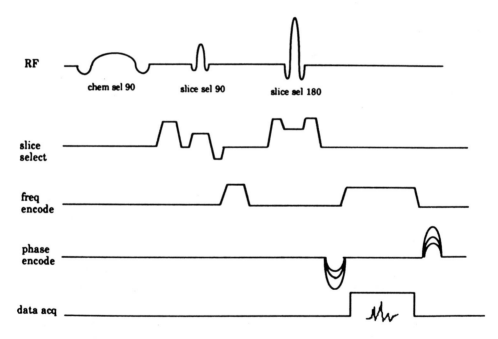

*Figure 20-14.* Diagram of a spin-echo pulse sequence incorporating a frequency-selective RF pulse for fat saturation. The chemical-shift-selective RF pulse is placed at the frequency of fat prior to the slice-selective 90° RF pulse. Following this RF pulse, the routine spin-echo pulse sequence ensues. chem sel 90 = chemical-shift-selective 90° pulse; slice sel 180 = slice-selective 180° RF refocusing pulse; slice select = slice-selective gradient pulses; freq encode = frequency-encoding gradient pulses; phase encode = phase-encoding gradient pulses; data acq = spin-echo data acquisition.

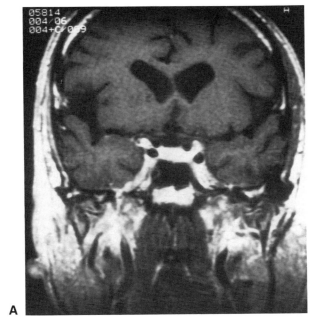

SE 600/15

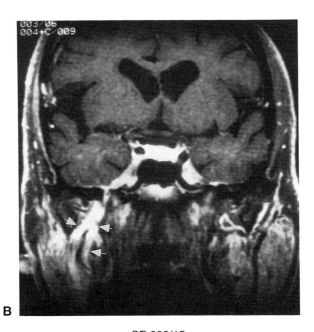

SE 600/15

*Figure 20-15.* Squamous cell carcinoma extending along the third division of the fifth cranial nerve. (A) Coronal contrast-enhanced T1-weighted MR image without fat saturation demonstrates no obvious abnormality in the region of the right foramen ovale or masticator space. (B) Coronal contrast-enhanced T1-weighted MR image with fat saturation demonstrates abnormal enhancement of the branches of the third division of the fifth cranial nerve (arrows) consistent with perineural extension of squamous cell carcinoma toward the cavernous sinus.

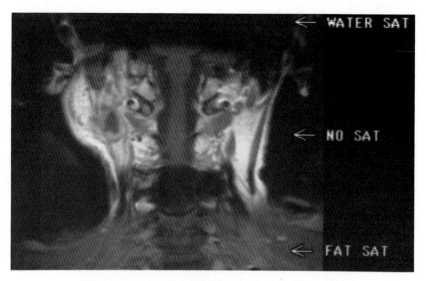

SE 600/15

*Figure 20-16.* Susceptibility artifact with the fat-saturation technique. Coronal contrast-enhanced T1-weighted MR image through the skull base and thoracic inlet shows three bands of saturation heterogeneity. Fat has been saturated inferiorly near the thoracic inlet. There is no fat saturation or water saturation in the mid-neck. There is increased susceptibility artifact and saturation of water protons through the skull base. These bands of saturation heterogeneity are due to the position-dependent changes in spectral frequency of fat and water protons. When a fat-saturation pulse is then applied to a particular frequency, it may result in fat saturation, no saturation, or water saturation, depending on the location within the body.

Some cases of chemical-shift fat saturation are associated with an interesting but annoying artifact. In these instances, the fat saturation is incomplete and magnetic susceptibility artifacts are increased over those in routine spin-echo sequences **(Option (C) is false).** This problem is most likely to occur at areas of changing body contour such as the junctions of the neck and head and of the neck and chest (Figure 20-16). At these sites, the change in body volume results in magnetic susceptibility gradients, which in turn cause a shift of the frequencies of hydrogen protons within fat and water. The protons within fat in one part of the body (e.g., the neck) may therefore resonate at a different frequency from those in an adjacent part of the body (e.g., the head). The frequency range of the saturation pulse may therefore not include all of the fat protons, and thus some will escape saturation. An additional problem that results from the shift of these frequencies is that the chemical-shift frequency of

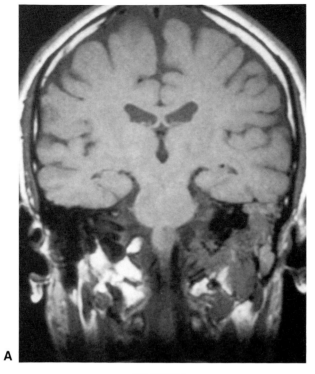

SE 600/15

*Figure 20-17.* Squamous cell carcinoma of the temporal bone with fat-saturation artifact. (A) Coronal noncontrast T1-weighted MR image demonstrates a soft tissue mass involving the left temporal bone. (B) Coronal contrast-enhanced T1-weighted MR image without fat saturation demonstrates diffuse enhancement of the neoplasm involving the left temporal bone (arrows). (C) Coronal contrast-enhanced T1-weighted MR image following an RF fat-saturation pulse shows that susceptibility artifacts near the skull base have resulted in a spectral shift of water and fat protons, resulting in "water saturation" rather than fat saturation. This has caused a diminution of the signal of the neoplasm (arrows). Thus it is possible that enhancing lesions may actually be obscured with fat-saturation techniques.

the hydrogen protons in water in one area of the body overlaps the frequency of the fat protons in another area of the body. If this occurs, the saturation pulse will saturate both the hydrogen protons in water at the first site and the fat protons in the other site (Figure 20-16). Gadolinium may also be obscured by this process. This effect is especially severe for enhancing lesions at the skull base and at the thoracic inlet (Figure 20-17). These artifacts can be reduced by placing water bags

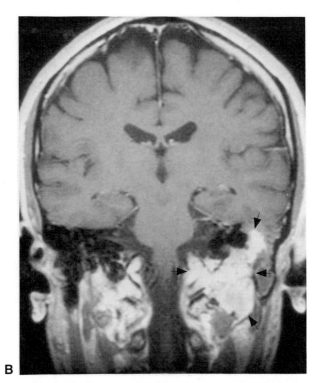

B

SE 600/15

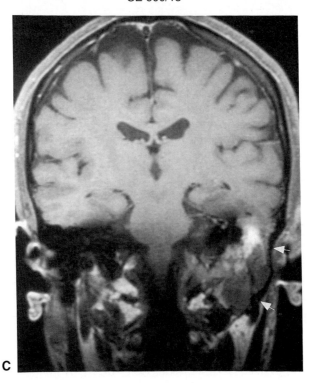

C

SE 600/15

468

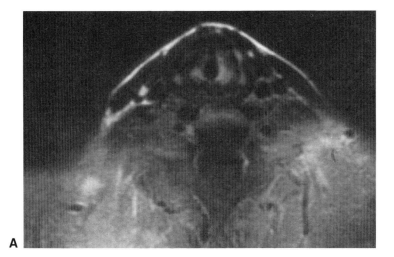

SE 600/15

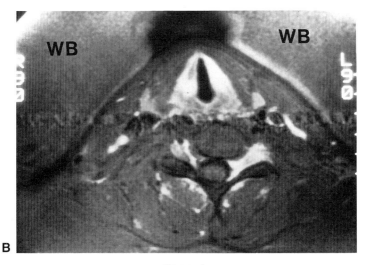

SE 600/15

*Figure 20-18.* The use of water bags to reduce fat-saturation artifacts. (A) Transaxial T1-weighted MR scan with fat saturation demonstrates water saturation rather than fat saturation through the larynx, resulting in a decrease in signal intensity of muscles as well as laryngeal soft tissues. (B) Same slice as panel A after contrast medium administration and positioning of water bags (WB) overlying the anterior neck. The use of a volume-filling substance such as small intravenous solution bags placed over the neck results in a diminution in the artifacts related to fat saturation, and thus more homogeneous fat saturation is achieved.

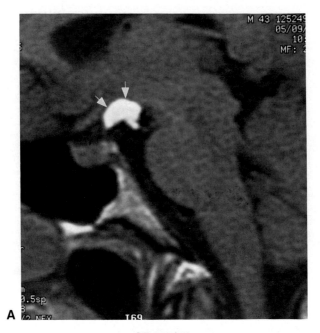

SE 600/15

*Figure 20-19.* Lipoma of the tuber cinereum simulating an aneurysm. This 45-year-old man presented with headache and an MR study suggestive of a thrombosed basilar tip aneurysm. (A) Sagittal T1-weighted MR image without fat saturation demonstrates a focal area of high signal intensity near the tip of the basilar artery in the suprasellar cistern (arrows). The lack of an obvious chemical-shift artifact made the diagnosis of lipoma exceedingly difficult. (B) Axial T2-weighted MR image through the suprasellar cistern demonstrates a hypointense mass adjacent to the tip of the basilar artery (arrows), suggesting either a thrombosed aneurysm or possibly a lipoma. (C) Sagittal T1-weighted MR image following fat saturation demonstrates absence of signal within the suprasellar cistern (arrows), indicating the lipomatous nature of this mass. This obviated further investigation for aneurysm and established the diagnosis of lipoma of the tuber cinereum.

(small intravenous bags) around the patient's neck in an attempt to make the volume of the neck similar to that of either the head or the chest (Figure 20-18).

The utility of fat-saturation techniques is primarily in the detection of gadolinium-enhancing abnormalities adjacent to or within fat. However, another valuable use of this technique is in the verification of fatty lesions that are too small to demonstrate a chemical-shift artifact. For instance, a small lipoma may be confused with a focal area of hemorrhage on

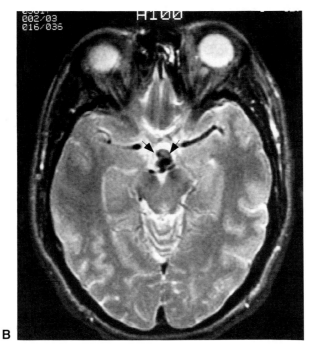

SE 2,800/80

T1-weighted images of the brain. If the fat-saturation pulse is used in this case, hemorrhagic lesions will not be saturated and will remain high in signal intensity while fatty lesions will be saturated and will show a decreased signal intensity (Figure 20-19). Thus the diagnosis of lipoma can be verified by using the fat-saturation technique **(Option (D) is true).**

*William P. Dillon, M.D.*

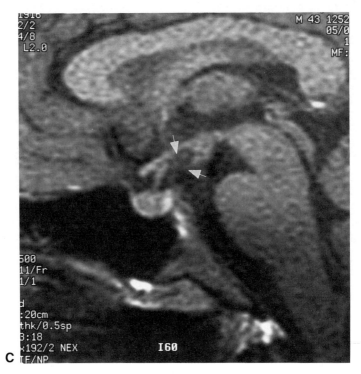

SE 600/15

## SUGGESTED READINGS

### SINONASAL CARCINOMAS

1. Batsakis JG. Tumors of the head and neck: clinical and pathological considerations, 2nd ed. Baltimore: Williams & Wilkins; 1984:177–187
2. Parsons JT, Mendenhall WM, Mancuso AA, Cassisi NJ, Million RR. Malignant tumors of the nasal cavity and ethmoid and sphenoid sinuses. Int J Radiat Oncol Biol Phys 1988; 14:11–22
3. Som PM. The role of CT in the diagnosis of carcinoma of the paranasal sinuses and nasopharynx. J Otolaryngol 1982; 11:340–348
4. Som PM, Dillon WP, Sze G, Lidov M, Biller HF, Lawson W. Benign and malignant sinonasal lesions with intracranial extension: differentiation with MR imaging. Radiology 1989; 172:763–766
5. Som PM, Shugar JM. The significance of bone expansion associated with the diagnosis of malignant tumors of the paranasal sinuses. Radiology 1980; 136:97–100

### CONCHA BULLOSA

6. Calhoun KH, Waggenspack GA, Simpson CB, Hokanson JA, Bailey BJ. CT

evaluation of the paranasal sinuses in symptomatic and asymptomatic populations. Otolaryngol Head Neck Surg 1991; 104:480–483

7. Lidov M, Som PM. Inflammatory disease involving a concha bullosa (enlarged pneumatized middle nasal turbinate): MR and CT appearance. AJNR 1990; 11:999–1001
8. Lloyd GA. CT of the paranasal sinuses: study of a control series in relation to endoscopic sinus surgery. J Laryngol Otol 1990; 104:477–481
9. Yousem DM, Kennedy DW, Rosenberg S. Ostiomeatal complex risk factors for sinusitis; CT evaluation. J Otolaryngol 1991; 20:419–424
10. Zinreich SJ, Mattox DE, Kennedy DW, Chisholm HL, Diffley DM, Rosenbaum AE. Concha bullosa: CT evaluation. J Comput Assist Tomogr 1988; 12:778–784

## INVERTED PAPILLOMA

11. Benninger MS, Roberts JK, Sebek BA, Levine HL, Tucker HM, Lavertu P. Inverted papillomas and associated squamous cell carcinomas. Otolaryngol Head Neck Surg 1990; 103:457–461
12. Lawson W, Le Benger J, Som P, Bernard PJ, Biller HF. Inverted papilloma: an analysis of 87 cases. Laryngoscope 1989; 99:1117–1124
13. Lund VJ, Lloyd GA. Radiological changes associated with inverted papilloma of the nose and paranasal sinuses. Br J Radiol 1984; 57:455–461
14. Myers EN, Fernau JL, Johnson JT, Tabet JC, Barnes EL. Management of inverted papilloma. Laryngoscope 1990; 100:481–490
15. Segal K, Atar E, Mor C, Har-El G, Sidi J. Inverting papilloma of the nose and paranasal sinuses. Laryngoscope 1986; 96:394–398
16. Weissler MC, Montgomery WW, Turner PA, Montgomery SK, Joseph MP. Inverted papilloma. Ann Otol Rhinol Laryngol 1986; 95:215–221

## SINONASAL VASCULAR TUMORS

17. Bryan RN, Sessions RB, Horowitz BL. Radiographic management of juvenile angiofibromas. AJNR 1981; 2:157–166
18. Deschler DG, Kaplan MJ, Boles R. Treatment of large juvenile nasopharyngeal angiofibroma. Otolaryngol Head Neck Surg 1992; 106:278–284
19. Mehra YN, Mann SB, Dubey SP, Suri S. Computed tomography for determining pathways of extension and a staging and treatment system for juvenile angiofibromas. Ear Nose Throat J 1989; 68:576–589

## FAT SUPPRESSION

20. Atlas SW, Grossman RI, Hackney DB, Goldberg HI, Bilaniuk LT, Zimmerman RA. STIR MR imaging of the orbit. AJR 1988; 151:1025–1030
21. Barakos JA, Dillon WP, Chew WM. Orbit, skull base, and pharynx: contrast-enhanced fat suppression MR imaging. Radiology 1991; 179:191–198
22. Dixon WT. Simple proton spectroscopic imaging. Radiology 1984; 153:189–194
23. Hendrix LE, Kneeland JB, Haughton VM, et al. MR imaging of optic nerve lesions: value of gadopentetate dimeglumine and fat-suppression technique. AJR 1990; 155:849–854

24. Simon JH, Szumowski J. Chemical shift imaging with paramagnetic contrast material enhancement for improved lesion depiction. Radiology 1989; 171:539–543

25. Tien RD. Fat-suppression MR imaging in neuroradiology: techniques and clinical application. AJR 1992; 158:369–379

26. Tien RD, Chu PK, Hesselink JR, Szumowski J. Intra- and paraorbital lesions: value of fat-suppression MR imaging with paramagnetic contrast enhancement. AJNR 1991; 12:245–253

27. Yousem DM, Som PM, Hackney DB, Schwaibold F, Hendrix RA. Central nodal necrosis and extracapsular neoplastic spread in cervical lymph nodes: MR imaging versus CT. Radiology 1992; 182:753–759

*Notes*

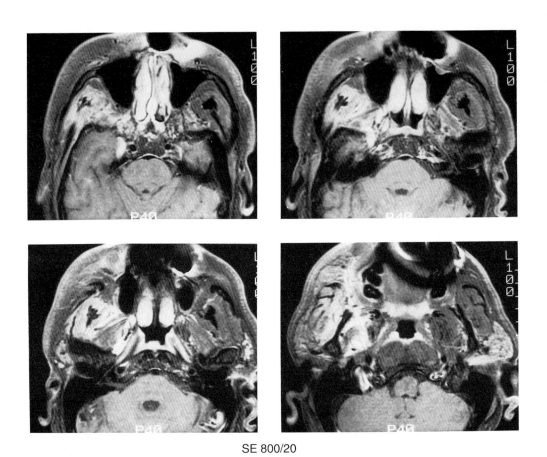

SE 800/20

*Figure 21-1*

*Figures 21-1 and 21-2.* This 38-year-old man has painful swelling of the right side of his face and numbness in the right side of his jaw and chin. You are shown axial (Figure 21-1) and coronal (Figure 21-2) MR images with gadolinium DTPA enhancement and fat saturation.

# Case 21: Masticator Space Malignant Schwannoma

## Question 85

Which *one* of the following is the MOST likely diagnosis?

(A) Lipoma
(B) Denervation atrophy
(C) Malignant schwannoma
(D) Lymphangioma
(E) Abscess

The T1-weighted postcontrast axial and coronal images (Figures 21-1 and 21-2) show an enhancing mass in the right trigeminal ganglion; this mass extends forward and downward through an expanded right foramen ovale (see Figures 21-3 and 21-4). There is extensive enhancement of the muscles in the right masticator space, including the medial and lateral pterygoid, masseter, and temporalis muscles. There is expansion of both sides of the masticator space, laterally toward the face and medially toward the pharynx. The enhancing mass follows the course of the mandibular nerve or the third division of the right trigeminal nerve as it spreads through the masticator space. There is a (pathologic) fracture of the right mandibular ramus, suggesting an aggressive neoplastic process. These findings are most likely due to a malignant schwannoma of the right mandibular nerve with extension along the nerve into the trigeminal ganglion **(Option (C) is correct)**.

Lipomas of the head and neck (Option (A)) are well-encapsulated benign lesions in the subcutaneous tissues, and nearly 50% involve the buccal mucosa. They are histologically identical to normal adipose tissue and, if large, may present as a mass and even cause nerve compression. Hemorrhage can occur within a lipoma but is rare.

Uncomplicated lipomas and the fat pads of the buccal regions have low attenuation on CT (Figure 21-5). On MRI, they have high signal intensity on the T1-weighted images; however, they do not enhance. They also are

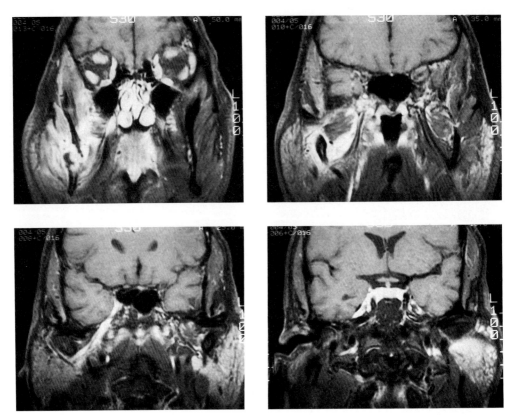

SE 800/20

*Figure 21-2*

not associated with fractures. The enhancement of the lesion in the test images, the mandibular fracture, and the extension into the trigeminal ganglion all make lipoma an unlikely diagnosis.

Denervation atrophy of the muscles of mastication (Option (B)) may occur with lesions of the brain, trigeminal ganglion, or peripheral trigeminal nerve branches. This atrophy is often secondary to metastasis or iatrogenic injury to the trigeminal nerve branches following surgery for head and neck tumors. Other causes of denervation atrophy include generalized inflammatory disease (rheumatoid arthritis and secondary temporomandibular joint [TMJ] dysfunction), biochemical denervation (such as myasthenia gravis), and trauma. Accompanying muscle atrophy is muscular fatty replacement and a high signal intensity on T1-weighted images, with obvious loss of the muscle mass. There is also muscle edema

A                                                                                          B

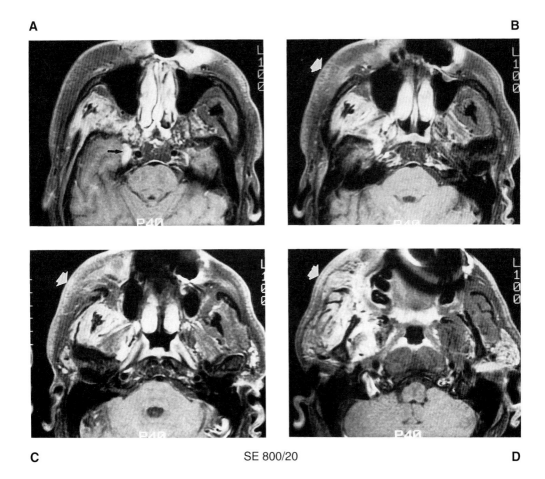

C                                          SE 800/20                                          D

*Figure 21-3*

*Figures 21-3 and 21-4* (Same as Figures 21-1 and 21-2, respectively).
Malignant schwannoma of the right inferior mandibular nerve and
trigeminal ganglion. Figure 21-3 shows axial postcontrast MR images
with fat saturation. The enhancement in the right trigeminal ganglion
is clearly seen (arrow, panel A). There is tubular expansion of the right
foramen ovale. The tumor expands the muscles of mastication and soft
tissues. Note the swelling overlying the right cheek (arrow, panels B
through D). The highly invasive tumor mass causes disruption of the
fascial planes and extends into the sockets of the teeth and buccal space.
Figure 21-4 shows coronal postcontrast MR images with fat saturation.
The transcranial course of the tumor through the foramen ovale is clearly
visible (arrow, panels C and D). The widespread disruption of the muscles
by the tumor is evident on these enhanced images. Note the pathologic
fracture of the right mandibular ramus (arrow, panels A and B).

A                                                                                    B

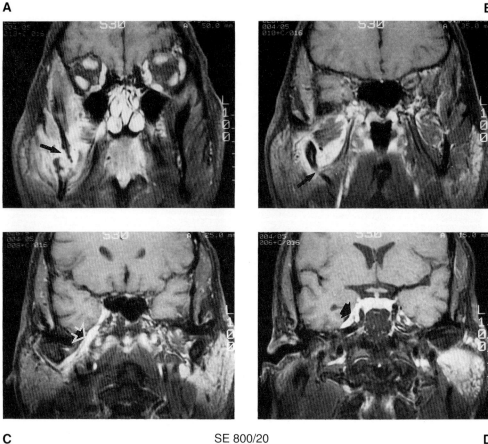

C                                    SE 800/20                                       D

*Figure 21-4*

with T2 lengthening (increased signal intensity) on the T2-weighted images during the active phase of resorption (usually within 6 weeks of injury). There is volume loss and more-extensive fatty replacement in the chronic stage (Figure 21-6). There is, however, no expansion of the masticator space as seen in the test images.

Lymphangiomas (Option (D)) of various sizes may be found in the masticator space of children and young adults. These lesions are probably congenital. There is usually a long history of facial and pharyngeal swelling, with skin and mucosal discoloration. This is in contrast to the test patient, whose facial swelling did not develop until adulthood. When masticator space lymphangiomas expand, they often extend into the adjacent deep cervical spaces, not necessarily along the course of a par-

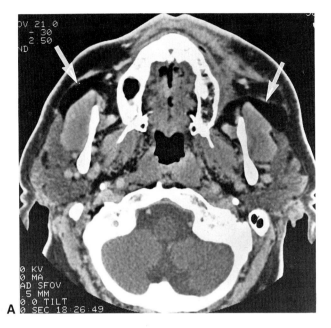

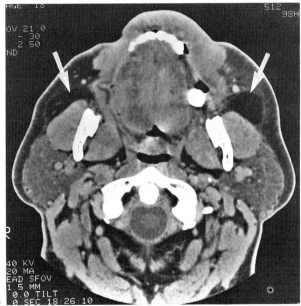

*Figure 21-5.* (A and B) Axial postcontrast CT images of buccal fat pads. There are bilateral hypointense masses anterior to the masseter muscles. These buccal fat pads lie within the buccomasseteric spaces (arrows). Note the location of the rami of the mandible, which are centered between the lateral and medial compartments of the masticator spaces.

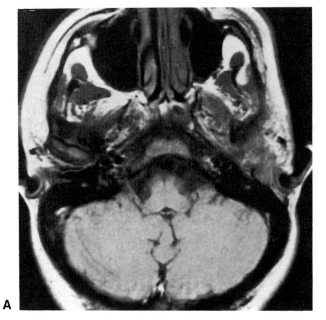

SE 1,000/20

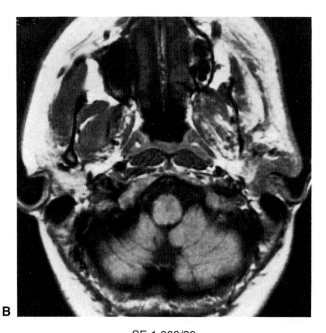

SE 1,000/20

*Figure 21-6.* (A and B) Axial MR images showing denervation atrophy in the left muscles of mastication. This 19-year-old woman underwent resection of a left facial plexiform neurofibroma. She now complains of weakness in her left jaw. Note the small size of the masticator muscles, both laterally and medially, in the left masticator space. There is fat replacement of the muscle fibers, consistent with denervation atrophy.

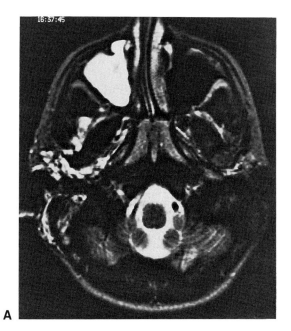

SE 2,500/90

*Figure 21-7.* Multicompartmentalized lymphangioma. (A and B) Axial MR images. This 12-year-old girl presented with a soft tissue mass in the right side of the face and the right oropharynx. There is a heterogeneous but predominantly bright soft tissue lesion encompassing the right masticator, parapharyngeal, and parotid spaces. The lesion extends through fascial boundaries and shows multiple septations, with low-intensity areas representing fibrosis, hemorrhage, or calcifications. (C and D) Coronal postcontrast MR images with fat saturation. The widely infiltrating and dramatically enhancing lesion extends in both the lateral and medial compartments of the masticator space. There is medial extension into the right parapharyngeal space, with lobular distortion of the upper pharyngeal airway. No specific areas of flow void are evident; however, the widespread enhancement suggests a highly vascular lesion.

ticular cranial nerve or its branches (Figure 21-7). The multicompartmentalized appearance of masticator space lymphangioma is unlike the unicompartmentalized lesion in the test images.

Masticator space abscesses (Option (E)) are typically secondary to odontogenic infections, penetrating injuries, or septic arthritis of the TMJ (Figure 21-8A and B). These abscesses are associated with severe cellulitis, soft tissue swelling, and disruption of the fascial boundaries within the masticator space. The pus within a well-formed masticator space ab-

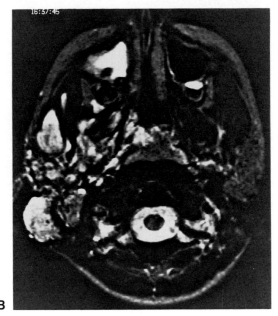

B

SE 2,500/90

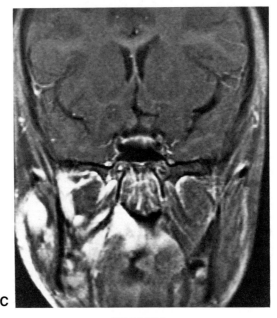

C

SE 500/20

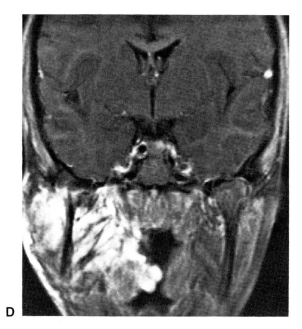

D

SE 500/20

scess would demonstrate a relatively homogeneous area of low attenuation with peripheral enhancement following contrast agent administration. There may be adjacent osteomyelitis with destruction of the bony structures (Figure 21-8C and D). The test images depict a widely infiltrating and enhancing process, without a focal area of necrosis or abscess formation, and so masticator space abscess is an unlikely diagnosis.

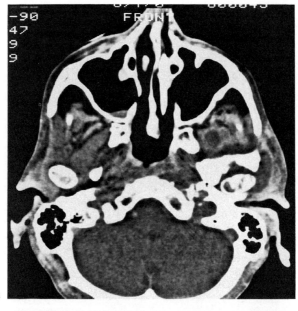

A

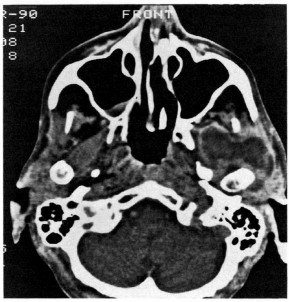

B

*Figure 21-8.* (A and B) Axial postcontrast CT scans showing TMJ septic arthritis and osteomyelitis with masticator space abscess. There is a low-attenuation lesion, which surrounds the left TMJ and extends into the adjacent parotid gland and masticator space. The lesion traverses through the condylar notch between the condyle and coronoid process. There is ill-defined surrounding soft tissue enhancement consistent with a cellulitis. (C and D) Axial bone-window CT images of masticator space abscess. There is irregular destruction of the margins of the left TMJ and of the condyle of the left mandible (arrow).

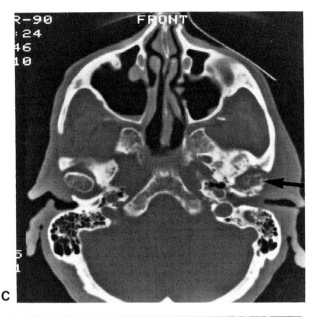

C

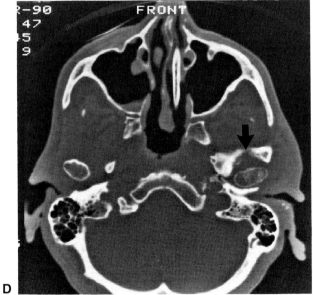

D

# Question 86

Concerning malignant schwannomas of the head and neck,

(A) they often arise in the trigeminal nerve
(B) they follow the course of a cranial nerve
(C) they rarely cause pain
(D) they are usually sensitive to radiation therapy

The masticator space is formed by a splitting of the superficial layer of the deep cervical fascia along the inferior aspect of the mandible, thereby creating a fascial sling that defines this space. The medial limb of the sling courses along the border of the medial pterygoid muscle from the caudal aspect of the mandible to the scaphoid fossa of the sphenoid bone, which is located medial to the foramen ovale. The lateral limb of the sling covers the masseter muscle from the caudal aspect of the mandible to the zygomatic arch. This fascia then continues cephalad over the temporalis muscle to attach to the skull. In the coronal plane, the zygoma divides the masticator space into a cranial or suprazygomatic portion and a caudal or infrazygomatic portion. The masticator space is readily identified on coronal sectional imaging through the mandible (Figure 21-9), and in the axial plane the mandible also divides this space into medial and lateral compartments (Figure 21-5).

The masticator space contains the four muscles of mastication, namely the masseter, the medial pterygoid, the lateral pterygoid, and the temporalis muscles. These muscles surround the central bony structure of this space, which is composed of the posterior body and ramus of the mandible, including the condylar fossa and TMJ. The nerves traversing the masticator space are all branches of the mandibular division of the trigeminal nerve (V3), which enters the masticator space through the foramen ovale. These nerves include the masticator nerve (V3 motor branch), which innervates the muscles of mastication, and the inferior alveolar, buccal, and lingual nerves (V3 sensory branches). The inferior alveolar nerve courses in the ramus of the mandible from the mandibular foramen to the mental foramen. The blood supply to the masticator space is via the maxillary branch of the external carotid artery and its branches.

The spaces adjacent to the masticator space are the buccal space anteriorly, the parapharyngeal space posteromedially, and the parotid space directly posteriorly. The buccal space has no true fascial boundaries and is therefore often simultaneously involved by masticator space abnormalities. It contains the buccal fat pad, the facial artery and vein, the buccinator muscle, and the distal portion of the parotid duct.

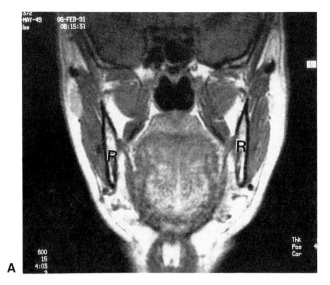

SE 600/15

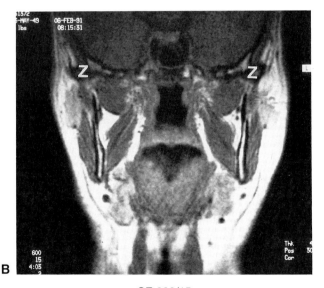

SE 600/15

*Figure 21-9.* (A through C) Coronal MR images showing normal anatomy of the masticator space. The masticator space is divided into lateral and medial compartments in relation to the rami of the mandible (R). The zygomatic arches (Z) divide the masticator spaces into superior and inferior compartments. The parapharyngeal spaces lie medial to the masticator spaces. Note the position of the parotid glands (P) posterior and lateral to the masticator spaces.

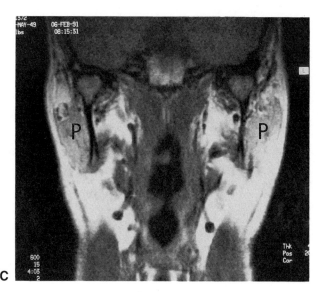

C

SE 600/15

Radiographically, a lesion is considered to arise within the masticator space when it is centered within the muscles of mastication. If the lesion is large and extends beyond the boundaries of the masticator space, it is considered to originate from the masticator space if the center of its volume is anterior to the parapharyngeal space, within the muscles of mastication or the mandible.

Imaging of the masticator space requires assessment of the entire course of V3 from the mental foramen of the mandible through the mandibular ramus to the mandibular foramen, upward into the foramen ovale and posteriorly into Meckel's cave near the petrous apex. There is frequent involvement of the adjacent buccal space, which lacks fascial boundaries, and so it is essential to image the entire buccal space, including the distal course of the parotid duct.

Primary malignant tumors of the masticator space include soft tissue sarcomas originating from the muscles of mastication, chondrosarcomas from the mandible or the TMJ, and osteosarcomas from the mandible. Malignant schwannomas of the head and neck typically originate in the masticator space from branches of the trigeminal nerve **(Option (A) is true).**

The incidence of malignant schwannomas is approximately 5 to 10% of all sarcomas and 2 to 12% of all nerve sheath tumors. Patients with neurofibromatosis type 1 (NF-1) have a 5 to 30% chance of developing a *de novo* malignant neurogenic tumor. The typical NF-1 patient with a malignant neural tumor is 20 to 50 years old, and most malignant schwannomas arise in the extremities or trunk, with the head and neck location accounting for fewer than 10% of the cases.

The most common clinical complaint in a patient with a malignant trigeminal nerve tumor is painful swelling or a discrete mass **(Option (C) is false).** Trismus occurs with a large lesion whenever the tumor restricts motion of the TMJ. Numbness in the jaw or chin, paresthesias, and muscle atrophy or weakness may develop if a major nerve trunk is affected. The tumor initially causes a fusiform, nodular swelling of the involved nerve and ultimately diffusely infiltrates the nerve, spreads into the surrounding soft tissues, and often contains areas of hemorrhage or necrosis. Approximately 30% of malignant schwannomas are between 5 and 10 cm in diameter, and another 30% are larger than 10 cm in diameter. Many malignant schwannomas contain interlacing fascicles of spindle cells with a herringbone pattern as typically seen in fibrosarcomas. The nuclei demonstrate various degrees of pleomorphism and hyperchromia.

Malignant schwannomas of the masticator space usually involve the inferior alveolar or masticator nerves. CT and MRI demonstrate a tubular mass within the nerve distribution and widening or erosion of the associated foramina of the mandible or skull base. Perineural spread proximally into the trigeminal ganglion or distally beyond the mental foramen occurs in over 50% of cases **(Option (B) is true).** On MRI, these lesions are isointense with muscle on T1-weighted scans and hyperintense to muscle on T2-weighted scans. They exhibit marked enhancement following paramagnetic contrast agent infusion (Figures 21-3 and 21-4).

Malignant schwannomas are highly malignant lesions that recur following local excision in 50 to 80% of cases. The 5-year survival rate is 50 to 75% in patients without NF and 15 to 30% in patients with NF-1. Recurrences and metastases may occur as late as 5 to 10 years following treatment. Small tumors (less than 5 cm in diameter) are associated with a better prognosis. Generally, patients with head and neck malignant schwannomas have a poorer prognosis than do those with similar tumors of the extremities, which can be treated with amputation. One factor contributing to the poor prognosis of this tumor is its resistance to radiation therapy **(Option (D) is false).**

# Question 87

Concerning hemangiomas and lymphangiomas of the head and neck,

(A) lymphangiomas typically disseminate along the drainage pathways of the cervical lymphatics
(B) large ones usually involve multiple spaces
(C) hemangiomas are typically pulsatile
(D) lymphangiomas typically destroy adjacent bone
(E) the presence of phleboliths indicates the cavernous variety of hemangioma

Hemangiomas within the head and neck present in cutaneous, mucosal, or intramuscular locations. The cutaneous variety is the classic strawberry nevus; is usually self-limited; and occurs in the skin of the scalp, neck, or face. The mucosal variety usually involves the oral or nasal cavities and presents as a palpable mass. If invasive, this form of the tumor may result in cosmetic deformity or respiratory embarrassment. Whereas cutaneous and mucosal hemangiomas are the most common tumors of the head and neck in children and are five times as common in girls as in boys, the intramuscular form of hemangioma is uncommon in the head (7%) or neck (4%).

Hemangiomas are divided into capillary and cavernous types depending on the size of the vessels. The more common form is the capillary hemangioma, which is composed of capillary-sized vessels. It occurs in the first few years of life and typically involutes by age 5 or 6 years. Because of this, many clinicians initially choose a conservative, watchful approach. If some therapy is deemed necessary, the current treatment is by steroids, compression mask, or laser therapy. Cavernous hemangiomas are also common in childhood and are composed of large, endothelium-lined vascular spaces. Thrombosis of these vascular spaces may result in calcifications, which are readily identified on CT as phleboliths. These phleboliths indicate the cavernous variety **(Option (E) is true).** Cavernous hemangiomas occur in the same location as capillary hemangiomas, although they are larger, more invasive, and less likely to regress. Unlike arteriovenous malformations or fistulas, there are no palpable pulsations or thrills **(Option (C) is false).**

The radiographic appearance of hemangiomas is variable. The classic appearance is a mass of water or soft tissue density, infiltrating through tissue planes in the cutaneous or deep soft tissue structures of the head and neck. The surrounding bony structures are not destroyed. At most, some bone remodeling may occur when a hemangioma presses against the bone for many months or years. MRI is superior to CT in defining the

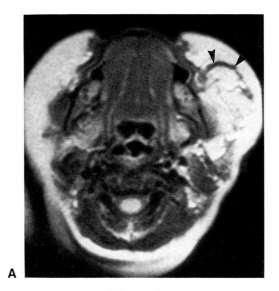

SE 2,200/30

*Figure 21-10.* (A) Axial MR image showing capillary hemangioma of the left masticator space. The lesion in the left masticator space is nearly isointense with fat on this proton-density image. There is significant contrast differential between the lesion and the muscles of the face and neck. Note the circumferential area of flow void in the anterior margin of the tumor (arrowheads). (B) Axial T2-weighted MR image of capillary hemangioma of the left masticator space. The difference in signal intensity between the lesion and the surrounding fat and soft tissues is dramatic. Again, note the area of signal void anteriorly, which represents either an arterial or a venous structure (arrowheads).

precise extent, size, and location of these lesions. CT typically underestimates their extent, since the margins are less clearly seen. Hemangiomas are isointense with muscle on T1-weighted images and hyperintense to muscle on T2-weighted images. These T2-weighted images permit clear definition of the extent of the lesion and its margins as a result of the superb contrast difference between the hemangioma and muscle (Figure 21-10). Typically, the lesion has a heterogeneous pattern because of the presence of fat, fibrosis, thrombosis, or calcifications. Cavernous hemangiomas do not contain large vessels, and so there are no signal voids on MR images as typically seen in patients with hypervascular arteriovenous malformations. Occasionally, a serpiginous channel of low signal intensity is seen within the lesion; this most probably represents a feeding or draining vessel (Figure 21-10).

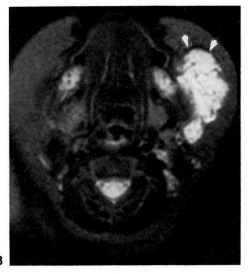

SE 2,200/80

Lymphangiomas develop from sequestered lymphatic sacs that fail to communicate with the peripheral draining lymphatic channels. These lesions are classified into three groups on the basis of the size of the lymphatic channels. The lymphangioma simplex is composed of capillary-sized, thin-walled lymphatic channels. The cavernous lymphangioma is made up of dilated lymphatics with fibrous adventitia. The cystic lymphangioma or cystic hygroma is formed by cysts ranging from a few millimeters to several centimeters in diameter. All three types often co-exist in the same lesion; therefore, they are collectively referred to as lymphangiomas. Larger lesions tend to disseminate widely in the head and neck along the cervical lymphatic channels **(Option (A) is true)**.

Nearly 75% of lymphangiomas occur in the neck, generally in the posterior triangle. Other, less common, sites are the parapharyngeal, submandibular, and masticator spaces. Surgical resection is the only effective treatment, and the success rate depends on the accurate delineation of the extent, size, and location of the lesions. Recurrence is common whenever the tumor is only incompletely removed.

CT with intravenous contrast enhancement can show the relationship of lymphangiomas to surrounding vessels but may not be able to separate the mass from the neighboring soft tissue structures of similar density. As is true for hemangiomas, MRI is superior to CT in defining the nature and extent of lymphangiomas. The typical MR appearance of a lymphangioma is of a heterogeneous lesion, isointense with muscle on T1-

weighted images and hyperintense on T2-weighted images. This reflects the predominance of the fluid-filled spaces. If the lesion is filled with concentrated proteinaceous fluid, it may be hyperintense to muscle on the T1-weighted scans. The focal heterogeneities, appearing as low-intensity linear structures of variable thickness, correspond pathologically to fibrous septa. Lesions arising in areas of loose tissue, such as the neck or axilla, have well-defined borders. Those arising in areas of more compact tissue have poorly defined borders, but there is never evidence of bone destruction **(Option (D) is false).** Differentiation between lymphangiomas and hemangiomas on MRI is impossible, unless there is specific identification of feeding arteries or draining veins. Therefore, these lesions are often lumped together and referred to as hemangiolymphangiomas. These lesions may attain considerable size and extend through the fascial boundaries into several compartments of the neck **(Option (B) is true).**


## Question 88

Concerning an abscess of the masticator space,

(A) it is commonly associated with dental infections
(B) it presents as a mass in the cheek
(C) trismus is rarely present
(D) it rarely spreads to the buccal space

An odontogenic abscess is the most common serious infection of the masticator space. Such an abscess most often results from dental infections of the second or third molar teeth **(Option (A) is true).** Common clinical symptoms and signs include cheek swelling **(Option (B) is true),** pain, and trismus **(Option (C) is false).** The infection is confined to the masticator space early in the course of the disease and may be treated by intraoral abscess drainage. When a masticator space odontogenic infection breaks out, it usually spreads from the main compartment upward to the suprazygomatic portion of the masticator space (temporal compartment) since there are no fascial barriers between the compartments of the masticator space. Simultaneous involvement of the adjacent buccal spaces, via contiguous spread to the buccal fat pad anterior to the masseter and lateral to the buccinator muscles, is common **(Option (D) is false)** (Figure 21-11). Less frequently, infections can spread inferiorly,

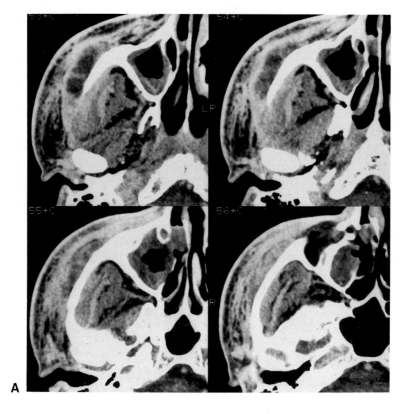

*Figure 21-11.* Abscess. (A and B) Multiple postcontrast axial CT scans showing odontogenic buccomasseteric space abscess with cellulitis. The widespread cellulitis encompassing the buccomasseteric space and masseter muscle is clearly seen. There is soft tissue disruption with enhancement of the fat and muscle structures. The well-defined abscess extends superiorly along the surface of the right zygomatic arch.

despite the existence of distinct fascial barriers, to involve the floor of the mouth and upper neck.

The roots of the teeth are related to the buccal space via the attachments of the buccinator muscle to the alveolar process of the mandible and maxilla. In most adults, the roots of the molar teeth are situated within the confines of the attachment of the buccinator muscle. In these cases, root abscesses are usually limited to the oral vestibule, medial to the cheek. However, in some adults with long roots and in children with incompletely erupted teeth, the roots extend beyond the insertion of the buccinator muscle, allowing the infection easier access to the buccal space. Involvement of multiple spaces in the head and neck

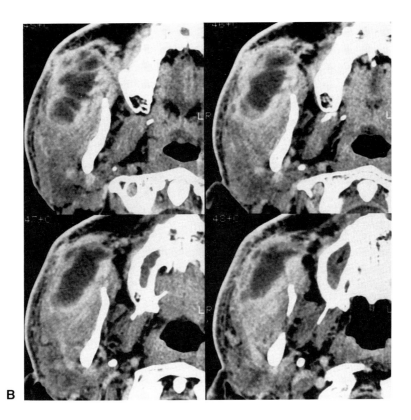

B

mandates more-extensive drainage procedures and long-term antibiotic therapy.

CT and MRI readily document both the pus collection within an abscess and the surrounding cellulitis. The extent of associated cellulitis is seen better on MRI than on CT, particularly if fat suppression imaging is used. If drainage of an infection of the masticator space is postponed, osteomyelitis of the neighboring osseous structures is likely, along with extension of the infectious process to adjacent contiguous areas including the parotid and parapharyngeal spaces. CT can accurately determine the extent of bony involvement (Figure 21-8C and D). Any bony irregularities adjacent to an abscess are strongly suggestive of osteomyelitis. When evident, osseous involvement requires subperiosteal drainage as well as soft tissue drainage of the abscess.

*Anton N. Hasso, M.D.*
*Thu-Anh Hoang, M.D.*

# SUGGESTED READINGS

## DISORDERS OF THE MASTICATOR SPACE

1. Braun IF, Hoffman JC Jr. Computed tomography of the buccomasseteric region: 1. Anatomy. AJNR 1984; 5:605–610
2. Braun IF, Hoffman JC Jr, Reede D, Grist W. Computed tomography of the buccomasseteric region: 2. Pathology. AJNR 1984; 5:611–616
3. Hardin CW, Harnsberger HR, Osborn AG, Doxey GP, Davis RK, Nyberg DA. Infection and tumor of the masticator space: CT evaluation. Radiology 1985; 157:413–417
4. Harnsberger HR. The normal and diseased masticator space. In: Harnsberger HR (ed), Handbooks in radiology: head and neck imaging. Chicago: Mosby-Year Book; 1990:46–60
5. Schellhas KP. MR imaging of muscles of mastication. AJR 1989; 153:847–855
6. Thawley SE, Panje WR. Comprehensive management of head and neck tumors. Philadelphia: WB Saunders; 1987:1253–1261
7. Tryhus MR, Smoker WR, Harnsberger HR. The normal and diseased masticator space. Semin US CT MR 1990; 11:476–485

## HEMANGIOMAS AND LYMPHANGIOMAS

8. Dillon WP. Vascular lesions of the head and neck. American Society of Head and Neck Radiology. 24th Annual Conference and Postgraduate Course, Boston, MA; 1991:125
9. Kaplan PA, Williams SM. Mucocutaneous and peripheral soft-tissue hemangiomas: MR imaging. Radiology 1987; 163:163–166
10. Siegel MJ, Glazer HS, St Amour TE, Rosenthal DD. Lymphangiomas in children: MR imaging. Radiology 1989; 170:467–470

*Notes*

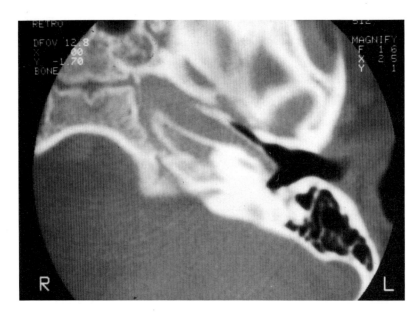

*Figure 22-1.* This 12-year-old boy presented with pulsatile tinnitus and a mass behind the left tympanic membrane. You are shown an axial CT scan.

# Case 22: Aberrant Carotid Artery

## Question 89

Which *one* of the following is the MOST likely diagnosis?

(A) Cholesterol granuloma (cholesterol cyst)
(B) Glomus tympanicum
(C) Aberrant carotid artery
(D) Dehiscent jugular fossa
(E) Facial nerve sheath tumor

Figure 22-1 shows a mass in the left middle ear (white arrow, Figure 22-2) in continuity with the petrous portion of the carotid canal (arrowheads); that is, there is no bony separation of the mass from the carotid canal. The lateral wall of the carotid canal is not seen in its normal position (Figure 22-3). Rather, it is lateral to its usual position and protrudes into the middle ear. This lesion would be visible through the tympanic membrane. The appropriate diagnosis, therefore, is an aberrant carotid artery (Figure 22-4) **(Option (C) is correct)**.

The terms "cholesterol cyst" and "cholesterol granuloma" (Option (A)) have in recent years been applied to a lesion that occurs almost exclusively in the petrous apex. The lesion begins as an obstructed air cell, and a combination of small hemorrhages, granulomatous reaction, and perhaps continuing mucosal secretion results in expansion of the air cell. Such a cholesterol cyst has sharp margins, and the lesion can erode into the carotid artery. The lesion in the test case extends directly from, rather than erodes into, the carotid canal. Therefore, this is not the most likely diagnosis. There is an additional entity also called a cholesterol granuloma, which occurs in both the middle ear and the petrous apex. This lesion is found in association with chronic inflammatory disease of the ear. Although such cholesterol granulomas also contain cholesterol clefts and granulation tissue, unlike the cholesterol cysts they do not usually result in an expansile mass in the petrous apex.

Glomus tympanicum tumor (Option (B)) can be excluded because, by definition, it arises in and is limited to the middle ear (Figure 22-5). A

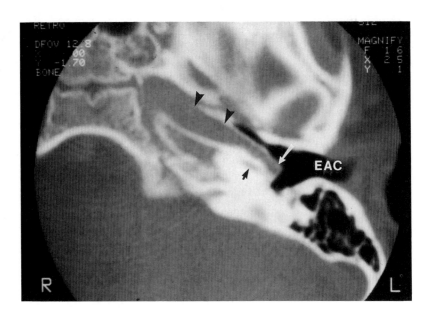

*Figure 22-2* (Same as Figure 22-1). Aberrant carotid artery. Axial CT scan. The abnormality (white arrow) can be followed directly into the carotid canal (arrowheads). There is no bony separation between the carotid artery canal and the middle ear mass, which represents a lateral position of the aberrant carotid artery. Note that it extends lateral to the basilar turn of the cochlea (black arrow). This mass would be visible through the external auditory canal (EAC).

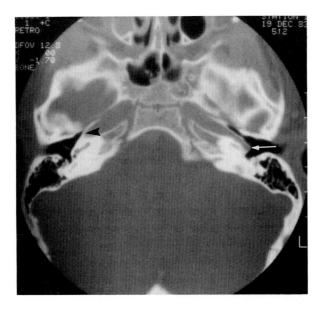

*Figure 22-3.* Same patient as in Figures 22-1 and 22-2. Axial CT scan including the opposite side. Note the position of the lateral wall of the carotid artery canal (arrowhead) on the normal right side; it is anterior to the basilar turn of the cochlea. The arrow indicates the aberrant carotid artery on the abnormal left side. (Reprinted with permission from Curtin [1].)

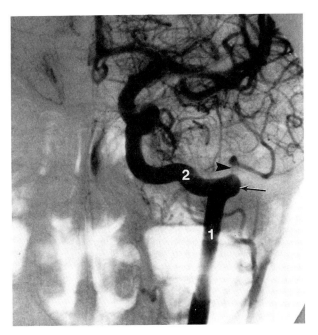

*Figure 22-4.* Coronal subtraction angiogram of an aberrant carotid artery. The vertical (1) and horizontal (2) segments should form a gradual curve. In this case there is a lateral deviation (arrow) of the carotid artery at the transition point. This part of the carotid artery lies in the middle ear. The persistent stapedial artery (arrowhead) is seen extending from the aberrant portion of the internal carotid artery. (Illustration courtesy of J. Moret, Fondation Ophthalmologique Adolphe de Rothschild, Paris, France.)

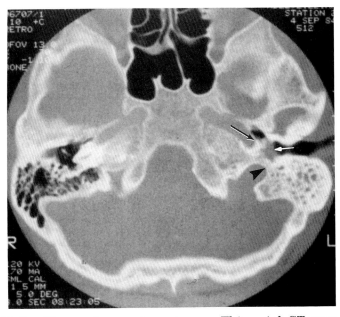

*Figure 22-5.* Glomus tympanicum tumor. This axial CT scan shows a small lesion (white arrow) that would be visible through the external canal. Note that the lateral cortical plate of the jugular bulb (arrowhead) and the lateral cortical plate of the carotid canal (black arrow) are intact. These findings virtually exclude both glomus jugulare tumor and aberrant carotid artery.

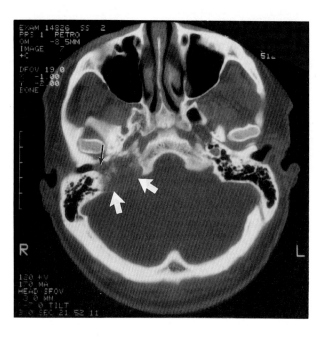

*Figure 22-6.* Glomus jugulare tumor. This axial CT scan shows the lesion protruding (white arrows) into the middle ear (black arrow). This lesion would be visible through the external auditory canal. The moth-eaten type of erosion of the walls of the jugular canal suggests that this is most probably a glomus jugulare tumor.

glomus tympanicum tumor (paraganglioma) arises on the promontory of the medial wall of the middle ear in the same region as the lesion in the test case. Indeed, both abnormalities present as a red "mass" behind the tympanic membrane. However, there would not be continuity of a glomus tympanicum tumor with the carotid artery canal. The wall of the carotid canal would be intact and in its normal position. If a glomus tumor erodes the bone, it is the jugular canal rather than, as in the test case, the carotid artery canal that is abnormal. When there is such bone erosion, the lesion is called a glomus jugulare tumor or jugulotympanicum tumor (Figure 22-6).

Dehiscent jugular fossa (Option (D)) can also be excluded. The defect in such a case is thinning or erosion of the bony wall between the middle ear and the jugular canal (Figure 22-7), not the carotid canal as in the test case. The lesion in the test case is not near the facial nerve canal; this excludes the diagnosis of facial nerve sheath tumor (Option (E)).

Clinically, an aberrant carotid artery, a dehiscent jugular fossa, a glomus tympanicum tumor, a glomus jugulare tumor, a hemangioma, or

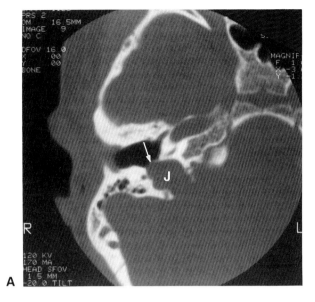

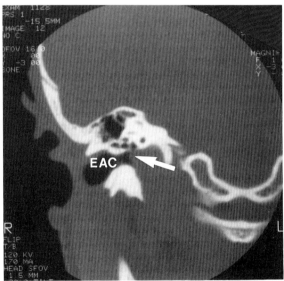

*Figure 22-7.* Dehiscent jugular fossa. (A) Axial CT scan showing a soft tissue mass (arrow) in the middle ear. This mass would be visible through the external auditory canal. A smoothly marginated extension from the jugular bulb (J) protrudes into the middle ear and represents a dehiscent jugular fossa. It is the intervening bony lateral wall of the jugular canal that is dehiscent. (B) Coronal CT scan showing the smooth-walled dehiscence (arrow) of the jugular fossa. Note its relationship to the external auditory canal (EAC).

other vascular malformations about the ear and in the posterior fossa can all present with pulsatile tinnitus. However, the CT finding of a laterally positioned carotid artery canal that projects into the middle ear is pathognomonic of an aberrant carotid artery.

## Question 90

Which *one* of the following is LEAST likely to cause a conductive hearing loss?

(A) Aberrant carotid artery
(B) Otosclerosis
(C) Acoustic neuroma
(D) Atresia of the external auditory canal
(E) Cholesteatoma

Hearing loss is usually categorized as either a conductive hearing loss or a sensorineural hearing loss. Sound travels through the ear, first as an actual physical vibration and then as an electrical signal. The physical vibration travels along the external auditory canal to the tympanic membrane. The malleus is attached to the tympanic membrane, and the sound vibration is relayed to it and then to the rest of the ossicular chain. The ossicles transmit the sound to the oval window, where the foot plate of the stapes passes the vibration to the perilymph. The sound wave passes through the perilymph along the turns of the cochlea until it reaches the hair cells in the spiral organ of Corti. Here the electrical neural impulse is generated, and thus the electrical signal representing the sound wave follows the cochlear nerve to the nuclei in the brain stem, where the sound is perceived. Conductive hearing loss results when there is an interference with the actual physical vibration through the external and middle ears. Since the sound wave is still an actual physical vibratory phenomenon as it travels along the turns of the cochlea, a conductive hearing loss could occur in the cochlea. However, this is very unusual; for practical purposes, a conductive hearing loss can be thought of as an abnormality that interferes with movement of the ossicles, the tympanic membrane, or the air vibrations in the external auditory canal. Thus conductive hearing loss is the result of a problem involving the oval window, middle ear, or external ear. A sensorineural hearing loss is the result of an interference with the generation of the electrical signal or the propagation of the neural impulse along the eighth nerve to the brain stem. Thus, it occurs only in problems central to the oval window.

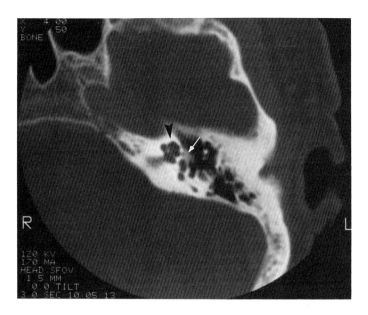

*Figure 22-8.* Otosclerosis. This axial CT scan shows abnormally thickened bone (arrow) at the anterior margin of the left oval window. The abnormal bone has a decreased density relative to the remainder of the otic capsule (arrowhead). This is called fenestral (oval window) otosclerosis.

When the patient presents with a conductive hearing loss, the radiologist should focus attention on both the middle ear and external ear. The causes of a conductive hearing loss include an aberrant carotid artery (Option (A)) that protrudes into the middle ear and can directly abut the ossicular chain. Often there is an associated anomaly called a persistent stapedial artery, which occurs with the aberrant carotid artery. This anomalous vessel passes through the stapes and thus, on this basis alone, can cause a conductive hearing loss.

Otosclerosis (Option (B)) is characterized by proliferation of abnormal bone at the margins of the oval window (Figures 22-8 and 22-9). This interferes with the movement of the stapes and so causes a conductive hearing loss. There may also be involvement of the cochlea, which produces a sensorineural hearing loss as well, but the conductive component almost always predominates.

An atresia of the external auditory canal (Option (D)) prevents the sound wave from reaching the tympanic membrane. Indeed, a severe external canal atresia will incorporate the tympanic membrane into the

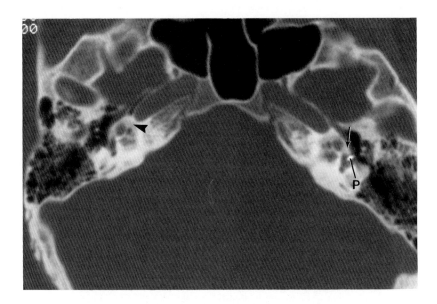

*Figure 22-9.* Otosclerosis. This axial CT scan of a more severe case of otosclerosis than that in Figure 22-8 demonstrates abnormal bone at the anterior margin of the left oval window (arrow). The demineralized bone (arrowhead) can be seen around the right cochlea as well. Note the metallic ossicular prosthesis (P) in the left ear.

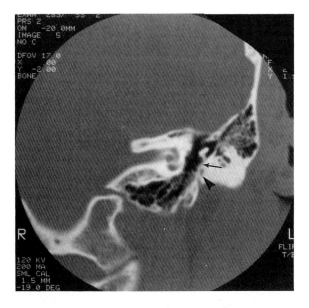

*Figure 22-10.* Atresia of the external auditory canal. This coronal CT scan shows that there is no external auditory canal. A bony atretic plate (arrowhead) is seen near the expected position of a normal external auditory canal. The malleus handle (arrow) is incorporated into the atretic plate. This patient would have a conductive hearing loss. (Reprinted with permission from Curtin [1].)

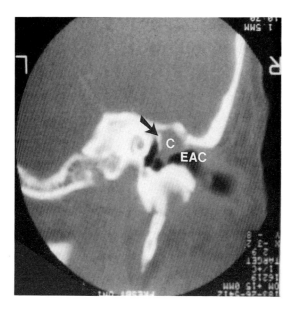

*Figure 22-11.* Cholesteatoma. This coronal CT scan shows a soft tissue mass (C) in the middle ear. This mass would be seen through the external auditory canal (EAC). The malleus (arrow) is displaced medially, and there is erosion of the scutum and lateral wall of the attic. Compare the position of the scutum with that in Figure 22-12B.

bony closure referred to as the atretic plate (Figure 22-10). The result is a conductive hearing loss.

A cholesteatoma (Option (E)) forms most frequently at the upper margin of the tympanic membrane (Figure 22-11). The cholesteatoma results when cells of the squamous epithelium from the external canal are trapped and isolated in the middle ear. They usually enter the middle ear through a perforation of the tympanic membrane, which occurs as a complication of chronic external and middle ear infection. The squamous epithelium sheds keratinous debris, which forms a small keratin ball or "pearl" if it cannot escape through the external canal. As the cholesteatoma grows, the resultant mass can touch or even erode the ossicular chain and thus cause a conductive hearing loss.

An acoustic neuroma involves the internal auditory canal and/or the cerebellopontine angle cistern. The lesion arises from the sheath of the eighth cranial nerve and interferes with the ability of the nerve to transmit an impulse. This causes a sensorineural hearing loss, not a conductive hearing loss **(Option (C) is correct).**

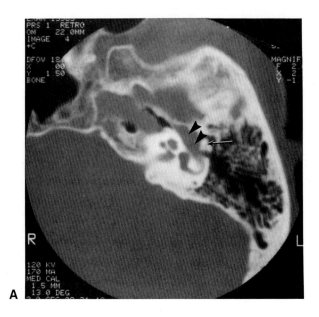

A

*Figure 22-12.*   Facial nerve lesion. (A) Axial CT scan. This case represents perineural extension along the facial nerve from an adenoid cystic carcinoma of the parotid. There is a soft tissue mass in the middle ear (arrowheads) that abuts the ossicular chain (arrow). This actually represents a concentrically enlarged facial nerve. The CT finding of enlargement of the facial nerve is the same as that seen with benign nerve sheath tumor (schwannoma) of the facial nerve. (B) Coronal CT section through the level of the cochlea (C) shows the soft tissue mass (arrow) in the position of the tympanic segment of the facial nerve canal. Note how it abuts the malleus (M). The scan shows a normal scutum (S) and the lateral wall of the attic (arrowhead). (C) Slightly posterior coronal CT scan at the level of the oval window (OW). There is concentric enlargement of the posterior tympanic segment of the facial nerve (arrow). The round window (RW) is also visible.

A facial nerve sheath tumor can cause either a conductive hearing loss or a sensorineural hearing loss, depending on the segment of the nerve from which it arises. Centrally, a lesion can arise in the internal auditory canal and cause a sensorineural hearing loss as the lesion presses on the eighth nerve. The tympanic segment of the facial nerve canal passes along the medial wall of the middle ear (Figure 22-12), and if a mass enlarges this segment, it may interfere with the ossicular chain and produce a conductive hearing loss. A facial nerve sheath tumor can actually present clinically as a conductive hearing loss without a facial paralysis.

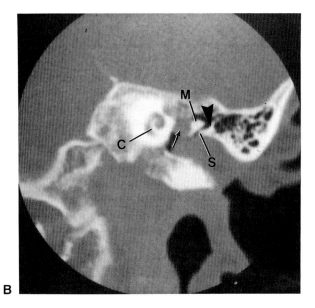

B

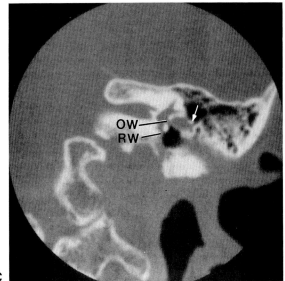

C

# Question 91

Concerning paragangliomas (glomus tumors),

(A) a glomus jugulare tumor is more likely to present with a conductive hearing loss than with a sensorineural hearing loss

(B) on CT, a glomus tympanicum tumor is differentiated from a glomus jugulare tumor by the demonstration of the intact bony lateral wall of the jugular bulb with the former

(C) most glomus jugulare tumors present with symptoms relating to the nerves that pass through the jugular foramen

(D) a glomus jugulare tumor has the same histology as a carotid body tumor

So-called glomus tumors that occur in the head and neck are more appropriately called paragangliomas. They arise from small nests of cells called the paraganglia, which are found in relation to cranial nerves or their ganglia. In the head and neck they arise primarily in four locations: carotid body tumors arise from the carotid bodies, which are near the carotid artery bifurcation; glomus vagale tumors arise in the region of the inferior or nodose ganglion of the vagus nerve and thus occur immediately below the skull base; glomus tympanicum tumors arise in association with Jacobson's nerve and the tympanic plexus on the promontory of the middle ear; and glomus jugulare tumors arise in the lateral wall of the jugular fossa. The different terms reflect only the differences in the anatomic locations. The various forms of glomus tumor in the head and neck share common histologic characteristics **(Option (D) is true)**.

Glomus tympanicum and glomus jugulare tumors can be confused clinically. Both can present as tumors that are visible through the tympanicum membrane. A glomus tympanicum tumor is, by definition, limited to the middle ear. A paraganglioma eroding the lateral wall of the jugular fossa is no longer limited to the middle ear and is classified as a glomus jugulare tumor (Figures 22-5 and 22-6) **(Option (B) is true)**. If the bony lateral wall of the jugular bulb is intact, the tumor is classified as a glomus tympanicum, whereas if the lateral wall is eroded the lesion is referred to as a glomus jugulare. Because most glomus jugulare tumors do extend into the middle ear, some authors refer to this type of lesion as a glomus jugulotympanicum.

When a glomus jugulare tumor enlarges, it tends to expand laterally into the middle ear, where the ossicular chain can be involved. This results in a conductive hearing loss. The middle ear component of the mass can also obstruct drainage into the eustachian tube, resulting in an effusion that can also cause a conductive hearing loss by damping the movement of the ossicular chain. Glomus jugulare tumors can erode into the cochlea or can extend medially into the interal auditory canal and cerebellopontine angle cistern. These larger tumors can cause a sensori-neural hearing loss, but this is much less frequent than a conductive hearing loss caused by middle ear involvement **(Option (A) is true).** If a glomus jugulare tumor extends medially, it will involve the pars nervosa region of the jugular fossa. Cranial nerves IX through XII may then be affected. Clinically demonstrable symptoms relating to these nerves occur only in large lesions, which account for less than 40% of such cases **(Option (C) is false).** A glomus vagale tumor can also grow into the pars nervosa as it follows the vagus nerve superiorly.

## Question 92

Aberrant carotid artery is frequently associated with absence of the:

(A) lateral wall of the jugular canal
(B) lateral wall of the carotid canal
(C) foramen spinosum
(D) facial nerve canal
(E) auditory ossicles

Both the carotid artery and its canal have vertical and horizontal segments in the temporal bone. The normal transition between the two segments is a curve directed anteromedially and passing just caudad to the cochlea. At this point, the wall of the carotid canal forms the anterior part of the medial wall of the middle ear.

An aberrant course of the carotid usually carries the vessel laterally so that it protrudes into the anterior middle ear (Figure 22-13; see also Figures 22-1 through 22-4). The vessel can be seen through the tympanic membrane, giving the characteristic appearance of a vascular mass. There have been a number of cases in which such a mass has been biopsied through the tympanic membrane with catastrophic results. Therefore, even though the anomaly is rare, this lesion becomes one of the most important entities to rule out both clinically and radiologically.

The diagnosis is most easily made by high-resolution CT. The lateral position of the vertical segment of the carotid artery or the transitional curve of the artery is readily seen, especially on coronal scans. The most important finding is that the lateral wall of the carotid canal is not

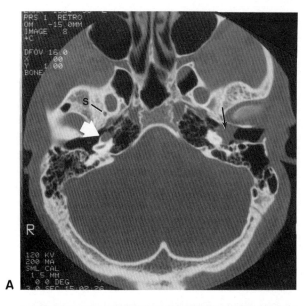

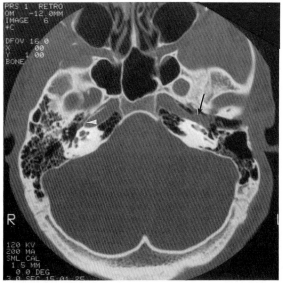

*Figure 22-13.* Aberrant carotid artery. Axial CT scans. (A) There is a soft tissue mass (arrow) in the left middle ear that would be visible through the external canal. Note that the carotid canal is not visualized on the abnormal left side but is seen in the normal position (arrowhead) on the right side. A foramen spinosum (S) is seen on the normal side but is absent on the left side. (B) Slightly higher (more cranial) level shows the connection (arrow) of the lesion to the transverse segment of the carotid artery. The lateral wall of the carotid canal is not demonstrated on the abnormal side but is visible (arrowhead) on the normal right side.

visualized in its normal position **(Option (B) is true).** The canal seems to pass directly into the middle ear, where the vessel can be seen along the promontory (lateral margin of the cochlea).

A second anomaly, persistence of the primitive stapedial artery, is frequently associated with an aberrant carotid artery. In the embryo, the primitive stapedial artery provides the original blood supply to areas that in the adult are in the distribution of the middle meningeal artery. Later in embryogenesis, the middle meningeal artery itself forms a connection with the external carotid arterial circulation and the stapedial artery regresses. If the stapedial artery persists, it usually passes from an aberrant carotid artery through the stapes and then enters the facial nerve canal. The vessel follows the facial canal to the region of the geniculate ganglion, where it exits onto the floor of the middle cranial fossa and continues as the middle meningeal artery. The vessel going through the stapes obviously interferes with the mobility of this small bone and causes a conductive hearing loss. The stapes and the other auditory ossicles are present, however **(Option (E) is false).** The tympanic segment of the facial canal may be larger than normal because the stapedial artery travels along it; however, it is not absent **(Option (D) is false).**

The middle meningeal artery originates from the aberrant vessel in the middle ear rather than from the external carotid artery below the skull base. The foramen spinosum is usually absent because the aberrant vessel travels through the facial canal rather than through the foramen spinosum **(Option (C) is true)** (Figure 22-14). The jugular canal is not involved by this anomaly and is expected to be normal **(Option (A) is false).**

*Hugh D. Curtin, M.D.*

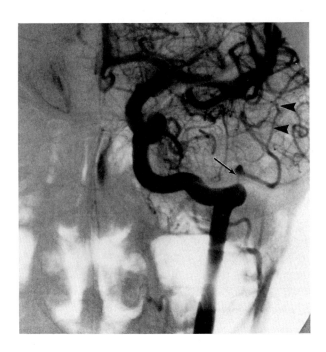

*Figure 22-14* (Same as Figure 22-4). Aberrant carotid artery. Coronal subtraction angiogram shows the middle meningeal distribution (arrowheads) deriving its blood supply from the aberrant vessel. The initial segment, the persistent stapedial artery (arrow), extends through the middle ear into the facial nerve canal.

## SUGGESTED READINGS

### ABERRANT CAROTID ARTERY

1. Curtin HD. Congenital malformations of the ear. Otolaryngol Clin North Am 1988; 21:317–336
2. Lasjaunias P, Moret J. Normal and non-pathological variations in the angiographic aspects of the arteries of the middle ear. Neuroradiology 1978; 15:213–219
3. Lo WW. Vascular tinnitus. In: Som PM, Bergeron RT (eds), Head and neck imaging, 2nd ed. Chicago: Mosby-Year Book; 1991:1108–1115
4. Lo WW, Solti-Bohman LG, McElveen JT Jr. Aberrant carotid artery: radiologic diagnosis with emphasis on high-resolution computed tomography. RadioGraphics 1985; 5:985–993

### TUMORS AND CYSTS OF THE TEMPORAL BONE

5. Curtin HD. CT of acoustic neuroma and other tumors of the ear. Radiol Clin North Am 1984; 22:77–105

6. Greenberg JJ, Oot RF, Wismer GL. Cholesterol granuloma of the petrous apex: MR and CT evaluation. AJNR 1988; 9:1205–1214

7. Jackson CG, Cueva RA, Thedinger BA, Glasscock ME III. Conservation surgery for glomus jugulare tumors: the value of early diagnosis. Laryngoscope 1990; 100:1031–1036

8. Lo WW. Tumors of the temporal bone and the cerebellopontine angle. In: Som PM, Bergeron RT (eds), Head and neck imaging, 2nd ed. Chicago: Mosby-Year Book; 1991:1046–1108

9. Lo WW, Solti-Bohman LG, Brackmann DE, Gruskin P. Cholesterol granuloma of the petrous apex: CT diagnosis. Radiology 1984; 153:705–711

10. Swartz J. Imaging of the temporal bone: a text/atlas. New York: Thieme; 1986:33–96

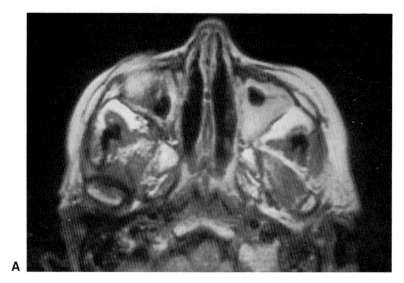

SE 1,800/30

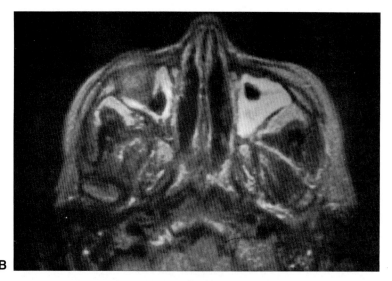

SE 1,800/90

*Figure 23-1.* This 38-year-old woman has left facial discomfort. You are shown axial proton-density (A) and T2-weighted (B) MR scans.

# Case 23: Intrasinus Low-Signal-Intensity Mass

## Question 93

Which *one* of the following is the LEAST likely diagnosis?

(A) Sinusitis with aeration
(B) Aspergilloma
(C) Sinusitis with dried secretions
(D) Subacute sinus hemorrhage
(E) Dentigerous cyst

The axial proton-density MR scan (Figure 23-1A) shows areas of inter-mediate signal intensity lining the walls of both maxillary sinuses. Centrally within each sinus is an area of signal void (see Figure 23-2A). On the T2-weighted MR scan (Figure 23-1B), the areas of the sinus that were intermediate in signal intensity on the axial proton-density MR scan have become areas of high signal intensity and the central regions within each sinus have remained signal voids (arrows, Figure 23-2B).

The signal intensity changes and the overall configuration of the soft tissues lining the sinuses suggest that they represent inflamed mucosa. Inflammation of the sinus mucosa has associated increased surface secretions and submucosal edema, both of which are usually composed of 95% water. Thus, the MR appearance of acute inflammation is that associated with water, namely a low T1-weighted, an intermediate proton-density, and a high T2-weighted signal intensity.

Working under the logical assumption that the MR changes represent inflammation and are consistent with all the options given, the problem then is to identify the possible causes of the signal void within each sinus.

Air (Option (A)), an aspergilloma (Option (B)), dried secretions (Option (C)), and a tooth in a dentigerous cyst (Option (E)) can all give areas of signal void and so are plausible diagnoses. Subacute sinus hemorrhage,

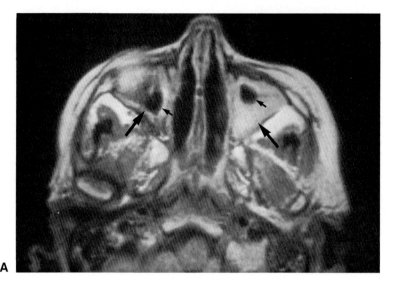

SE 1,800/30

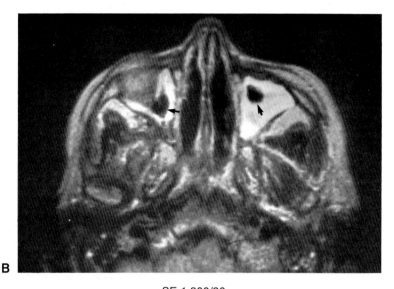

SE 1,800/90

*Figure 23-2* (Same as Figure 23-1). Axial proton-density MR scan shows areas of intermediate signal intensity lining the walls of both maxillary sinuses (large arrows). Centrally in each sinus is an area of signal void (small arrows), which represents residual sinus air. (B) Axial T2-weighted MR scan shows that the areas of intermediate signal intensity in panel A now have high signal intensity, whereas the central areas of signal void remain signal voids (arrows).

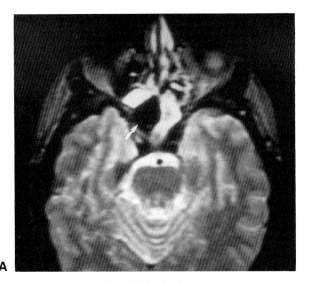

A

SE 2,000/100

*Figure 23-3.* Aspergilloma. Axial T2-weighted MR scan (A) and a CT scan (B). In panel A, an area of signal void (arrow) is seen in the right sphenoid sinus. There are secretions with high signal intensity in the left sphenoid sinus and the posterior right ethmoid sinuses adjacent to the signal void. Areas of signal void (apparently air-containing sinuses) are seen in the left ethmoid complex. However, in panel B, the left ethmoid sinuses and the right sphenoid sinus do not contain air. Instead, they are filled with relatively high-attenuation material (aspergilloma) (arrows). The lower-attenuation material in the remaining sinuses is inflamed mucosa and sinus secretions.

however, would have high signal intensities on all of the sequences **(Option (D) is therefore correct).**

Air gives a signal void because there simply are too few protons to give a detectable signal. Focal aeration within inflamed sinuses is the explanation for the signal voids seen in the test patient. An aspergilloma (Figure 23-3), dried secretions (Figure 23-4), and a tooth (Figure 23-5) give signal voids for a different reason. All are either rigid solids or semisolid structures. As a result, their molecules are relatively fixed in position and they have very low-frequency fluctuations of their magnetic fields, which result in a very pronounced shortening of the T2 relaxation times. Specifically, the T2 relaxation times of aspergillomas and dried secretions are on the order of a few milliseconds and the T2 relaxation time of a tooth (and also of bone) is only a few microseconds. Therefore,

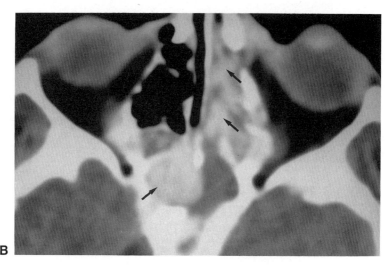

B

*Figure 23-3 (Continued)*

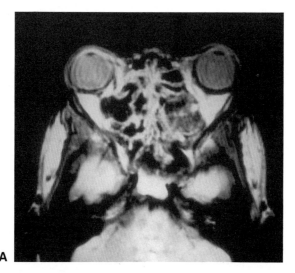

A

SE 2,000/90

*Figure 23-4.* Dried sinus secretions. (A) In the axial T2-weighted MR scan there is some high-signal-intensity mucosal thickening in the ethmoid and sphenoid sinuses, with apparent aeration (areas of signal void) in most of these sinuses. (B) However, in the CT scan the areas of signal void are high-attenuation dried secretions that opacify all of the sinuses. Widening of the ethmoid complexes is visible in both the MR and CT studies. This patient had chronic polyposis and dried sinus secretions.

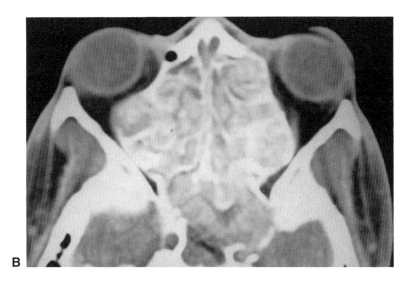

B

*Figure 23-4 (Continued)*

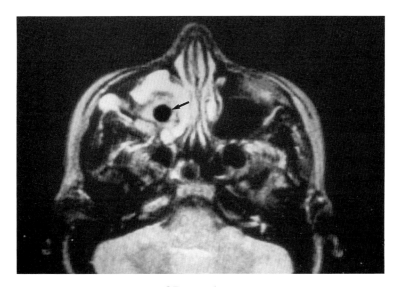

SE 1,800/90

*Figure 23-5.* Dentigerous cyst. An axial T2-weighted MR scan shows a central area of signal void (arrow) surrounded by a high-signal-intensity region. This appearance is similar to that of Figure 23-2; however, the signal void in this case is caused by a tooth in a dentigerous cyst.

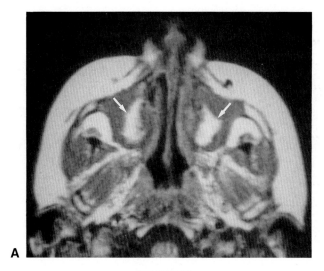

SE 500/20

*Figure 23-6.* Bilateral antral subacute hemorrhage. (A) In the axial T1-weighted MR scan there is a central area of high signal intensity in each maxillary sinus (arrows) surrounded by a zone of low signal intensity, which represents the sinus mucosa and secretions. (B) In the CT scan the central area (hemorrhage) has a high attenuation, whereas the surrounding mucosa and secretion have a lower attenuation.

whatever signal these substances give is completely dephased in an ultrashort time. When conventional clinical MR scanning is used, the shortest echo times available are too long to effectively refocus these brief signals. Thus, either little or no signal is detected and very low signal intensity or a signal void is seen.

Subacute hemorrhage, on the other hand, contains methemoglobin, which has high signal intensity on T1-weighted, proton-density, and T2-weighted studies as a result of its paramagnetic qualities and protein content (Figure 23-6).

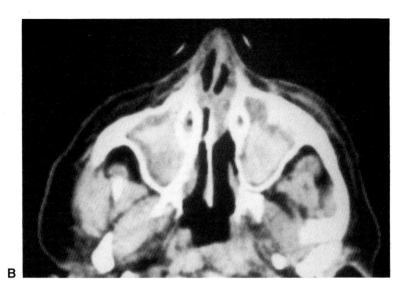

B

## Question 94

Concerning sinusitis,

(A) about 20% of cases of acute maxillary bacterial sinusitis are secondary to dental infections
(B) opacification of a sinus in a child under 2 years of age usually indicates the presence of infection
(C) acute disease is characterized on MRI by low and high signal intensities on T1- and T2-weighted images, respectively
(D) allergic disease usually involves just the maxillary sinus
(E) generalized headache is a common symptom

Sinusitis is a general term used to describe inflammation of the paranasal sinuses. Sinusitis can be caused by a virus, bacterium, fungus, allergy, or irritant. The most common etiology is probably allergy, and it is estimated that about 10% of the population has allergic rhinitis and sinusitis. The next most common cause is bacterial infection; bacterial sinusitis usually results from a rhinitis that has associated mucosal edema, which interferes with the sinus ostial drainage. Oxygenation within the sinus is altered, and this alters the flora, resulting in a bacterial sinusitis. The sinus obstruction can also be secondary to a benign or malignant mass; however, this is less common than obstruction due to swollen mucosa.

In most patients the roots of the molar teeth, and in some patients the premolar teeth, extend up into the floor of the maxillary sinus. Often only the sinus mucosa covers these roots. Infections of these roots can cause an antral sinusitis, and a carious tooth may present clinically as an antral sinusitis. Such maxillary dental infections are estimated to cause about 20% of the cases of acute maxillary sinusitis **(Option (A) is true).** Conversely, an acute antral sinusitis may present clinically as upper molar or premolar tooth pain, and a number of such teeth have been treated or extracted before the maxillary sinusitis was diagnosed and treated.

In children, the developing sinuses are small and the sinus mucosa is more redundant and boggy than in adults. Normal young children also tend to have more retained secretions than adults, and, in addition, children often cry immediately prior to or during a radiographic examination. Thus the presence of thickened mucosa and sinus secretions in an infant or young child may have no pathologic significance. There is some debate in the literature about how old a child should be before the paranasal sinuses are evaluated by the same criteria used for an adult. This transition age varies in the literature from 4 years of age to the mid-teens. However, it is clear that sinus opacification in a child under 2 years of age cannot be used as a reliable indicator of the presence of infection **(Option (B) is false).**

Acute sinusitis is characterized by vascular inflammation of the sinus mucosa, submucosal edema, and an increased amount of mucosal secretions. Since normal sinus secretions and the interstitial fluid associated with submucosal edema are both about 95% water, the MR characteristics are those associated with water. Thus there are low T1-weighted and high T2-weighted signal intensities, which reflect the long T1 and T2 relaxation times of water **(Option (C) is true)** (Figure 23-7).

Allergic disease is a systemic phenomenon, and when allergic sinusitis occurs it usually diffusely involves all of the paranasal sinuses and the nasal cavities **(Option (D) is false).** In fact, disease limited to a maxillary sinus is the classic presentation of an acute bacterial sinusitis.

Pain caused by sinusitis is usually local. The patient clearly points to the frontal region for frontal sinusitis, the cheek for maxillary sinusitis, and the area between the eyes for ethmoid sinusitis. Sphenoid sinusitis can be associated with orbital apex pain or suboccipital pain. Rarely, a generalized headache is caused by sinusitis; it is estimated that only 3% of the cases of sinusitis actually cause such a generalized headache **(Option (E) is false).**

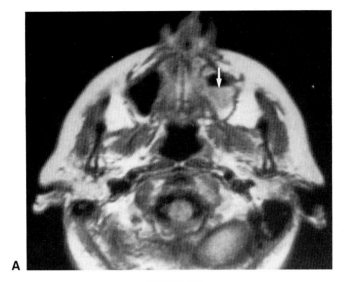

SE 700/20

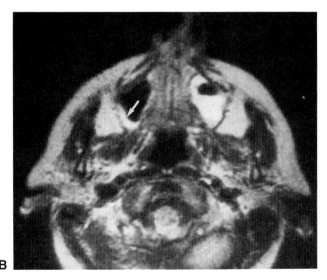

SE 2,000/90

*Figure 23-7.* Acute sinusitis. Axial T1-weighted (A) and T2-weighted (B) MR scans show mucosal thickening and an air-fluid level (arrow, panel A) in the left maxillary sinus and minimal mucosal thickening in the right maxillary sinus (arrow, panel B). These areas have low T1- and high T2-weighted signal intensities. These changes of acute sinusitis are thus characterized on MRI by signal intensities that reflect the high water content of the acute inflammatory process.

# Question 95

Concerning aspergillosis of the sinuses,

(A) it occurs in both immunosuppressed and otherwise healthy individuals
(B) it causes small-vessel thrombosis
(C) an aspergilloma has high signal intensity on both T1- and T2-weighted MR images
(D) the mucosal disease is easily distinguished from bacterial sinusitis on MRI
(E) it is often diagnosed as a result of its failure to respond to routine antibiotic therapy

Aspergillosis is a fungal infection that in humans is caused primarily by *Aspergillus fumigatus*, which accounts for nearly 90% of cases. When the paranasal sinuses are involved, most patients are otherwise healthy; in fact, such sinonasal disease is endemic in areas such as the Sudan. This paranasal sinus infection in most cases is unrelated to pulmonary aspergillosis, which occurs primarily in debilitated and immunosuppressed patients. However, sinus disease can also occur as part of a generalized infection in such debilitated patients. Aspergillosis also uncommonly occurs in an allergic form, with the patient reacting to the fungus itself. In either case, aspergillosis of the paranasal sinuses can occur in both immunosuppressed and otherwise healthy individuals **(Option (A) is true)**.

Pathologically, aspergillus infection, when invasive, can cause small-vessel thrombosis, which leads to areas of ischemic and hemorrhagic infarction that are similar to those found with mucormycosis **(Option (B) is true)**.

Aspergillus paranasal sinus infection has two main components: a reactive mucosal sinusitis and the formation of an aspergilloma. The mucosal disease is a nonspecific inflammatory reaction, which is characterized on MRI by low T1-weighted and high T2-weighted signal intensities, the same as are found in routine bacterial sinusitis **(Option (D) is false)**. The MR signal characteristics reflect the high water content associated with such inflammation. The aspergilloma is a semisolid, dehydrated mass of hyphae composed primarily of carbohydrates and macromolecular proteins. Primarily as a result of the semisolid nature of the aspergilloma, the T2 relaxation time is ultrashort and the MR signal intensities are either low or signal voids on both T1- and T2-weighted sequences (Figures 23-3, 23-8, and 23-9) **(Option (C) is false)**.

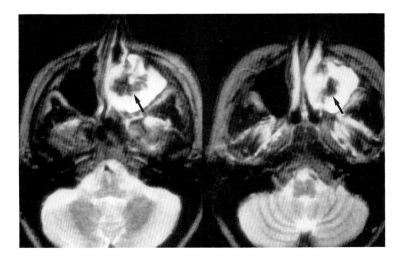

*Figure 23-8.* Aspergillosis. Axial T2-weighted MR scan shows the left maxillary sinus to be filled with high-signal-intensity material that surrounds a central region of low attenuation or signal void (arrows). The central region is an aspergilloma, and it had the same low signal intensity on T1-weighted scans. The surrounding zone of high signal intensity represents aspergilloma-induced sinusitis, and this area had a low T1-weighted signal intensity.

Because paranasal sinus aspergillosis usually occurs in otherwise healthy individuals, it often presents clinically as a routine sinusitis. As a result, the clinician initially treats these patients with decongestants, antihistamines, and antibiotics. It is only when the infection fails to respond to such a routine therapeutic regimen that the possibility of a fungal infection is clinically entertained **(Option (E) is true).** Surgery, in combination with antifungal medications, is then the treatment of choice.

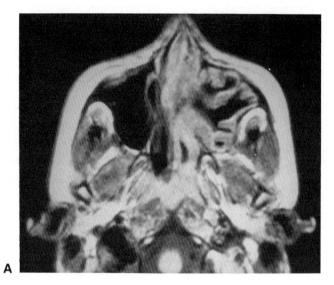

SE 2,000/20

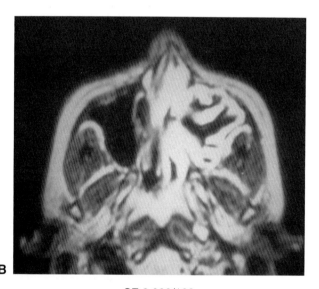

SE 2,000/100

*Figure 23-9.* Aspergillosis. Axial proton-density (A) and T2-weighted (B) MR scans show the presence in the left maxillary sinus of redundant, thickened mucosa that has low to intermediate signal intensity in panel A and high signal intensity in panel B. There is a central irregular area of signal void that simulates air; however, this central area was an aspergilloma that had high attenuation on CT (see Figures 23-3 and 23-8).

# Question 96

Concerning chronic sinonasal secretions,

(A) with time there is an increase in the bound-water fraction

(B) their protein content can be inferred from the signal intensities of T1- and T2-weighted MR scans

(C) dried secretions often give signal voids on T1- and T2-weighted MR scans

(D) on MRI, dried secretions can be routinely differentiated from an aspergilloma

(E) when they have low signal intensity on T1- and T2-weighted MR scans, they have high attenuation on CT

Normal sinonasal secretions are 95% water and only 5% solids. Most of these solids are macromolecular mucous glycoproteins. When a paranasal sinus becomes obstructed, the sinus mucosa that surrounds the entrapped secretions undergoes certain changes. With time, the mucosa develops more goblet cells, which produce the mucous glycoprotein. Thus, with time, there is increased production of this protein, and so the protein content of the secretions increases. Paralleling these changes, the sinus mucosa also slowly reabsorbs water from the secretions. The water in the secretions is in at least two forms. The first is referred to as free water and consists of water molecules whose magnetic fields are, at most, minimally affected by the macromolecular proteins. The second form is called bound water and consists of water molecules that are bound with various degrees of affinity to the macromolecular proteins. Such bound water behaves magnetically more like the macromolecular proteins than it does like free water. According to physicochemical models, there actually is a rapid exchange of water molecules between the free and bound states. The water that is absorbed by the surrounding sinus mucosa is the free water, and thus more and more of the water remaining in the secretions is in the bound-water fraction **(Option (A) is true).**

The combination of increased protein production and decreased free water results in a progressive increase in the protein content of the secretions. These changes in protein content, in turn, result in changes in the T1 and T2 relaxation times. These changes are summarized in Figure 23-10. By evaluating the T1- and T2-weighted signal intensities of MR scans, the protein content of these secretions can be inferred **(Option (B) is true).**

When the secretions become dried, the T2 relaxation times of such solids are ultrashort, on the order of microseconds. This reflects the fact that in such a solid the neighboring molecules exert maximal effect on

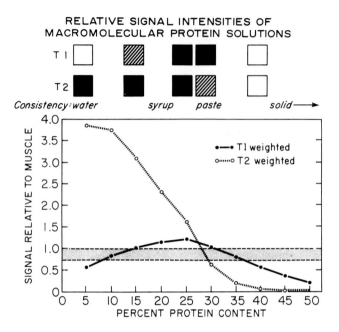

RELATIVE SIGNAL INTENSITIES OF
MACROMOLECULAR PROTEIN SOLUTIONS

*Figure 23-10.* Diagram of the T1- and T2-weighted signal intensities of sinonasal secretions as they change with protein concentration.

the magnetic field of the protons, resulting in a maximal dephasing of the protons. Thus, when excited, such solids have a signal, but it lasts only a few microseconds. At present, it is not possible with clinical MRI to obtain echo times short enough to refocus the signal from these solids, and thus no signal is detected. The resulting T2 shortening dominates the T1 relaxation time, which also becomes ultrashort, and hence signal voids are observed on T1- and T2-weighted MR scans (Figures 23-4 and 23-11) **(Option (C) is true)**.

In normal secretions the T1 relaxation time is long because of the 95% water content. With increasing protein content, the T1 relaxation time shortens and the signal intensity increases until the protein content is about 25 to 30%. Above this protein content, the signal intensity falls because of changes in the T2 relaxation time.

As discussed above, aspergillomas also give signal voids on T1- and T2-weighted MR scans, primarily because they are semisolid. The signal voids from dried secretions and from an aspergilloma cannot be differentiated on MRI **(Option (D) is false)**. Because both the dried secretions and the aspergilloma are routinely surrounded by inflamed mucosa, the

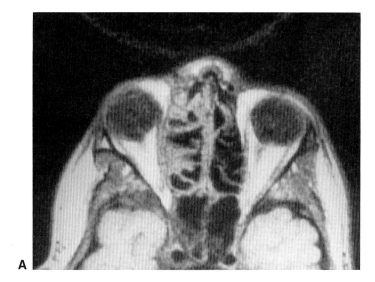

SE 700/20

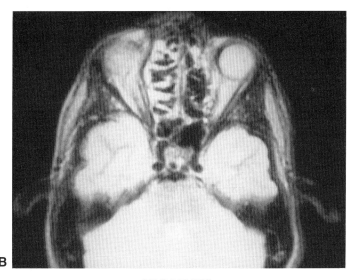

SE 2,500/100

*Figure 23-11.* Dried sinus secretions. Axial T1-weighted (A) and T2-weighted (B) MR scans and an axial CT scan (C), all performed on the same date. The MR images demonstrate moderate right ethmoid sinusitis with some mucosal thickening, which is characterized by low to intermediate T1- and high T2-weighted signal intensities. Some focal mucosal thickening is also present in the left anterior ethmoid sinuses. The remaining right ethmoid sinuses appear aerated, as does the right sphenoid sinus. However, in the CT image there is opacification of the entire right ethmoid and sphenoid sinuses. These sinuses were filled with hard, dried secretions in this patient with changes of chronic sinusitis.

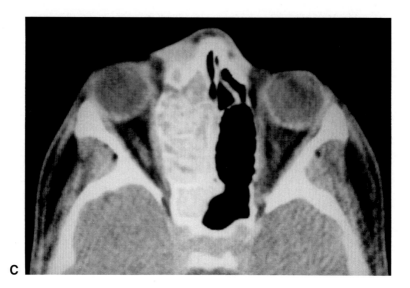

C

overall MR appearance is also similar (Figures 23-3, 23-4, 23-8, 23-9, and 23-11).

From the above discussion, it is clear that when secretions have low signal intensity on T1- and T2-weighted MR scans, they also have a very high protein content. This high concentration of protein also causes a high attenuation on CT scans because highly proteinaceous secretions are more dense (and thus attenuate X rays more) than less-proteinaceous soft tissues, secretions, or water **(Option (E) is true).**

## Question 97

Concerning sinus hemorrhage,

(A) it is a common finding in patients with hemophilia
(B) it is the cause of pain in barotrauma
(C) when subacute, it is usually distinguishable on MRI from secretions of acute sinusitis
(D) when subacute, it has a high attenuation on CT scans

Sinus hemorrhage is uncommon if unassociated with trauma. However, there are certain blood dyscrasias and diseases in which hemorrhage onto mucosal surfaces and into a paranasal sinus can occur; von Willebrand's disease and acute leukemias are examples of such blood abnormalities that can cause epistaxis. However, patients with hemophilia tend to bleed internally almost exclusively, with hemorrhage occurring primarily into joints; hemorrhage into the paranasal sinuses almost never occurs **(Option (A) is false).**

Barotrauma results from a sudden drop in intrasinus pressure, which causes submucosal and intrasinus hemorrhage. Such bleeding is most often found in parachutists and deep-sea divers. The hemorrhage causes the pain associated with barotrauma, and the most common clinical complaint in these patients is frontal sinus pain **(Option (B) is true).**

When sinus hemorrhage is subacute, there is a predominance of methemoglobin, which causes high signal intensity on T1- and T2-weighted MR scans (Figure 23-6). Acute sinusitis is associated with increased mucosal secretions and submucosal edema, both of which contain about 95% water. As a result, acute sinusitis has low T1-weighted and high T2-weighted signal intensities, reflecting the long T1 and T2 relaxation times of water (Figure 23-7) **(Option (C) is true).**

When hemorrhage is subacute, the overall protein concentration, especially within clotted blood, presumably accounts for the high attenuation seen on CT scans **(Option (D) is true).** This situation is similar to the high CT attenuation found with concentrated sinus secretions. In fact, subacute hemorrhage, concentrated secretions, and mycetomas all have high attenuation on CT scans and cannot be differentiated by CT (compare Figures 23-3, 23-4, 23-6, and 23-11). Subacute hemorrhage has high T1- and T2-weighted signal intensities on MRI, whereas mycetomas and dried secretions have low signal or signal voids on T1- and T2-weighted MR scans.

*Peter M. Som, M.D.*

SUGGESTED READINGS

1. Dillon WP, Som PM, Fullerton GD. Hypointense MR signal in chronically inspissated sinonasal secretions. Radiology 1990; 174:73–78
2. Som PM, Dillon WP, Curtin HD, Fullerton GD, Lidov M. Hypointense paranasal sinus foci: differential diagnosis with MR imaging and relation to CT findings. Radiology 1990; 176:777–781
3. Som PM, Dillon WP, Fullerton GD, Zimmerman RA, Rajagopalan B, Marom Z. Chronically obstructed sinonasal secretions: observations on T1 and T2 shortening. Radiology 1989; 172:515–520
4. Som PM, Dillon WP, Sze G, Lidov M, Biller HF, Lawson W. Benign and malignant sinonasal lesions with intracranial extension: differentiation with MR imaging. Radiology 1989; 172:763–766

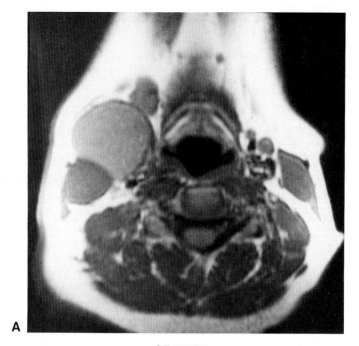

SE 500/30

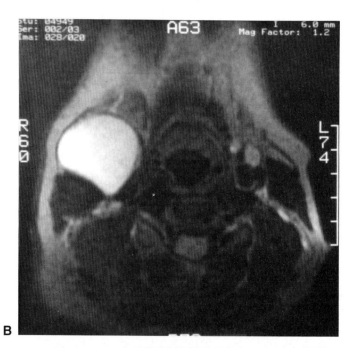

SE 2,500/100

*Figure 24-1.* This 38-year-old woman presented with fullness in the right neck. You are shown axial T1-weighted (A) and T2-weighted (B) MR scans.

# Case 24: Branchial Cleft Cyst

## Question 98

Which *one* of the following is the MOST likely diagnosis?

(A) Metastatic carcinoma
(B) Thyroglossal duct cyst
(C) Submandibular gland tumor
(D) Branchial cleft cyst
(E) Carotid body tumor

The test images (Figure 24-1) show an obvious abnormality in the right side of the neck (see Figure 24-2). The lesion has a smooth, thin wall, and the signal from the inside of the lesion is very homogeneous on both the T1- and T2-weighted sequences, with a low signal intensity on T1-weighted images and a high signal intensity on T2-weighted images. These signal characteristics suggest fluid.

These findings, combined with the very characteristic position just anterolateral to the carotid artery and jugular vein at the anterior margin of the sternocleidomastoid muscle, make branchial cleft cyst the most likely diagnosis **(Option (D) is correct).**

The position of the lesion can be used to eliminate several of the possibilities. Thyroglossal duct cyst (Option (B)) should not be considered. It is not a lateral neck mass; rather, it is expected to be nearly midline and should be inseparable from the strap muscles anterior to the thyroid cartilage (Figure 24-3). A thyroglossal duct cyst, when large, may extend to the side of the neck but would not be as far lateral as is the lesion in the test images, and its more medial component would be clearly identified on MR images.

The lesion in the test images is clearly separate from the submandibular gland, which is seen on the same images. Clinically a branchial cleft cyst and a submandibular gland mass can be confused, and CT or MR demonstration that the lesion is separate from the gland effectively excludes the diagnosis of a submandibular gland tumor (Option (C)). A

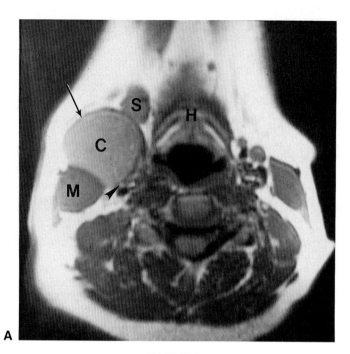

SE 500/30

*Figure 24-2* (Same as Figure 24-1). Branchial cleft cyst. (A) Axial T1-weighted MR image. The cyst (C) has a smooth thin wall (arrow) and low to intermediate signal intensity. The lesion is anterior to the sternocleido-mastoid muscle (M) and clearly separate from the submandibular gland (S). A narrow plane (arrowhead) separates the lesion from the carotid artery and the internal jugular vein. The hyoid bone (H) is also indicated. (B) Axial T2-weighted MR image shows a homogeneously high signal intensity in the cyst (C), indicating the presence of fluid. Again, the thin wall of the cyst is clearly seen and the submandibular gland is displaced anteriorly.

submandibular gland tumor would be embedded within the gland (Figure 24-4).

A carotid body tumor (paraganglioma) (Option (E)) does arise in this location and must be considered in the differential diagnosis. These tumors have a direct connection to the carotid bifurcation. This abnormality is very close to, but can be visually separated from, the carotid artery. The bifurcation would be seen on a scan slightly higher than the test image. A carotid body tumor is very vascular, and the large vessels cause flow voids, which would be easily demonstrable in a tumor of this size.

The abnormality that is perhaps the most difficult to differentiate from a branchial cleft cyst is lymphadenopathy. The location of the lesion in

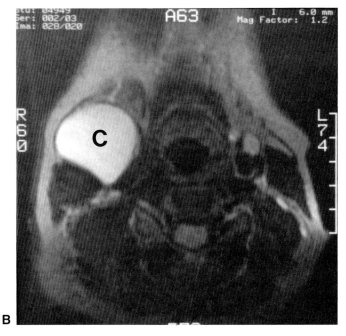

SE 2,500/100

the test patient's neck is a common site for a pathologically enlarged jugular chain lymph node (Figure 24-5). Nodes involved by metastatic carcinoma (Option (A)) can have central necrosis, and signal characteristics in the central necrotic region of the node may resemble those of fluid. In such a node, however, the signal is not usually as uniform as in the test case, and the wall of the node is usually irregular and thicker. Unless there is extracapsular tumor spread from the lymph node, the outer margin of the node is smooth, as in the test case. Although metastatic disease in a lymph node cannot be completely excluded on the basis of the images alone, the sharp, thin margin on the MR images makes this an unlikely diagnosis. The clinical picture would also help differentiate these entities. No mucosal lesion would be found on physical examination, and the branchial cleft cyst would not feel as hard as would a metastatic carcinoma.

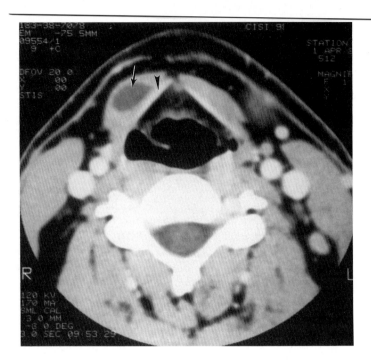

*Figure 24-3.* Thyroglossal duct cyst. Postcontrast axial CT scan shows this cystic lesion (arrow) to be firmly embedded in the strap muscles along the anterior surface of the thyroid cartilage (arrowhead). By comparison, a typical branchial cleft cyst would be more posterior and lateral in position and would not be situated deep to the strap muscles.

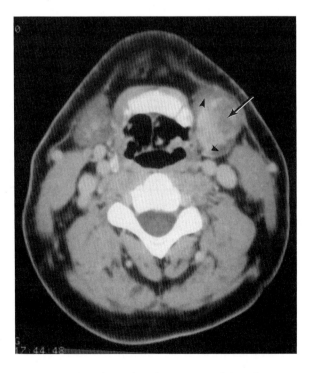

*Figure 24-4.* Submandibular gland tumor (adenoid cystic carcinoma). Postcontrast axial CT scan clearly shows the lesion (arrow) to be within the submandibular gland tissue (arrowheads) rather than separate from it (compare with Figures 24-1 and 24-2).

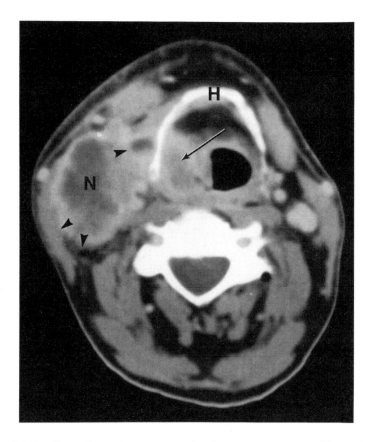

*Figure 24-5.* Lymph node metastasis from squamous cell carcinoma. Postcontrast axial CT scan shows an enlarged right cervical lymph node (N) with a low-attenuation center and a thick irregular wall. The outer margin (arrowheads) is irregular and unsharp, suggesting tumor extension through the capsule of the lymph node. The primary tumor is seen in the right pyriform sinus (arrow). Hyoid bone (H) is also indicated. (Reprinted with permission from Curtin HD. The larynx. In: Som PM, Bergeron RT (eds), Head and neck imaging, 2nd ed. St. Louis: Mosby-Year Book; 1991:593–692.)

# Question 99

Concerning cervical lymphadenopathy,

  (A) central necrosis is common in a node involved by Hodgkin's lymphoma
  (B) tuberculous adenitis rarely shows central necrosis
  (C) nodes involved by Castelman's disease nearly always enhance
  (D) extracapsular spread of tumor indicates a poor prognosis
  (E) by size criterion only, a 1-cm node in the jugulodigastric area is considered abnormal

The status of the cervical lymph nodes must be considered in two principal clinical situations. Either the patient has a known primary carcinoma and imaging is done to detect metastatic involvement of nodes, or the patient presents with neck fullness or a discrete mass and lymphadenopathy must be considered in the differential diagnosis.

In the first situation (a patient with a known primary tumor), certain criteria have been used to indicate whether a node is likely to be positive for metastatic tumor. The first criterion is size. If a node is larger than 1 cm, it is considered to be positive. The jugulodigastric area is an exception. The term "jugulodigastric" refers to the high jugular chain region, just posterior to the angle of the mandible. As the name indicates, this is the region where the digastric muscle crosses the jugular vein. In this area the maximum size for a node to be considered normal is 1.5 cm **(Option (E) is false)**.

More specific is the finding of a low-density internal defect within the node (Figure 24-5). This finding may represent necrosis or low-density tumor and is considered abnormal even if the node is of normal size.

Using density and size criteria, CT is more accurate than clinical evaluation. Many positive nodes will be found in a clinically negative neck; clinical evaluation has a false-negative rate of more than 25%. However, there may also be microscopic metastasis in a node that is normal by CT criteria. The false-negative rate is considered to be approximately 10% for CT.

The low-density internal defect is considered a common characteristic of nodes involved with metastatic squamous cell carcinoma. Central necrosis is rare in a node involved by Hodgkin's lymphoma **(Option (A) is false)**. The node is usually more homogeneous (Figure 24-6) and may have peripheral rim enhancement. Occasionally, central necrosis will occur in non-Hodgkin's lymphoma.

In the setting of squamous cell carcinoma, irregularity of the nodal margin on imaging is a very ominous sign. This appearance correlates

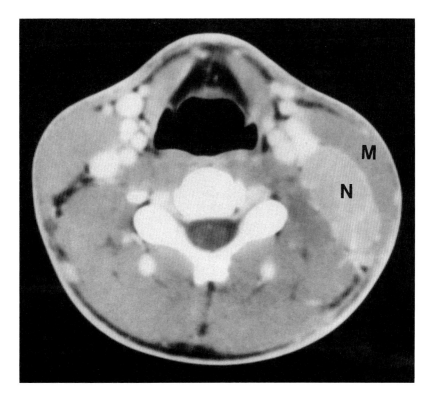

*Figure 24-6.* Hodgkin's lymphoma. Postcontrast axial CT scan shows enlarged lymph nodes (N) posterior to the internal jugular vein and deep to the sternocleidomastoid muscle (M). The nodes are fairly homogeneous and do not have necrotic centers.

well with tumor extension through the capsule of the node (so-called extranodal or extracapsular tumor spread). If the pathologist finds extracapsular spread when examining the lymph nodes of the surgical specimen, then the expected survival of the patient is only 50% of what would be expected if the metastatic nodes showed no extracapsular extension **(Option (D) is true).**

Abnormalities of the lymph nodes must also be considered even if there is no clinical or imaging evidence of a primary lesion in the upper aerodigestive tract. In a small number of cases (5 to 10%), an enlarging neck mass turns out to be a node involved by metastatic squamous cell carcinoma even though no primary tumor is found at endoscopy. However, especially when no primary tumor is evident, other abnormalities must be considered. Certainly other cancers, such as thyroid carcinoma,

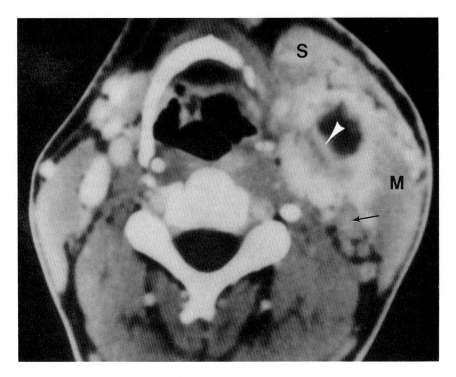

*Figure 24-7.* Tuberculosis. Postcontrast axial CT scan shows a large node situated between the submandibular gland (S) and the sternocleido-mastoid muscle (M). There is a low-attenuation necrotic center and a thick irregular wall (arrowhead). Other involved nodes (arrow) do not have necrotic centers. (Courtesy of Peter M. Som, M.D., Mount Sinai Medical Center, New York)

lymphoma, and primary tumors arising below the neck, must be considered, but there are also many nonmalignant causes of nodal enlargement.

Tuberculosis causing cervical lymph node enlargement is less common in the United States than in other regions of the world. However, its prevalence is high enough that it must be considered as a possible explanation of a neck mass. The appearance of nodes in tuberculosis and atypical mycobacterial infection can be variable. They can be fairly homogeneous, or they can have central necrosis and a thick wall (Figure 24-7). Both patterns can occur in the same patient, but central necrosis is quite common **(Option (B) is false).** In tuberculosis there is usually little of the surrounding infiltration of the fat planes that would be noted in cases of adenitis and cellulitis due to pyogenic bacteria.

Most pathologic lymph nodes have an intermediate or low density on CT. Enhancement of an enlarged lymph node is less common. A hypervascular metastasis from the thyroid or renal cell carcinoma, or, occasionally, a melanoma can give enhancing lymph nodes. Granulomatous disease, with its variability of appearance, can have a fairly homogeneous enhancing node, but usually other patterns will also be present in the same individual. Castelman's disease, a rare non-neoplastic lymphoid hyperplasia, can also have nodes that enhance on CT. Many names have been used to describe this disorder, including angiofollicular lymph node hyperplasia and angiomatous lymphoid hamartoma. As would be expected from these terms, the enlarged lymph nodes characteristic of this disease have vascular elements and almost always enhance **(Option (C) is true).** Castelman's disease or giant lymph node hyperplasia presents with an enlarging mass. The mass is usually in the thorax but occurs in the neck in approximately 15% of cases. Patients are usually asymptomatic but may have systemic manifestations such as fever and anemia. There is no evidence that Castelman's disease spreads to other sites, and surgical excision is considered curative when possible. There has been no instance of this disease developing into lymphoma. Although the disease is rare, it is important to recognize this entity because it can be confused with more significant malignant processes.

## Question 100

Concerning tumors of the submandibular gland,

- (A) they are more likely to be malignant than are those of the parotid gland
- (B) the most common tumor is squamous cell carcinoma
- (C) perineural extension of malignant tumors is uncommon
- (D) extraglandular extension involves the mylohyoid muscle more frequently than it does the lateral pterygoid muscle

The major salivary glands include the parotid, submandibular, and sublingual glands. The frequency of various types of tumors differs in each gland. Most parotid gland tumors are benign (about 80%), whereas a tumor of the submandibular gland is more likely to be malignant (about 50%) **(Option (A) is true).** Sublingual gland tumors are extremely rare but are usually malignant.

Squamous cell carcinoma accounts for the large majority of malignancies of the head and neck. However, the histology of malignancies arising in the salivary glands is significantly different. The most common malignant tumors of the parotid and submandibular glands are mucoepidermoid carcinoma and adenoid cystic carcinoma, respectively. Squamous cell carcinoma does occur but is rare (less than 10%) **(Option (B) is false).** Squamous cell carcinoma is uncommon because squamous epithelium is not usually found in normal salivary glands. Squamous metaplasia is, however, associated with chronic inflammation or may occur with certain salivary gland neoplasms. Squamous cell carcinoma may arise from this abnormal tissue. Indeed, primary squamous cell carcinoma of the salivary glands is so unusual that metastasis to the gland, usually from squamous cell carcinoma of the skin, occurs more frequently than a primary lesion.

Perineural tumor extension along a nerve is considered a hallmark of adenoid cystic carcinoma, which is the most frequent cancer of the submandibular gland. Therefore, perineural spread must always be considered **(Option (C) is false).** The most frequently involved large nerves in the region of the submandibular gland are the lingual and hypoglossal nerves.

Local direct tumor extension from the submandibular gland can involve the mandible or the adjacent musculature. The submandibular gland wraps around the posterior edge of the mylohyoid muscle, which can therefore be easily invaded once the tumor extends beyond the confines of the gland itself. The mylohyoid and digastric muscles are often removed along with the tumor. The lateral pterygoid muscle is significantly separated from the submandibular gland and is unlikely to be involved by extraglandular spread **(Option (D) is false).**

## Question 101

Concerning carotid body tumors,

(A) the internal carotid artery is frequently displaced anteriorly
(B) about 30% have symptomatic hypersecretion of catecholamines
(C) multiple lesions occur in approximately 50% of patients
(D) they usually have a homogeneous signal intensity on MRI

Paragangliomas are tumors of neural crest cell origin. They may arise in several locations in the head and neck. Temporal bone paragangliomas can be localized in the middle ear (glomus tympanicum), or they can involve the lateral wall of the jugular fossa (glomus jugulare or jugulotympanicum).

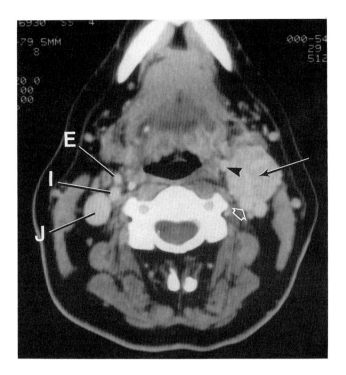

*Figure 24-8.* Left carotid body tumor. Postcontrast axial CT scan shows a brightly enhancing mass (solid arrow). Although the lesion is slightly eccentric compared with the carotid arteries, the external carotid artery (arrowhead) is displaced anteriorly and the internal carotid artery (open arrow) is displaced posteriorly. This is the characteristic CT appearance of a carotid body tumor. The internal (I) and external (E) carotid arteries are seen on the opposite side just above the level of the carotid bifurcation. The internal jugular vein (J) is indicated.

Beneath the skull base, paragangliomas can arise in two locations. The carotid body tumor arises at the carotid bifurcation. These tumors splay the bifurcation, pushing the internal carotid artery posteriorly and the external carotid artery anteriorly (Figure 24-8) **(Option (A) is false).** A vascular lesion pushing the internal carotid artery anteriorly would more likely be a glomus vagale tumor, which arises higher in the neck in association with the vagus nerve. Both the carotid body tumor and the glomus vagale tumor can present as neck masses. The glomus vagale tumor may also present as a submucosal bulge in the oropharynx.

Paragangliomas of the head and neck are almost never pharmacologically active. Although there have been reports of catecholamine secretion by head and neck paragangliomas, this does not occur in 30% of the cases **(Option (B) is false).**

Paragangliomas can occur in either a sporadic or familial pattern. In the more common sporadic nonfamilial cases, paragangliomas are multiple or bilateral in fewer than 10% of the cases. In the familial variety, this incidence has been reported to approximate 30%. In either case, 50% is too high a figure **(Option (C) is false).**

Carotid body tumors, like all paragangliomas, are very vascular and enhance intensely on CT. On MRI the many large vessels within paragangliomas are seen as flow voids within the tumor on both T1- and T2-weighted sequences. In addition, these lesions tend to have a "salt-and-pepper" appearance on T2-weighted images (Figure 24-9). Thus, these tumors do not have a homogeneous signal intensity **(Option (D) is false).**

*Hugh D. Curtin, M.D.*

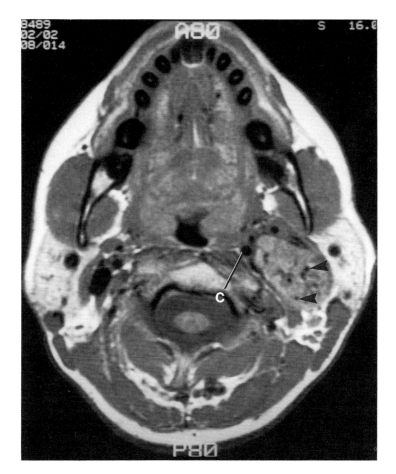

SE 700/30

*Figure 24-9.* Paraganglioma. Axial T1-weighted MR image shows a left (glomus vagale) paraganglioma. The position of this lesion is slightly unusual, since the internal carotid artery (C) is displaced medially rather than anteriorly. There are small flow voids (arrowheads) within the lesion, indicating the presence of large vessels within the tumor. These flow voids give the mass a heterogeneous appearance.

*SUGGESTED READINGS*

BRANCHIAL CLEFT CYSTS

1. Harnsberger HR, Mancuso AA, Muraki AS, et al. Branchial cleft anomalies and their mimics: computed tomographic evaluation. Radiology 1984; 152:739–748

## CERVICAL NODES

2. Harnsberger HR, Bragg DG, Osborn AG, et al. Non-Hodgkin's lymphoma of the head and neck: CT evaluation of nodal and extranodal sites. AJR 1987; 149:785–791

3. Lee YY, Van Tassel P, Nauert C, North LB, Jing BS. Lymphomas of the head and neck: CT findings at initial presentation. AJR 1987; 149:575–581

4. Mancuso AA, Harnsberger HR, Muraki AS, Stevens MH. Computed tomography of cervical and retropharyngeal lymph nodes: normal anatomy, variants of normal, and applications in staging head and neck cancer. II. Pathology. Radiology 1983; 148:715–723

5. Smoker WRK, Harnsberger HR, Reede DL, Holliday RA, Som PM, Bergeron RT. The neck. In: Som PM, Bergeron RT (eds), Head and neck imaging, 2nd ed. St. Louis: Mosby-Year Book; 1991:497–592

6. Som PM. Lymph nodes of the neck. Radiology 1987; 165:593–600

7. Suen JY. Cancer of the neck. In: Myers EN, Suen JY (eds), Cancer of the head and neck, 2nd ed. New York: Churchill Livingstone; 1989:221–254

## SUBMANDIBULAR TUMORS

8. Peel RL, Gnepp DR. Diseases of the salivary glands. In: Barnes L (ed), Surgical pathology of the head and neck, vol 1. New York: Marcel Dekker; 1985:533–645

9. Som PM. Salivary glands. IV. Tumors and tumorlike conditions. In: Som PM, Bergeron RT (eds), Head and neck imaging, 2nd ed. St. Louis: Mosby-Year Book; 1991:497–592

## PARAGANGLIOMAS

10. Olsen WL, Dillon WP, Kelly WM, Norman D, Brant-Zawadzki M, Newton TH. MR imaging of paragangliomas. AJR 1987; 148:201–204

11. Vogl T, Bruning R, Schedel H, et al. Paragangliomas of the jugular bulb and carotid body: MR imaging with short sequences and Gd-DTPA enhancement. AJR 1989; 153:583–587

*Notes*

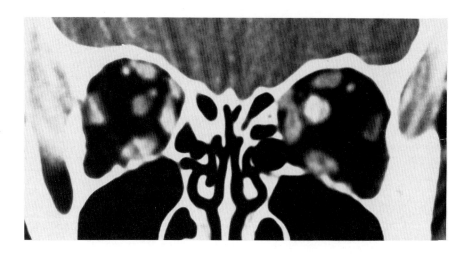

*Figure 25-1*

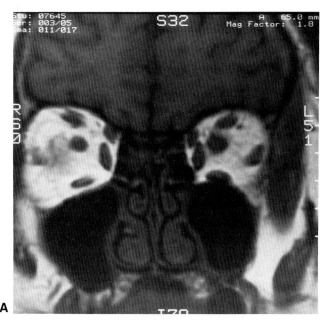

SE 600/20

*Figure 25-2*
*Figures 25-1 and 25-2.* This 65-year-old woman has a long-standing history of progressive loss of vision in her left eye. A fundoscopic examination revealed an elevated pale disk with optociliary shunt vessels. The right eye was normal. You are shown a postcontrast coronal CT scan (Figure 25-1), a T1-weighted coronal MR scan (Figure 25-2A), and a T1-weighted postcontrast axial MR scan (Figure 25-2B).

# Case 25: Optic Nerve Sheath Meningioma

## Question 102

Which *one* of the following is the MOST likely diagnosis?

- (A) Optic nerve sheath meningioma
- (B) Optic nerve glioma
- (C) Optic neuritis
- (D) Optic nerve sarcoidosis
- (E) Orbital pseudotumor

The postcontrast coronal CT scan (Figure 25-1) shows marked enhancement of the enlarged left optic nerve (arrow, Figure 25-3), and the T1-weighted coronal MR scan (Figure 25-2A) shows enlargement of the left optic nerve (arrow, Figure 25-4A). The T1-weighted axial MR scan obtained after administration of gadolinium DTPA (Figure 25-2B) shows enlargement, as well as enhancement, along the entire intraorbital portion of the left optic nerve (arrows, Figure 25-4B). Enlargement and enhancement of the optic nerve on CT or MR scans are characteristic of all of the listed diagnostic options; however, the age of the test patient, the long-standing history of progressive visual loss, and the presence of optociliary shunt vessels detected on fundoscopic examination suggest optic nerve sheath meningioma **(Option (A) is correct).** Optociliary shunts are vessels that develop from preexisting optic disk capillaries in compensation for chronic retinal venous obstruction caused characteristically by optic nerve meningioma.

Optic nerve gliomas (Option (B)) are usually found in children (2 to 8 years of age) and have an increased incidence in patients with neurofibromatosis 1. They do occur in adults; however, those seen in patients without a history of neurofibromatosis have been reported to be very aggressive (glioblastoma multiforme), and they usually extend intracranially and rapidly progress to cause bilateral blindness. The long-

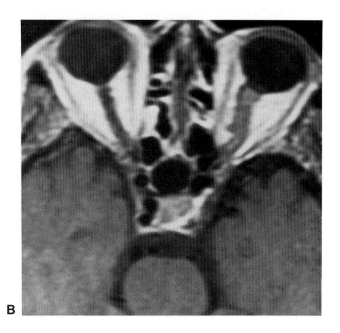

B

SE 800/20

*Figure 25-2 (Continued)*

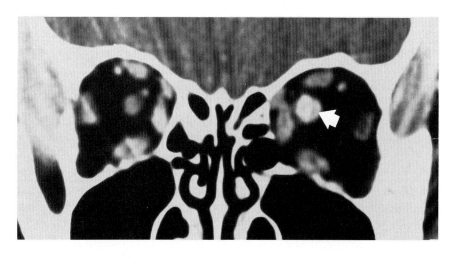

*Figure 25-3* (Same as Figure 25-1).    Optic nerve sheath meningioma. Postcontrast coronal CT scan shows marked enhancement of the enlarged left optic nerve (arrow).

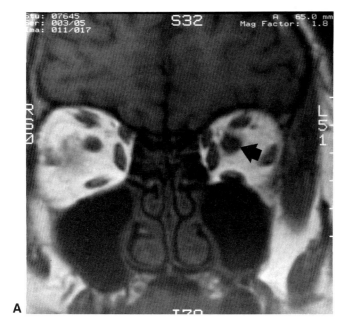

SE 600/20

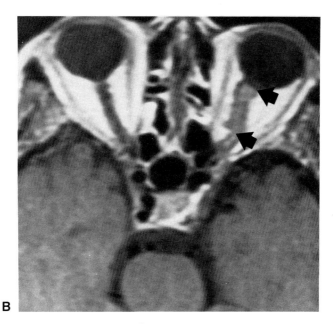

SE 800/20

*Figure 25-4* (Same as Figure 25-2).  Optic nerve sheath meningioma. (A)
T1-weighted coronal MR scan shows enlargement of the left optic nerve
(arrow). (B) T1-weighted axial MR scan obtained after administration of
gadolinium DTPA shows enlargement, as well as enhancement, along
the entire intraorbital portion of the left optic nerve (arrows).

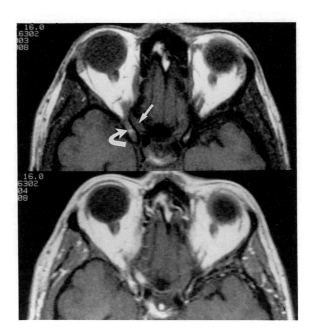

*Figure 25-5.* Optic neuritis. T1-weighted MR scans before (top) and after (bottom) administration of gadolinium DTPA show enhancement of only the intracanalicular portion of the right optic nerve (straight arrow). The left optic nerve shows no enhancement. The curved arrow points to the marrow portion of the anterior clinoid process.

standing history of progressive, unilateral loss of vision in the elderly test patient makes the diagnosis of an optic nerve glioma unlikely.

Optic neuritis (Option (C)) is frequently an acute demyelinating disease of the optic nerve. The typical clinical profile consists of a sudden loss of vision followed by spontaneous improvement over several months. Optic neuritis usually occurs in patients with confirmed multiple sclerosis or as an isolated clinical finding, in which case it may represent a *forme fruste* of multiple sclerosis. The CT and MR findings are subtle, and enhancement is often in a small segment of the optic nerve, best demonstrated by comparing pre- and postcontrast T1-weighted MR images (Figures 25-5 and 25-6). CT is far less sensitive than MRI in detection of optic nerve enhancement in patients with optic neuritis. In addition, diffuse, intense enhancement of the optic nerve, as seen in the test case, is quite rare in patients with optic neuritis.

Optic nerve sarcoidosis (Option (D)) can present as abrupt or very slow visual loss, with or without disk changes. In most cases of optic nerve sarcoidosis, CT and MR findings are very subtle and only infrequently

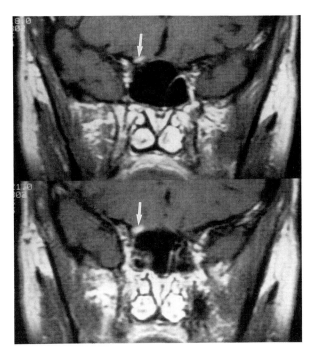

SE 600/20

*Figure 25-6.* Same patient as in Figure 25-5. Postcontrast T1-weighted coronal MR scans show enhancement of the intracanalicular segment of the right optic nerve (arrows).

show an enlarged nerve or an expanded optic canal. However, when a biopsy of an enlarged enhancing optic nerve is performed, granulomas are often found (Figures 25-7 through 25-13). In the test case, sarcoidosis cannot be excluded on the basis of the CT and MR findings alone; however, the age of the patient, lack of history of sarcoidosis, lack of clinical and imaging findings of disk changes compatible with sarcoidosis (disk granuloma) (Figure 25-9), and presence of optociliary shunt vessels all speak against optic nerve sarcoidosis. Sarcoidosis also frequently involves the central nervous system and lacrimal glands. The lack of enlargement of the lacrimal glands on both the CT and MR images, as well as the lack of abnormal findings in the brain, are other points militating against the diagnosis of optic nerve sarcoidosis.

The optic nerve may be secondarily involved by various inflammatory lesions of adjacent tissues, including the sinonasal cavities, the base of the skull, and the meninges. In patients with idiopathic inflammatory

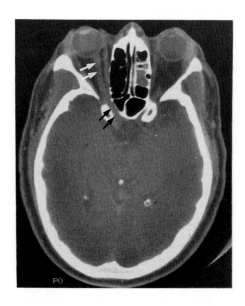

*Figure 25-7.* Sarcoidosis of the optic nerve. Axial CT scan shows slight diffuse enlargement of the right optic nerve (white arrows) in this 40-year-old black man. Notice enlargement of the right optic canal (black arrows).

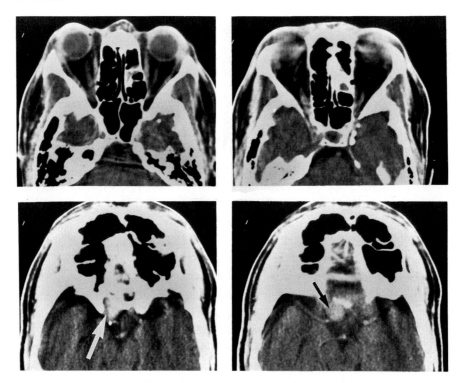

*Figure 25-8.* Same patient as in Figure 25-7. Sarcoidosis of the optic nerve. Serial postcontrast CT scans show enhancement of the intracanalicular and intracranial segments of the right optic nerve (white arrow), as well as an enhancing granuloma (black arrow) along the anterior aspect of the chiasmatic cistern. At surgery, sarcoid granulomas were found.

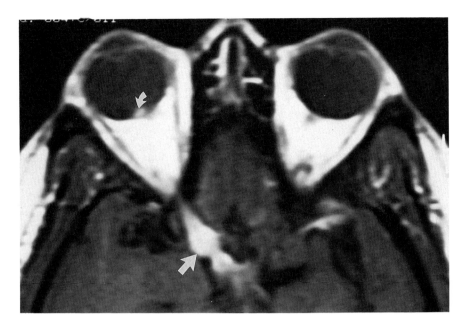

*Figure 25-9.* Sarcoidosis of the optic nerve. Postcontrast T1-weighted MR scan shows marked enhancement of the intracanalicular and intracranial segments of the right optic nerve (straight arrow). There is also an enhancing intraocular mass (curved arrow), indicative of intraocular granuloma. These MR findings were initially felt to be compatible with either optic nerve glioma or meningioma in this 28-year-old black woman. However, because of the enhancing lesion in the globe and the clinical setting, sarcoidosis was suggested as the primary consideration, and the patient was placed on steroid therapy. Follow-up MR images are shown in Figures 25-10 through 25-13.

orbital pseudotumor (Option (E)), especially in the subacute or chronic forms, there may be visual loss or disk swelling, suggesting an optic neuritis or perineuritis. In these cases, inflammatory cuffing of the optic nerve may mimic optic nerve sheath meningioma or optic nerve glioma on CT and MR scans. In patients with idiopathic inflammatory optic neuritis, visual impairment is rarely an early symptom, as it was in the test patient, and other clinical signs usually evolve before vision is disturbed. In patients with pseudotumor neuritis, the optic nerve is rarely seen as an isolated, enlarged, and enhancing image on CT and MR scans. There are other CT and MR findings characteristic of pseudotumors. Even in the rare situations when the optic nerve involvement is the predominant feature of the orbital pseudotumor, the optic nerve usually appears irregular, with a ragged, fluffy border, on CT and MR scans.

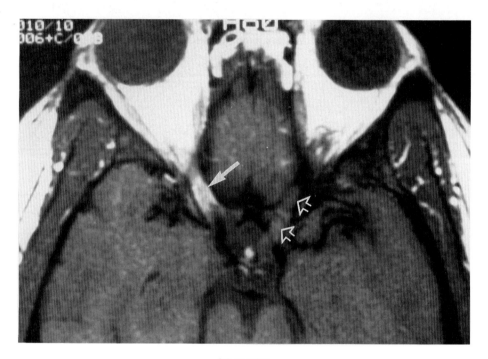

SE 612/25

*Figure 25-10.* Same patient as in Figure 25-9. Sarcoidosis. Postcontrast T1-weighted MR scan, taken a few weeks after initiation of steroid therapy, shows decreased enhancement of the right optic nerve (solid arrow) and normal left optic nerve (open arrows).

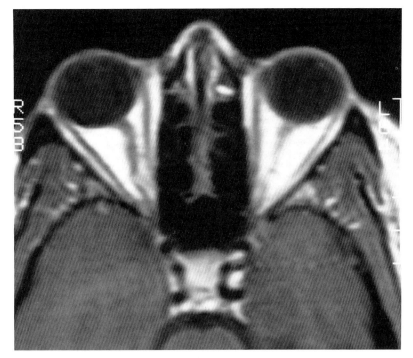

SE 600/20

*Figure 25-11.* Same patient as in Figure 25-9. Sarcoidosis. Postcontrast T1-weighted MR scan taken after about 16 weeks of steroid therapy shows a normal appearance of both optic nerves. The response to steroid therapy is better seen in coronal MR scans (Figures 25-12 and 25-13).

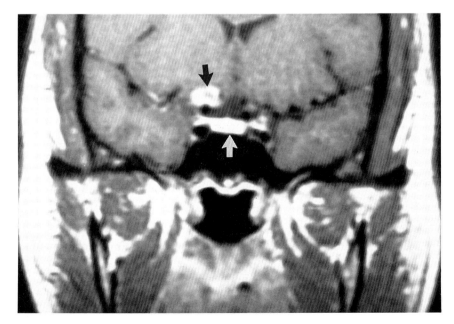

SE 600/20

*Figure 25-12.* Same patient as in Figure 25-9. Sarcoidosis. Postcontrast T1-weighted coronal MR scan shows marked enhancement of the intracranial portion of the right optic nerve (black arrow). Enhancement of the pituitary gland (white arrow) is normal.

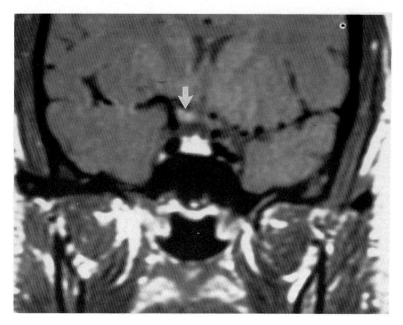

SE 967/25

*Figure 25-13.* Same patient as in Figure 25-9. Sarcoidosis. Postcontrast T1-weighted coronal MR scan following steroid therapy, showing marked improvement. There is asymmetry and slight thickening and enhancement of the right side of the chiasm (arrow).

## Question 103

Concerning optic nerve sheath meningiomas,

- (A) they usually occur in middle-aged women
- (B) those occurring in children behave aggressively
- (C) bilateral lesions are diagnostic of neurofibromatosis
- (D) the presence of tumoral calcification allows their distinction from optic nerve gliomas

An optic nerve sheath meningioma arises either from the meningothelial cells of the arachnoid that are situated along the optic nerve sheath or from an extension of an intracranial meningioma into the orbit. Another rare group of meningiomas consists of tumors that arise from ectopic arachnoid cells within the orbital cavity, either in the muscle cone or in the walls of the orbit. These ectopic, intraorbital, "extradural" men-

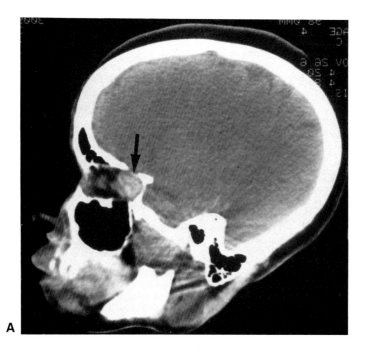

*Figure 25-14.* Presumed fibrous meningioma. (A) Sagittal CT scan shows an enhancing mass (arrow) in the left orbital apex. (B) Sagittal T1-weighted MR scan shows a hypointense mass (arrow) in the left orbital apex. (C) Postcontrast axial CT scan shows marked but inhomogeneous enhancement of the left orbital apex mass (arrow). (D) Proton-density axial MR scan shows a hypointense left orbital apex mass (arrow). (E) T2-weighted axial MR scan shows a hypointense left orbital apex mass (arrow).

ingiomas do not appear to have any connection to the optic nerve sheath or the optic canal and do not appear to originate intracranially. Their origin is uncertain. However, they probably arise from congenitally displaced nests of meningothelial cells along the orbital walls or within the muscle cone. They are frequently associated with characteristic, localized expansion of adjacent ethmoid air cells, the so-called blistering. Some investigators believe that ectopic meningiomas could also arise from the small nerves within the orbit that possess arachnoid cells along their sheaths. Others believe that many lesions presumed to represent primary intraorbital, extraoptic fibromatous or angiomatous meningiomas may not have arisen from meningeal tissue and could be fibroxanthomas (Figures 25-14 and 25-15).

Meningiomas are usually seen in middle-aged and elderly women (median age of 38 years; 80% in women) **(Option (A) is true).** Childhood

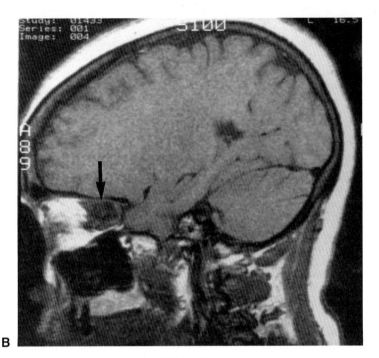

SE 600/25

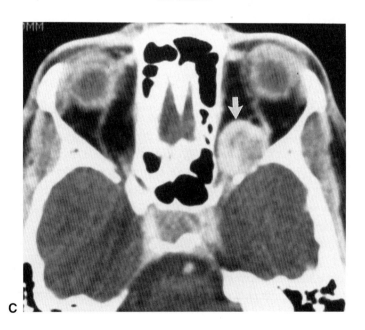

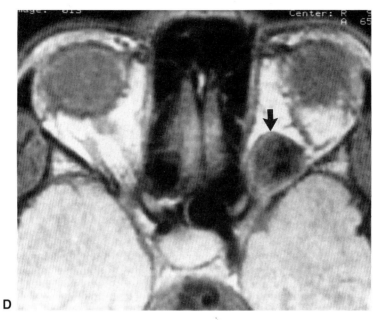

D

SE 2,000/20

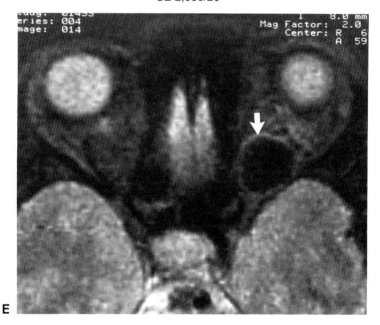

E

SE 2,000/80

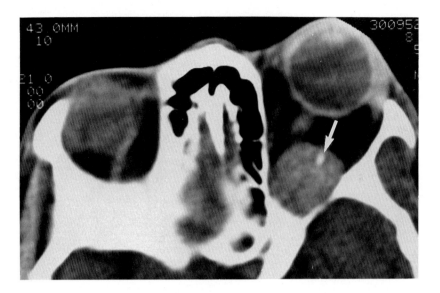

*Figure 25-15.* Same patient as in Figure 25-14. Presumed fibrous meningioma. The patient underwent a biopsy of the orbital mass under CT guidance. This CT scan shows the tip of the biopsy needle (arrow). The biopsy specimen showed dense fibrous connective tissue. The presumptive diagnosis was intraorbital extra-optic fibromatous meningioma. The patient underwent total excision of the mass. The final diagnosis was neurofibroma.

optic nerve sheath meningioma is often associated with neurofibromatosis 2 and is usually much more aggressive than the adult form; children have a higher recurrence rate and a poorer survival rate than adults **(Option (B) is true).** Bilateral optic nerve sheath meningiomas may occur in patients with or without neurofibromatosis **(Option (C) is false).** Bilateral optic nerve gliomas, however, always occur in patients with neurofibromatosis 1. Optic nerve sheath meningiomas present as very slowly progressing axial proptosis and loss of vision. Characteristic symptoms and signs of optic nerve sheath meningioma include very slow visual loss with preservation of the central visual field for years. The presence of optociliary venous shunts on the disk, when accompanied by disk pallor and visual loss, is highly suggestive of indolent nerve sheath meningioma. These vessels are known by a variety of names, including retinochoroid venous collaterals, retinal-venous-to-ciliary-venous bypass channels, retinociliary or opticociliary veins, or opticociliary (optociliary) shunt vessels. They are vessels that develop from preexisting optic disk capillaries in compensation for chronic retinal venous obstruction caused by central retinal vein occlusion. These venous channels detour blood flow from the retinal venous circulation to the choroidal venous circulation at the optic nerve head to bypass the partially obstructed central vein in the distal optic nerve. Opticociliary shunt vessels occur with perioptic nerve meningiomas as well as spheno-orbital meningiomas; however, they have also occasionally been found in patients with optic nerve glioma, glaucoma, chronic papilledema, or perioptic nerve arachnoid cyst.

In patients with optic nerve sheath meningioma, surgical procedures generally do not preserve vision. With indolent tumors there may be no advantage to any form of surgical intervention. When the intracanalicular segment of the optic nerve and the intracranial segment of the optic nerve are involved, transfrontal craniotomy for tumor resection may be advisable to prevent involvement of the chiasm and the contralateral optic nerve. Optic nerve sheath meningiomas in children are more aggressive than those in adults, and tissue diagnosis is imperative to prevent clinical confusion with orbital glioma. Meningeal hemangiopericytoma is an uncommon, aggressive tumor of the orbital nerve sheath that may be clinically and histologically confused with perioptic meningioma.

CT is an excellent imaging study for evaluating optic nerve sheath meningioma. CT scans are best obtained both before and after infusion of iodinated contrast medium. Thin sections (1.5 to 3 mm) are essential to visualize the actual extent of the tumor. Optic nerve sheath meningioma is confined to the dura mater, and so it often appears as a well-defined, tubular thickening of the optic nerve (Figure 25-16). Optic nerve sheath meningiomas are commonly seen as a diffuse, tubular enlargement or as a localized, eccentric expansion of the optic nerve, often at the orbital apex. After injection of contrast medium, meningiomas often show homogeneous and well-defined enhancement (Figure 25-17). The "tram-track" sign originally described with optic nerve sheath meningioma, in which enhanced CT scans show lucency (optic nerve) in the center of an enlarged and enhanced optic nerve-sheath complex, is not a specific finding of optic nerve sheath meningioma but may also be seen in CT scans of pseudotumors and optic neuritis. On CT scans, linear, plaquelike, or granular calcifications within or along an optic nerve mass are highly suggestive of an optic nerve sheath meningioma (Figures 25-18 and 25-19). Meningiomas surround the optic nerve, and thus the caliber of the nerve itself is attenuated within the surrounding tumor. This is in contrast to gliomas, where the nerve itself appears expanded. This feature is best appreciated on MRI (Figure 25-20). Calcification is more common in meningiomas; however, in rare instances, optic nerve gliomas show calcification on CT scans **(Option (D) is false).**

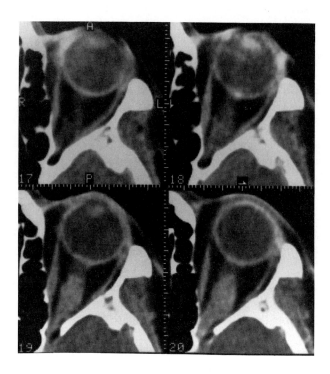

*Figure 25-16.* Optic nerve sheath meningioma. Postcontrast serial axial CT scans show tubular enlargement, as well as moderate enhancement, of the left optic nerve.

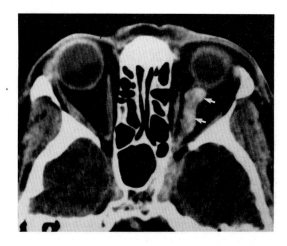

*Figure 25-17.* Optic nerve sheath meningioma. Serial postcontrast axial CT scan shows marked enhancement of the enlarged left optic nerve (arrows).

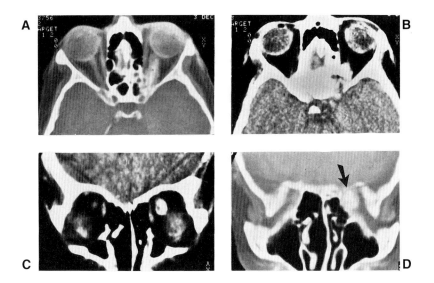

*Figure 25-18.*   Optic nerve sheath meningioma. Serial axial (A and B) and coronal (C and D) CT scans show enlargement, as well as calcification, of the left optic nerve. Note the postoperative changes of the left sphenoid wing (arrow).

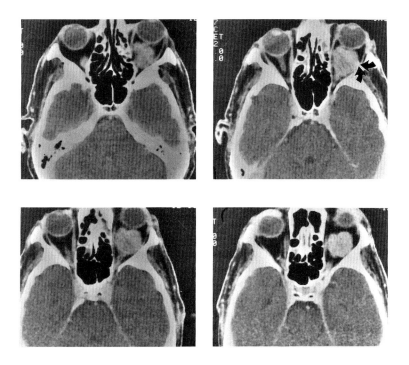

*Figure 25-19.*   Optic nerve sheath meningioma. Serial postcontrast CT scans show marked fusiform enlargement of the left optic nerve. A small, faint area of calcification (arrows) is present.

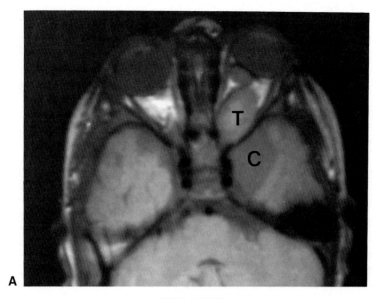

SE 2,000/20

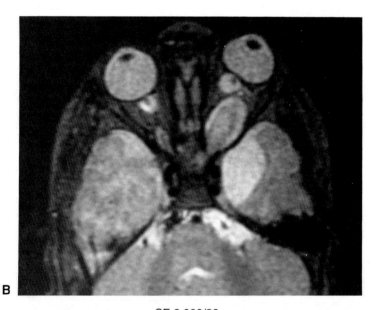

SE 2,000/80

*Figure 25-20.* Optic nerve glioma. (A) Proton-density axial MR scan shows marked enlargement of the left optic nerve. The tumor (T) is isointense to the brain. There is an arachnoid cyst (C) medial to the left temporal lobe. (B) T2-weighted axial MR scan shows the tumor expanding the optic nerve, which is characteristic of optic glioma. The optic nerve sheath is displaced to the sides. The glioma is isointense to the brain. (C) Proton-density sagittal MR scan shows extension of the tumor within the optic canal (arrow). (D) Proton-density axial MR scan shows involvement of the chiasm (arrows). (Courtesy of Allen Putterman, M.D., Department of Ophthalmology, University of Illinois, Chicago.)

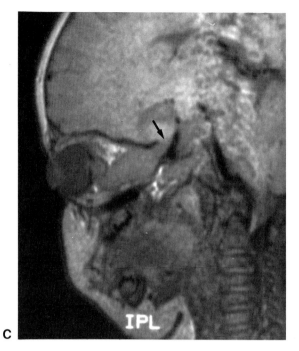

C

SE 2,000/20

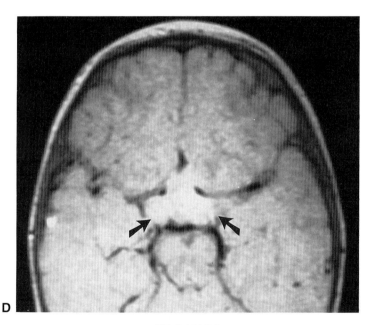

D

SE 2,000/20

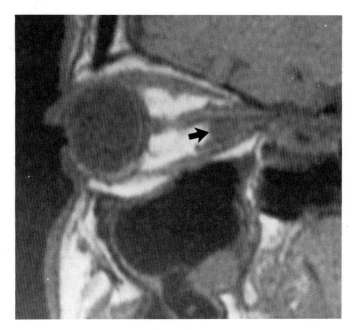

SE 800/20

*Figure 25-21.* Optic nerve sheath meningioma. T1-weighted sagittal MR scan shows an apical mass (arrow). At surgery this was found to be a meningioma. The lesion is almost isointense to the optic nerve and brain.

MRI can make significant contributions to the imaging evaluation of optic nerve sheath meningiomas. On MR images, meningioma can be seen as a localized (Figure 25-21) or fusiform (Figure 25-22) enlargement of the optic nerve. The tumor retains an isointense appearance to the optic nerve and brain tissue on most MR pulse sequences. The T1- and T2-weighted images usually show no definite change in the intensity of the meningiomas compared with that of the normal optic nerve or brain tissue. However, compared with the brain, meningiomas may also be hypointense on T1-weighted and proton-density images and hyperintense on T2-weighted images. Images obtained after intravenous injection of gadolinium-DTPA disclose marked or moderate enhancement of meningiomas. Typical CT and MR characteristics of optic nerve sheath meningioma are demonstrated in Figures 25-23 and 25-24, respectively. When intravenous gadolinium is used, additional T1-weighted fat-suppression pulse sequences may prove valuable for better defining an enhancing meningioma (Figure 25-24C). Intraorbital extension of an intracranial

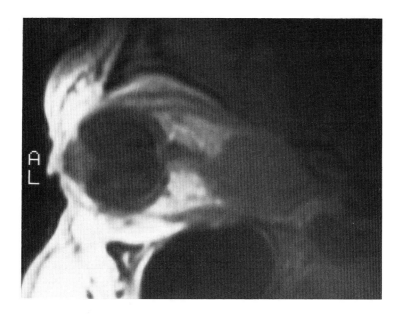

*Figure 25-22.* Optic nerve sheath meningioma. T1-weighted MR scan, obtained with a surface coil, shows a large, hypointense mass along the superior aspect of the optic nerve.

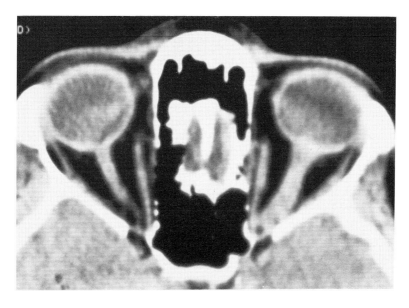

*Figure 25-23.* Optic nerve sheath meningioma. Postcontrast CT scan shows diffuse enlargement of the left optic nerve with moderate to marked enhancement.

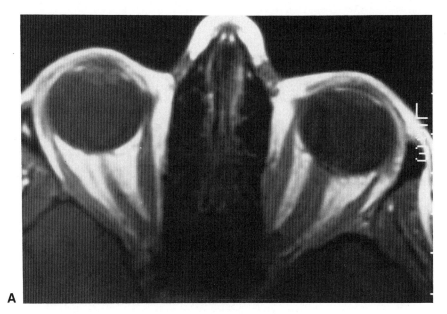

A

SE 500/20

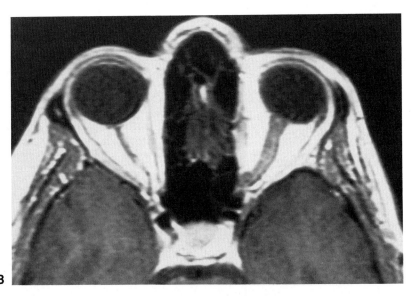

B

SE 400/20

*Figure 25-24.* Same patient as in Figure 25-23. Optic nerve sheath meningioma. (A) T1-weighted transaxial MR scan shows the mass, which is hypointense to fat and isointense to the normal contralateral optic nerve. (B) Postcontrast T1-weighted axial MR scan shows moderate to marked enhancement of the left optic nerve sheath meningioma. (C) Post-contrast T1-weighted fat suppression axial MR scan shows marked enhancement of the left optic nerve sheath meningioma. (D) STIR MR scan shows marked hyperintensity of the left optic nerve sheath meningioma.

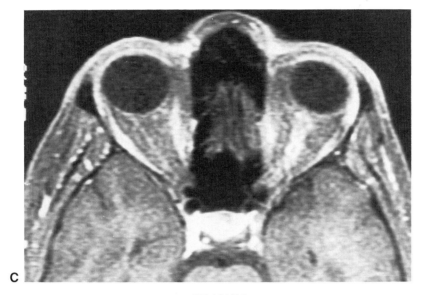

SE 400/15

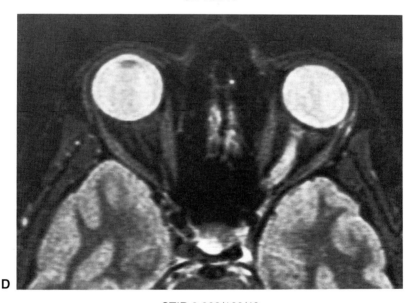

STIR 2,000/160/40

meningioma may easily be demonstrated on postcontrast CT or MR scans (Figure 25-25). Intracanalicular meningiomas usually represent either extensions of posterior orbital tumors or invasion into the canal by periforaminal meningiomas arising in the vicinity of the anterior clinoid.

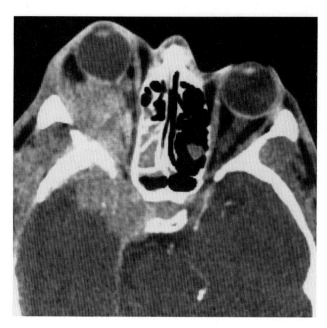

*Figure 25-25.* Sphenoid wing meningioma. Postcontrast CT scan shows a recurrent sphenoid wing meningioma with marked extension into the right orbit, as well as into the right temporal fossa.

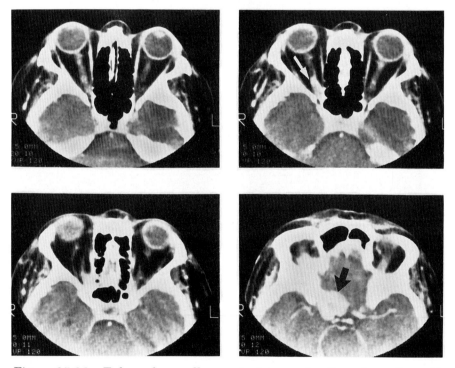

*Figure 25-26.* Tuberculum sella meningioma extending along the optic nerve. Serial postcontrast CT scans show marked enhancement of the tuberculum sella meningioma (black arrow). Note its extension along the optic nerve (white arrow).

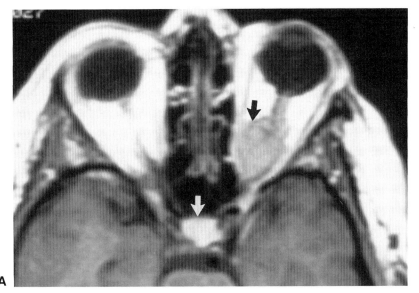

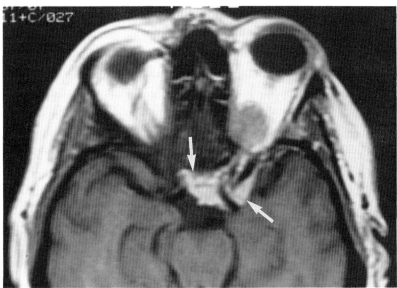

*Figure 25-27.* Chiasmatic-paraclinoid meningioma extending along the optic nerve. (A) Postcontrast T1-weighted MR scan shows intense enhancement (white arrow) adjacent to the chiasmatic cistern and an enhancing mass along the optic nerve (black arrow). (B) Postcontrast T1-weighted MR scan shows the infiltrative chiasmatic-paraclinoid meningioma (arrows) with extension into the left orbital apex.

Purely midcanalicular meningiomas are extremely rare (Figures 25-26 and 25-27).

# Question 104

Concerning optic nerve gliomas,

   (A) they occur most frequently in children
   (B) those occurring in adults are frequently high-grade astrocytomas
   (C) bilateral lesions are characteristic of neurofibromatosis 1
   (D) kinking and buckling of the enlarged optic nerve are frequently present

Optic nerve glioma is a tumor arising from the neuroglia (glial cells) of the optic nerve. It is usually a tumor of childhood (2 through 8 years of age) **(Option (A) is true).** However, it can be seen at birth and in adults. Nine of ten cases are symptomatic in the first two decades of life. Childhood gliomas are controversial lesions both clinically and pathologically; there are questions about their natural course and growth potential and the effectiveness of therapy. In general, optic nerve glioma in children is regarded as a benign, well-differentiated, and slowly growing, noninvasive pilocytic astrocytoma.

The fact that most optic nerve gliomas manifest in early childhood strongly suggests that they are really congenital in origin and are due to some kind of abnormality in the embryonic development of the neuroglia of the nerve. On the other hand, optic nerve glioma in adults is a rare but invasive malignant astrocytic tumor (usually glioblastoma multiforme) **(Option (B) is true).** With the exception of visual loss and anatomic location, the childhood and adult optic gliomas have little in common. Children with optic gliomas present with insidious proptosis and diminished vision, although remarkably well-preserved vision is not uncommon. Adults with optic gliomas present with rapid, severe, unilateral visual loss, at times mimicking optic neuritis. The course of the disease is very rapid, with bilateral visual deterioration and other intracranial signs. Death follows within a few months to 2 years.

The natural history of childhood optic glioma does not involve malignant transformation or systemic metastasis. Adulthood optic gliomas may metastasize. In childhood glioma, local invasion into the extraocular muscles rarely occurs. The primary sequela of childhood glioma is atrophy resulting from damage to the optic nerve fibers and the optic nerve nutrient arteries.

Bilateral optic nerve gliomas are characteristic of neurofibromatosis 1 **(Option (C) is true).** Adulthood optic gliomas have no relationship with neurofibromatosis. The association of von Recklinghausen's neurofibromatosis and optic glioma is well known. The frequency of this association is not known, but it is more common than generally recognized.

Orbital gliomas may be contiguous with astrocytic proliferation extending posteriorly into the optic canal, the intracranial optic nerve, and the chiasm itself, that is, in the configuration of an "optochiasmatic" glioma (see Figure 25-20C and D). Optic glioma may also be part of a more extensive pathologic process that involves the hypothalamus: "optohypothalamic glioma," with or without a congenital or juvenile diencephalic syndrome. Posterior continuation with involvement of optic tracts and hemispheres may also be present.

The American Cancer Society has proposed a clinical staging system for optic pathway gliomas: T1, involvement of one optic nerve, intraorbital or intracranial; T2, involvement of both optic nerves; T3, involvement of the optic chiasm; and T4, involvement of the hypothalamus or thalamus. Diencephalic syndrome of early childhood has been extensively described; it consists of emaciation (despite adequate nutritional intake), hypotension, hypoglycemia, optic nerve atrophy, sexual precocity, and laughing seizures. Most cases of diencephalic syndrome are due to low-grade astrocytomas of the hypothalamus or adjacent chiasm, and almost all patients are younger than 2 years at presentation. In general, primary astrocytic tumors of the anterior visual pathways in children tend to behave as relatively pilocytic astrocytomas with limited growth potential. The level of visual impairment at initial diagnosis does not change appreciably thereafter.

An optic nerve glioma is seen on CT as a well-defined, fusiform enlargement of the optic nerve. Diffuse, tortuous enlargement of the optic nerve with a characteristic kinking and buckling (sinusoid) appearance is a characteristic feature of the childhood form of optic glioma (Figure 25-28) **(Option (D) is true).** Many orbital gliomas involve the optic canal. Calcification is rare in optic nerve gliomas. Following intravenous contrast administration, they may show homogeneous (Figure 25-28) or heterogeneous enhancement. The heterogeneity is the result of tumor infarction, secondary to obliteration, of the small nutrient arteries of the optic nerve.

MRI also readily demonstrates an enlarged fusiform and kinked optic nerve (Figure 25-20). On T1-weighted images, the optic glioma appears isointense or slightly hyperintense compared with the white matter. On T2-weighted images, the lesion may show greater variability in intensity; however, it may appear hyperintense compared with the white matter (Figure 25-20B). Many orbital gliomas involve the optic canal; this is best appreciated by MRI (Figure 25-20C). Intracranial extension of optic nerve gliomas often can be better appreciated on MRI than on CT (Figure 25-20D).

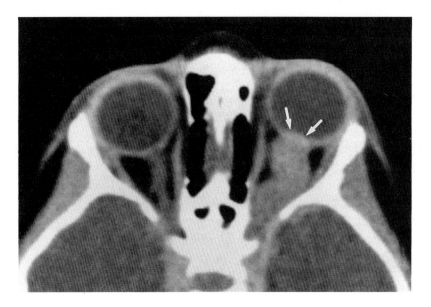

*Figure 25-28.* Optic nerve glioma. Postcontrast CT scan shows moderate to marked enhancement of the enlarged left optic nerve. There is characteristic kinking and buckling of the enlarged optic nerve. Also note the marked enlargement of the optic disk (arrows).

MRI is superior to CT in demonstrating the posterior extent of optic pathway gliomas and often detects focal areas of T2 hyperintensity in the basal ganglia, internal capsule, cerebellum, and white matter that are not detected by CT. Dural ectasia (optic hydrops) is a rare condition that may result in apparent enlargement of the optic nerve. This condition may be seen in patients with neurofibromatosis, and therefore on CT and MRI it may mimic optic nerve tumors. In this situation, MRI is more sensitive than CT in differentiating the conditions (Figure 25-29). The use of paramagnetic contrast media results in enhancement of gliomas, although less than that seen in meningiomas (Figures 25-30 and 25-31).

The diagnosis and management of childhood optic nerve glioma depend on the clinical constellation of signs and the findings on CT and MRI. If the diagnosis is nearly certain, surgical exploration for biopsy is not advised. Surgical intervention for total excision of the tumor is contemplated when the tumor shows evidence of progressive enlargement. If proptosis in a child with a blind or near-blind eye as a result of optic glioma is cosmetically unacceptable, resection of the tumor from the globe to the orbital apex via a frontal craniotomy is recommended. Enucleation or exenteration is not indicated. Care should be taken not to injure the

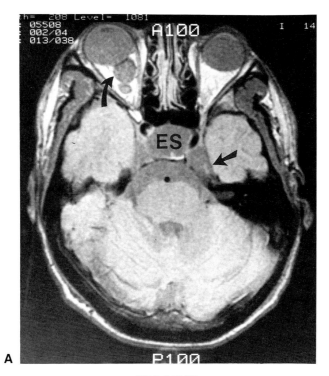

SE 2,000/20

*Figure 25-29.* Optic nerve hydrops. (A) Proton-density axial MR scan shows enlargement of the right optic nerve (curved arrow), mimicking an optic nerve tumor. Note the empty sella (ES), the enlarged cisterns of the gasserian ganglions (straight arrow), and the enlarged prepontine cistern. (B) T2-weighted axial MR scan shows that the enlarged optic nerve is due to expansion of the subarachnoid space around the nerve (dural ectasia). The CT scans of this patient were interpreted as optic nerve meningioma or glioma.

motor nerves and arteries at the globe. The efficacy of radiation therapy for orbital gliomas is unsubstantiated. In practical terms, patients with neurofibromatosis and evidence of a multifocal or diffuse optic nerve glioma are probably best left untreated and simply observed (Figures 25-29 and 25-30).

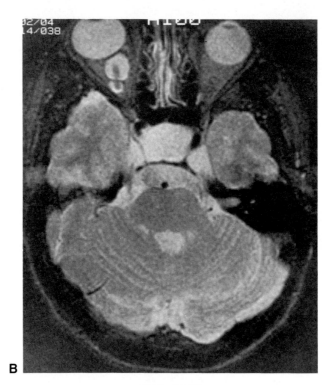

SE 2,000/80

SE 2,000/20

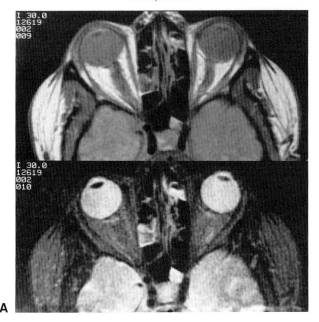

SE 2,000/80

SE 600/20

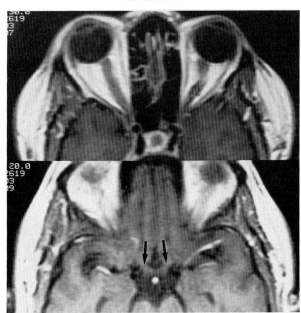

SE 600/20

*Figure 25-30.* Neurofibromatosis and optic nerve glioma. (A) Proton-density (top) and T2-weighted (bottom) MR scans show irregular enlargement of the right optic nerve. The tumor is isointense to the brain in the proton-density image and hypointense to the brain in the T2-weighted image. (B) T1-weighted MR scans obtained after administration of gadolinium DTPA show minimal enhancement along the right optic nerve glioma. The intracranial portions of the optic nerves appear normal (arrows).

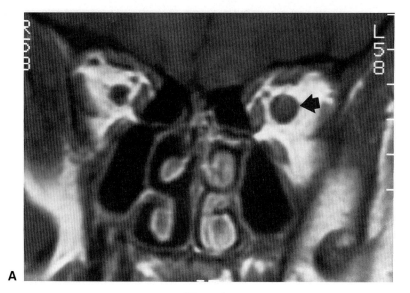

SE 600/20

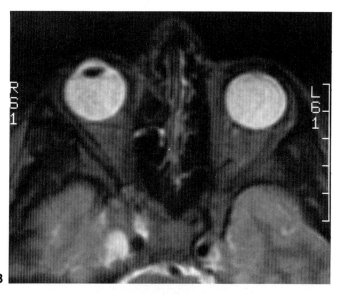

SE 2,000/80

*Figure 25-31.* Neurofibromatosis and optic nerve glioma. (A) Postcontrast T1-weighted coronal MR scan shows enlargement of the central
portion of the left optic nerve (arrow) characteristic of optic nerve glioma.
There is no significant enhancement. (B) T2-weighted axial MR scan
shows the left optic nerve glioma. The lesion is hypointense to the brain,
similar to the lesions in Figures 25-24B and 25-34A.

# Question 105

Concerning optic neuritis,

(A) it is commonly a manifestation of multiple sclerosis
(B) it occurs in patients with malnutrition
(C) it occurs in both the acute and chronic forms of sarcoid involvement of the nervous system
(D) it commonly causes diffuse enlargement of the optic nerve

Optic neuritis is a clinical syndrome rather than a specific disease. It is often described as an acute, inflammatory process involving the optic nerve. However, this definition fails to convey the complex nosologic spectrum, which includes idiopathic, immune-mediated, metabolic, and infective optic neuritis. The term papillitis refers to the intraocular form of optic neuritis in which disk swelling is observed. When the optic nerve is damaged by vascular, compressive, or unknown mechanisms, the more general term optic neuropathy is preferable.

Multiple sclerosis is the most common cause of optic neuritis (**Option (A) is true**). Visual loss is typically unilateral in patients with demyelinative optic neuritis. Optic neuropathies following chickenpox, rubella, rubeola, mumps, herpes zoster, mononucleosis, and viral encephalitis are referred to as parainfectious, as opposed to those caused by direct tissue infiltration by microorganisms. Visual loss is typically bilateral, occurring 10 to 14 days after the primary illness. This delay suggests a cascade of autoimmune mechanisms. Postinfectious radiculopathy of the Guillain-Barré type tends to spare the central nervous system, but both optic neuritis and otic neuritis have been reported. Optic neuritis in patients with systemic lupus erythematosus or other autoimmune states is referred to as autoimmune optic neuritis.

Infective causes of optic neuritis include syphilis (neuroretinitis, papillitis, and perineuritis), toxoplasmosis, toxocariasis (papillitis), and, uncommonly, borreliosis (Lyme disease). The spectrum of optic neuropathies that occurs with human immunodeficiency virus (HIV) infection includes syphilitic optic perineuritis; papillitis or neuroretinitis of cytomegalovirus, syphilis, and hepatitis B infections; or acute retinal necrosis syndrome (herpesviruses). Cytomegalovirus inclusions have been found in all layers of the retina and glial cells of the optic nerve. The role of HIV itself as an etiologic agent in optic nerve disease is unknown. Occasionally, herpes zoster ophthalmicus is associated with optic neuritis, either in the retrobulbar form or with a severe ischemic papillitis. Histopathologically, herpes zoster involves the optic nerve as an inflammatory arteritis with associated mild leptomeningitis. Insidious and slowly progressive bilateral loss of function in the central fields, with resultant diminished acuity, should alert the physician to the possibility of nutritional and toxic optic neuropathy (neuritis) related to dietary deficiencies of B-complex vitamins, particularly thiamin, folic acid, and vitamin $B_2$ **(Option (B) is true).** Optic neuritis may accompany acute meningitis in children or adults. Purulent leptomeningitis spreads to invade the optic nerve sheath. The optic nerve may also be involved in granulomatous and fungal meningitis, including that due to syphilis, tuberculosis, aspergillosis, and cryptococcosis.

The average annual incidence of optic neuritis has been reported to be 6.4 cases per 100,000 in Olmsted County, Minn.; this is the only U.S. population for which such epidemiologic data are available. About half the cases are idiopathic, and the other half are associated with multiple sclerosis. There is ample evidence that optic neuritis is a manifestation of multiple sclerosis. Isolated idiopathic optic neuritis is considered a *forme fruste* of multiple sclerosis. The typical clinical presentation consists of sudden loss of vision, which can vary in severity from a slight deficit in the field of vision to complete loss of light perception, followed by spontaneous improvement over several months. Most patients have lasting symptoms of visual impairment, and even when visual acuity returns to normal, abnormalities in the visual field, color vision, and contrast sensitivity are common. Optic neuritis is found in persons of all ages, with the peak incidence in the third and fourth decades of life. Cases in women outnumber those in men by 2:1. The disorder is overwhelmingly monocular in adults. Pain is present and characteristically aggravated by touching or moving the eye. Untreated patients generally recover even if visual acuity is severely impaired at the peak of the episode. In fact, the vast majority of patients will recover their original acuity within several months.

The association of optic neuritis with multiple sclerosis has long been recognized. Lesions in the anterior visual pathway are always found in the brains of patients who die of multiple sclerosis. Electrophysiologic abnormalities, compatible with optic nerve lesions, are frequent in patients with multiple sclerosis even in the absence of visual symptoms. Most patients with acute idiopathic optic neuritis and with no other neurologic disorder have the same areas of high-intensity signal in the cerebral white matter on T2-weighted MR images that are found in patients with multiple sclerosis. A prospective investigation of patients with idiopathic optic neuritis but no previous or concurrent neurologic abnormalities showed that clinical symptoms and signs of multiple sclerosis developed in 74% of the women and 34% of the men by the 15th year after the onset of visual loss. Moreover, the clinical characteristics of idiopathic optic neuritis and the optic neuritis associated with multiple sclerosis are identical. Acute optic neuritis thus appears to exemplify an attack of acute multiple sclerosis.

The efficacy of corticosteroids and corticotropin for the treatment of optic neuritis is controversial. Although numerous reports have suggested that they are effective, this is not uniformly true. For example, Herishanu et al. reported that multiple sclerosis may develop at an increasing rate among patients with optic neuritis who receive intravenous methylprednisolone. Although controlled studies in England in the 1960s and 1970s show that neither corticotropin nor retrobulbar corticosteroid injections improved visual outcome, most ophthalmologists and neurologists still treat acute optic neuritis with corticosteroids. The agent prescribed is generally oral prednisone. Beck et al. have recently performed a prospective, randomized comparative study of the efficacy of oral prednisone and intravenous methylprednisolone, each compared with an oral placebo, for acute unilateral optic neuritis in 457 adults. The results of their investigations confirmed that oral prednisone had no advantages over placebo. Furthermore, recurrences of optic neuritis were more frequent in the group treated with oral prednisone. Visual acuity recovered faster in the patients who received intravenous methylprednisolone than in the controls, but after 6 months the placebo group had caught up. Beck et al. concluded that oral prednisone not only is ineffective against optic neuritis but also increases the risk of new episodes. Intravenous methylprednisolone followed by oral prednisone will speed the recovery of visual loss due to optic neuritis and result in slightly better vision at 6 months. Although the authors could not offer a biologic explanation for the higher rate of new episodes in the group given oral prednisone, they thought that this finding was very unlikely to be a chance occurrence.

In patients with optic neuritis, CT may show enlargement of the optic nerve with some degree of contrast enhancement. MRI is more sensitive than CT in the detection of optic neuritis. On CT and MRI, the optic nerve may infrequently appear diffusely enlarged **(Option (D) is false)**. On T2-weighted MR images, the involved optic nerve may be slightly or moderately more hyperintense than the one on the normal side (Figure 25-32). In general, in patients with optic neuritis, contrast enhancement on CT and MRI is often subtle (Figure 25-33) or present in a short segment of the optic nerve; it is best demonstrated by comparing pre- and postcontrast T1-weighted MR images (Figures 25-5 and 25-6). MR

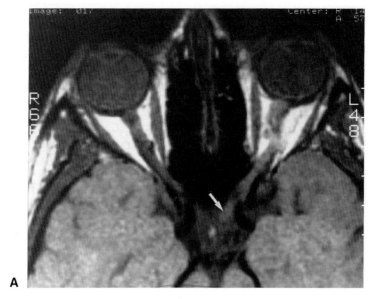

SE 2,000/20

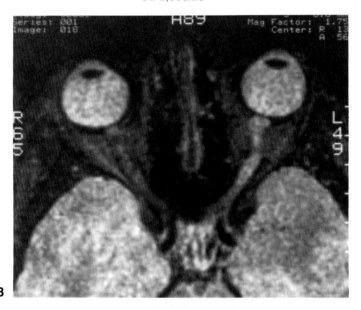

SE 2,000/80

*Figure 25-32.* Left optic neuritis in a 14-year-old girl. (A) Proton-density MR scan shows slight thickening, as well as a slight increase in signal intensity, of the left optic nerve, including its intracranial portion (arrow). (B) T2-weighted MR scan shows slight thickening and increased signal intensity of the left optic nerve. The patient responded to steroid therapy and made a full recovery. This MR appearance of diffuse thickening of the optic nerve is infrequent in patients with optic neuritis.

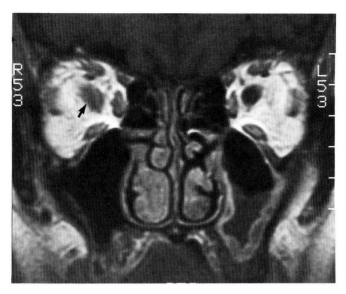

SE 400/20

*Figure 25-33.* Optic neuritis. Postcontrast T1-weighted MR scan shows irregular thickening of the right optic nerve with moderate enhancement (arrow).

visualization of plaques in cases of demyelinating optic neuritis is infrequent; however, at times it may be accentuated by short-tau inversion-recovery (STIR) pulse sequences (Figure 25-34). At times, postcontrast T1-weighted fat-suppression MRI shows the segmental or focal enhancement of the optic nerve in optic nerve neuritis more clearly.

*Optic nerve sarcoidosis.* Certain inflammatory conditions, such as syphilis, tuberculosis, or sarcoidosis, may be responsible for a chronic and progressive loss of vision. Chronic optic neuropathy, however, is more frequently due to a compressive lesion such as meningioma (intracanalicular or tuberculum sellae), pituitary tumor, or paraclinoid aneurysm.

Sarcoidosis frequently involves the nervous system and can present as abrupt or very chronic visual loss, with or without disk changes. In one series of 11 cases of sarcoidosis of the optic nerve in patients ranging in age from 16 to 48 years, only two patients were previously known to have the disorder. Four patients showed disk granulomas, four had optic nerve granulomas, and five had posterior uveitis and retinitis. In this series, chest radiographs were characteristically abnormal in 8 of 11 patients. Only one-third had elevated serum levels of angiotensin-converting enzyme (ACE). CT scans in these 11 patients infrequently

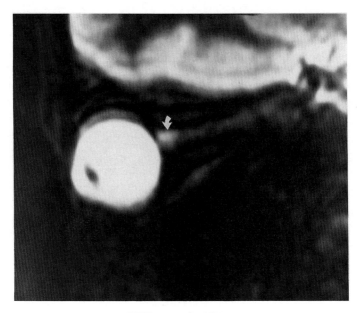

STIR 2,000/250/70

*Figure 25-34.* Optic neuritis. STIR sagittal MR scan shows a focal area of increased signal intensity (arrow) along the optic nerve in this patient with known multiple sclerosis.

showed enlarged nerves or other findings. Although sarcoidosis is classically believed not to involve the optic nerves commonly, we have seen increasing numbers of cases of presumed optic nerve sarcoidosis on MR and CT scans, some of them with histologic confirmation.

Sarcoidosis is an idiopathic, multisystem, granulomatous inflammation, often involving the mediastinal and peripheral lymph nodes, the lungs, liver, spleen, bone marrow, parotid glands, eyes, lacrimal glands, and many other organs. In the United States, the disease is more prevalent in young adult blacks and more common in women than men. In ophthalmologic series, up to 50% of patients with sarcoidosis have ocular involvement. Thirty percent of cases of posterior uveitis are associated with sarcoidosis. Neurologic involvement with sarcoidosis takes two forms. In acute sarcoidosis, there tends to be involvement of a peripheral nerve, especially a cranial nerve and in particular the facial nerve. The optic nerve (which is not a peripheral nerve) is involved next most frequently. Sarcoid uveitis, in combination with a facial nerve palsy and fever, is known as Herford's syndrome or uveoparotid fever. The second form of nervous system sarcoid occurs in the chronic form of the disease, with central nervous system (CNS) involvement. Involvement of the optic nerve is more common in this form. The involvement may be at the chiasm or in the intracanalicular or intraorbital segments of the optic nerve. Optic neuritis, granulomatous protrusions from the optic nerve head into the vitreous, and optic atrophy are manifestations of CNS and optic nerve sarcoid disease **(Option (C) is true).** Apart from the involvement of the lacrimal gland, involvement of the orbital tissues by true systemic sarcoidosis is extremely rare.

Orbital pseudotumor may have an epithelial or granulomatous pattern, which could easily be mistaken for sarcoidosis. Sarcoidosis-like lesions can be found in patients with syphilis, lymphogranuloma venereum, leprosy, tularemia, torulosis, histoplasmosis, blastomycosis, and coccidioidomycosis.

The early lesions of sarcoidosis are much more likely to respond to corticosteroid therapy than are the late, fibrotic hyalinized lesions. Lesions that demand systemic corticosteroid therapy are uveitis, optic neuritis, diffuse pulmonary and CNS lesions, persistent facial palsy, persistent hypercalcemia, and cutaneous lesions.

*Diagnostic imaging in optic nerve sarcoidosis.* When an ophthalmologist or neurologist suspects that an optic nerve is involved by sarcoidosis or that there is sarcoid of the CNS, a chest radiograph can be very useful. Active pulmonary sarcoidosis characteristically shows bilateral hilar adenopathy, with or without parenchymal disease. The nodes characteristically stand out from the right heart border, and there is associated right paratracheal nodal involvement. Chest abnormalities are found in about 80% of patients with ocular sarcoidosis (uveitis). Gallium scintigraphy is more sensitive than chest radiography for showing pulmonary involvement in patients with sarcoidosis. It lacks specificity, however, because other pulmonary diseases also show similar uptake. Lacrimal gland uptake of Ga-67 also occurs in more than 80% of patients with active sarcoidosis. This uptake is also nonspecific.

CT and MR scans in patients with optic nerve sarcoidosis may show no significant findings; however, not infrequently, they may show enlargement of the optic nerve, as well as expansion of the optic canal, mimicking an optic nerve sheath meningioma on orbital imaging (Figures 25-7 through 25-13).

# Question 106

Concerning optic nerve pseudotumor (perineuritis),

(A) it presents clinically as a painful eye associated with decreased vision
(B) it is rarely associated with involvement of the adjacent retrobulbar fat
(C) CT shows enhancement of the optic nerve
(D) MRI shows ragged, edematous enlargement of the optic nerve-sheath complex

The optic nerve may be secondarily involved by various inflammatory lesions of surrounding tissues, including the orbit, paranasal sinuses, base of the skull, and meninges. Idiopathic inflammatory cuffing of the orbital and intracranial optic nerve may present with progressive visual deterioration and thus mimic an optic nerve sheath meningioma clinically. In general, acute and subacute idiopathic inflammatory orbital syndromes have been designated as pseudotumors, a clinically and histologically ill-defined category of lesions, which are discussed in detail in Case 10. In patients with orbital pseudotumor, the main focus of inflammation may involve the anterior orbit and adjacent globe with and without perineural infiltration (cuffing). The major features on presentation are pain, proptosis, lid swelling, injection, and decreased vision **(Option (A) is true)**. Other findings may include uveitis, sclerotenonitis, papillitis, and exudative retinal detachment. The characteristic CT and MR findings are of a diffuse anterior orbital infiltration intimately related to the globe, producing thickening of the choroid, sclera, and Tenon's capsule. There may be a fluid (exudate) in Tenon's space, producing a characteristic semilunar configuration around the posterior globe with obscuration of the junction of the globe and the optic nerve, and there may be variable extension along the optic nerve sheath. The optic nerve involvement may be seen in patients with other types of orbital pseudotumors, including diffuse, myositic, and apical types of pseudotumors, as well as in those with orbital lymphoma and orbital leukemic infiltration (Figure 25-35). In patients with optic nerve pseudotumor (perineuritis), optic nerve involvement is rarely an isolated finding. There are other CT and MR findings in the retrobulbar and extraconal spaces characteristic of pseudotumor **(Option (B) is false)**. CT shows variable enhancement **(Option (C) is true)**. MRI shows a ragged, edematous enlargement of the optic nerve sheath complex, as well as enhancement **(Option (D) is true)**. Rapid steroid responsiveness is almost pathognomonic for pseudotumors. CT and MR scanning are useful, particularly for assessing

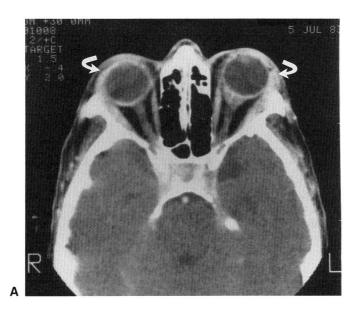

*Figure 25-35.* Orbital pseudotumor with involvement of the optic nerve. (A) Postcontrast CT scan shows enlargement of both lacrimal glands (curved arrows), as well as enlargement of both lateral rectus muscles. Note the effacement of the orbital fat lateral to the lateral rectus muscles as a result of cellular infiltration. Also notice the perioptic cuffing on the left side. (B) Postcontrast CT scan following steroid therapy shows that the process is progressing, with marked enlargement of the left optic nerve. The left lacrimal gland (arrow) remains enlarged. There is slight improvement on the right side, with visualization of orbital fat lateral to the right lateral rectus muscles (arrowheads). A biopsy specimen taken at this time showed lymphoma.

resolution after therapy. Failure of resolution should suggest alternative diagnoses, and a biopsy may be necessary.

*Mahmood F. Mafee, M.D.*

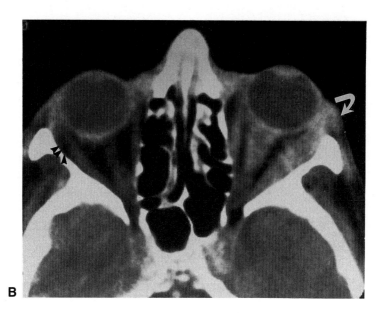

B

*SUGGESTED READINGS*

## OPTIC NERVE SHEATH MENINGIOMA

1. Ellenberger C. Perioptic meningiomas. Syndrome of long-standing visual loss, pale disk edema, and optociliary veins. Arch Neurol 1976; 33:671–674
2. Frisen L, Royt WF, Tengroth BM. Optociliary veins, disc pallor and visual loss. A triad of signs indicating spheno-orbital meningioma. Acta Ophthalmol 1973; 51:241–249
3. Schatz H, Green R, Talamo JH, Hoyt WF, Johnson RN, McDonald HR. Clinicopathologic correlation of retinal to choroidal venous collaterals of the optic nerve head. Ophthalmology 1991; 98:1287–1293
4. Zakka KA, Summerer RW, Yee RD, Foos RY, Kim J. Optociliary veins in a primary optic nerve sheath meningioma. Am J Ophthalmol 1979; 87:91–95

## OPTIC NERVE GLIOMA

5. Glaser JS. Topical diagnosis: prechiasmal visual pathways. In: Duane TD (ed), Clinical ophthalmology. Philadelphia: JB Lippincott; 1990; 2; 5:1–85
6. Hershey BL, Peyster RG. Imaging of cranial nerve II. Semin US CT MR 1987; 8:164–184
7. Rootman J, Robertson W. Neurogenic tumors. In: Rootman J (ed), Diseases of the orbit. Philadelphia: JB Lippincott; 1988:281–334

## OPTIC NEURITIS

8. Beck RW, Cleary PA, Anderson MM Jr, et al. A randomized, controlled trial of corticosteroids in the treatment of acute optic neuritis. The Optic Neuritis Study Group. N Engl J Med 1992; 326:581–588

9. Ebers GC. Optic neuritis and multiple sclerosis. Arch Neurol 1985; 42:702–704

10. Gould ES, Bird AC, Leaver PK, McDonald WI. Treatment of optic neuritis by retrobulbar injection of triamcinolone. Br Med J 1977; 1:1495–1497

11. Herishanu YO, Badarna S, Sarov B, Abarbanel JM, Segal S, Bearman JE. A possible harmful late effect of methylprednisolone therapy on a time cluster of optic neuritis. Acta Neurol Scand 1989; 80:569–574

12. Lessell S. Corticosteroid treatment of acute optic neuritis. N Engl J Med 1992; 326:634–635

13. Percy AK, Nobrega FT, Kurland LT. Optic neuritis and multiple sclerosis. An epidemiologic study. Arch Ophthalmol 1972; 87:135–139

14. Rawson MD, Liversedge LA, Goldfarb G. Treatment of acute retrobulbar neuritis with corticotrophin. Lancet 1966; 2:1044–1046

15. Rizzo JF III, Lessell S. Risk of developing multiple sclerosis after uncomplicated optic neuritis: a long-term prospective study. Neurology 1988; 38:185–190

## SARCOIDOSIS

16. Beardsley TL, Brown SV, Sydnor CF, Grimson BS, Klintworth GK. Eleven cases of sarcoidosis of the optic nerve. Am J Ophthalmol 1984; 97:62–77

17. Crick RP, et al. The eyes in sarcoidosis. Br J Ophthalmol 1961; 45:461–481

## ORBITAL PSEUDOTUMOR

18. Jakobiec FA, Jones IS. Orbital inflammations. In: Clinical ophthalmology. Philadelphia: JB Lippincott; 1990; 2; 35:1–75

19. Mafee MF. The orbit proper. In: Som P, Bergeron RT (eds), Head and neck imaging. St. Louis: CV Mosby; 1991:747–813

20. Rootman J, Robertson W, Lapointe JS. Inflammatory diseases. In: Rootman J (ed), Diseases of the orbit. Philadelphia: JB Lippincott; 1988:143–204

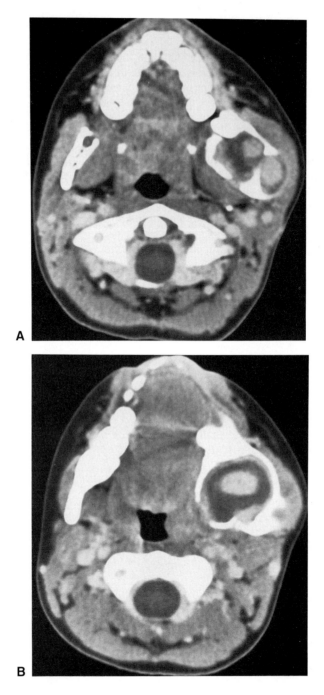

*Figure 26-1.* This 8-year-old boy has an enlarging mass in the left side of the mandible. You are shown two transaxial postcontrast CT scans filmed with soft tissue windows (A and B) and transaxial and coronal postcontrast CT scans filmed with bone windows (C and D).

# Case 26: Aneurysmal Bone Cyst

## Question 107

Which *one* of the following is the MOST likely diagnosis?

(A) Ameloblastoma
(B) Dentigerous cyst
(C) Aneurysmal bone cyst
(D) Actinomycosis
(E) Metastatic neuroblastoma

The test images document an expansile, multilocular, cystic-appearing lesion in the left side of the ramus and body of the mandible (Figures 26-1 and 26-2). This lesion contains several well-defined dense collections that may represent portions of fluid-fluid levels. The unerupted molar tooth is displaced but is at the periphery of the cyst and is not included in the lesion. Overall, the findings are most likely to represent an aneurysmal bone cyst **(Option (C) is correct).**

Ameloblastoma (Option (A)) is a neoplasm arising from the remnants of either the dental lamina or the enamel organ. This tumor accounts for about 1% of all tumors and cysts in the mandible and maxilla. It can present at many ages, usually in patients 20 through 50 years of age, with a peak incidence at about age 35 years. About 80% of ameloblastomas occur in the mandible and involve chiefly the molar-ramus region. Maxillary lesions constitute 20% of cases and are also generally found in the molar region. Ameloblastomas are slow growing and may achieve substantial size before they become clinically apparent. The most common clinical presentation is swelling of the jaw with minimal pain.

Because ameloblastomas are the most common of the cystic odontogenic malignancies, the diagnosis can often be suggested based on the imaging findings even though these findings are nonspecific and are compatible with a variety of less common odontogenic lesions. Typically, there is a multilocular radiolucency with large multicystic areas, and there is often resorption of the roots of adjacent teeth. Areas of cortical

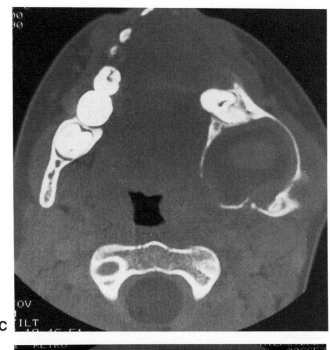

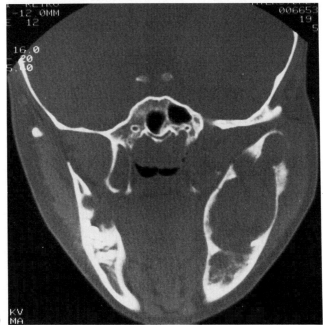

*Figure 26-1 (Continued)*

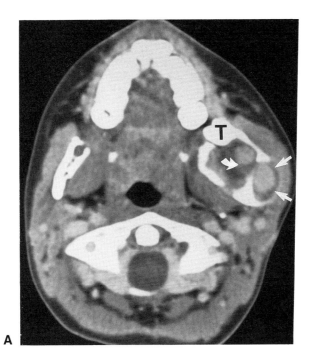

*Figure 26-2* (Same as Figure 26-1, panels A, B, and C). Aneurysmal bone cyst of the mandible. Axial soft tissue-windowed (A and B) and transaxial bone-windowed (C) postcontrast CT scans of the mandible in a child with an enlarging lesion along the left side of the face show a multilocular cystic mass that expands the medullary cavity of the left hemimandibular ramus and angle. The soft tissue images (panels A and B) document heterogeneous cyst contents with a possible fluid-fluid level (arrowheads). There is expansion of the cortex of the ramus of the mandible, and the lesion has broken through the cortex laterally near the condylar process (arrows in panel A). Despite the cortical extension, there is a well-defined rim around the cyst and no extension into the adjacent soft tissues. The adjacent tooth (T) is displaced, without evidence of resorption of the roots.

erosion may be present, and tumor extension into adjacent soft tissues can occur, although this usually occurs in the larger, more advanced lesions (Figures 26-3 and 26-4). The small lesions are frequently unilocular, and this form represents an early stage of tumor development. When an ameloblastoma presents as a small unilocular cystic mass, it may be radiographically indistinguishable from other cysts and biopsy may be the only way to make a diagnosis. The presumption that unilocular lesions expand to become multilocular lesions is supported by the fact that

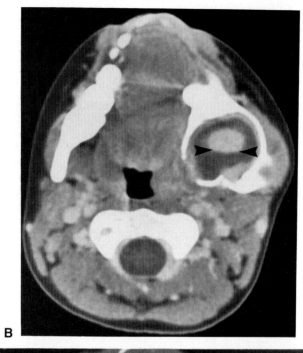

B

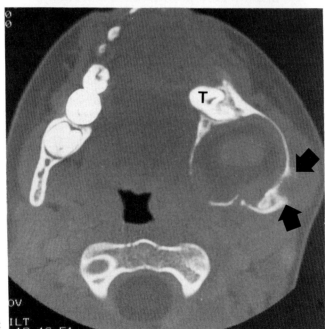

C

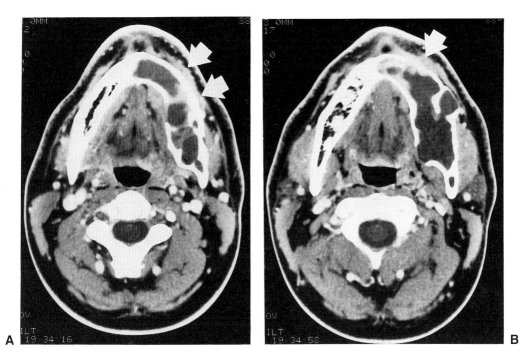

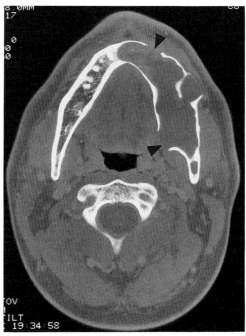

*Figure 26-3.* Ameloblastoma. Axial postcontrast CT scans of the mandible in an adult man with deformity of the face as a result of expansion of the left side of the mandible show a multilocular expansile lesion in the body and angle of the left hemimandible that has intermixed enhancing (solid) components and large lower-density (cystic) components. The tumor has broken through the cortex anteriorly near the mentum and has extended into the overlying subcutaneous tissues. (A and B) There is thickening of the platysma muscle as a result of tumor invasion (arrows in panels A and B). On the bone-windowed image (C), it is apparent that the cortex is destroyed focally both anteriorly and posteromedially (arrowheads).

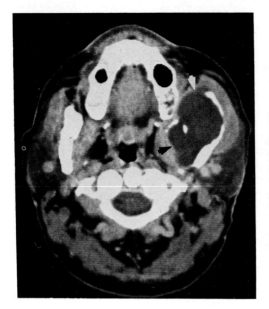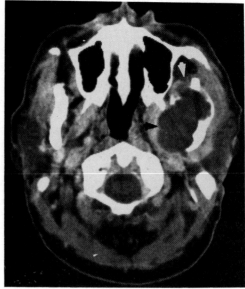

*Figure 26-4.* Ameloblastoma. Axial postcontrast CT scans of the mandible show a large tumor in the left mandibular ramus with a heterogeneous, primarily "cystic" appearance. The tumor has broken through the cortex at multiple sites into the surrounding muscles of mastication (arrowheads). (Reprinted with permission from Hasso [5].)

unilocular ameloblastomas are found in much younger patients than are multilocular lesions. The test patient is a young boy with a large expansile multilocular lesion, which shows no evidence of extension into the surrounding soft tissues. Therefore, ameloblastoma is an unlikely diagnosis.

The radiographic appearance of a dentigerous cyst (Option (B)) is that of a well-defined, typically unilocular cyst that contains a displaced but otherwise normal unerupted tooth. The tooth is clearly within the cyst and is actually attached to the cyst wall (Figure 26-5). The growth of the cyst drags the tooth to its abnormal position. Dentigerous cysts may range in size from a slightly enlarged dental follicle to a lesion that occupies most of the jaw. They arise most commonly in the mandible and involve primarily the molar teeth. There is typically displacement of the adjacent teeth, with minimal if any resorption of their roots. The roots of the adjacent tooth in the test images are deviated, but there is no evidence of resorption. However, there is no tooth within the lesion and, furthermore, the test images document a multilocular lesion, making a dentigerous cyst an unlikely diagnosis.

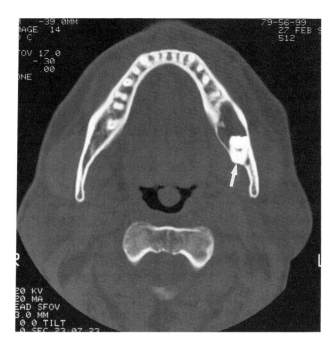

*Figure 26-5.* Dentigerous cyst. There is an isolated cystic lesion involving the body and ramus of the left hemimandible. The cystic lesion contains a fully developed tooth, most probably the left third molar. There is slight resorption of the roots of the tooth (arrow).

Actinomycotic infections (Option (D)) were common before the advent of modern antibiotic therapy. The genus *Actinomyces* contains organisms that have characteristics of both bacteria and fungi. It is now recognized that *Actinomyces* species are true bacteria. They are gram-positive, microaerophilic, non-spore-forming bacteria. They lack the nuclear membrane found in the eucaryotic fungi, and, more significantly, they are sensitive to certain antibacterial antibiotics but not to antifungal agents.

Several *Actinomyces* species, including *A. israelii*, the pathogen responsible for human disease, are found in the human oral cavity as part of the normal flora. They are found in the tonsillar crypts and the oropharyngeal mucosa of healthy individuals. The most common area to be involved by actinomycotic infection (about half of all cases) is the cervicofacial region. The organisms cannot penetrate intact mucosa, and so infection occurs only when normal tissue integrity has been disrupted, usually by minor oral trauma, dental manipulation, or gingivitis. These insults to the affected tissues allow the bacteria to proliferate in concert with other oral organisms such as *Bacteroides* species. Other predisposing conditions include immunosuppression, diabetes, chronic illness, and cancer. When established, actinomycosis spreads slowly by direct extension without regard for fascial planes. Actinomycosis spreads by direct invasion, and so reactive adenopathy is unusual.

Actinomycosis should be considered when a firm jaw mass, which is thought to be infectious, does not respond to conventional antibiotic therapy. Mandibular actinomycosis is characterized by prolonged morbidity and multiple recurrences. The classic course is chronic, but an acute form characterized by suppuration, tenderness, and abscess formation suggestive of an acute pyogenic infection may occur. When there is bone involvement, the mandible is the most common site (Figure 26-6). The disease is often undetected in the mandible until the infection spreads to the adjacent soft tissues, and associated fistulas and sinus tracts occur in the neck. The test patient has no specific signs or symptoms of an infectious process, nor is there evidence of any soft tissue infection. Also, actinomycosis would not typically cause a multilocular expansile mandibular lesion. Hence, actinomycosis is an unlikely diagnosis.

Neuroblastoma (Option (E)) is a malignant tumor originating from neural crest cells. It is one of the most common cancers of childhood, making up 8% of all pediatric tumors. Most cases occur before the age of 4 years, with a peak incidence around 2 years of age. Fewer than 10% of tumors occur in patients older than 10 years. Up to 70% of neuroblastomas occur in the retroperitoneal space below the diaphragm in the adrenal glands or sympathetic ganglia.

The presenting symptoms of neuroblastoma are variable and include abdominal pain or mass, weight loss, bone pain, fever, and anemia. These tumors are frequently biologically active and produce excessive amounts of catecholamines. This may lead to episodes of hypertension, headaches, and gastrointestinal symptoms. Early metastasis is common, and most patients have disseminated disease at the time of diagnosis. Frequently involved areas are the liver, lymph nodes, long bones, and skull. The facial bones are also commonly involved.

The radiologic findings of metastatic neuroblastoma include "smudgy" indistinctness of the bony margins, which may be irregularly destroyed. The smudgy appearance is due to radial bone spiculation extending into the soft tissues or sinuses (Figure 26-7). Metastasis to suture margins can produce characteristic widening with irregular margins. There is usually an associated extraosseous soft tissue mass, which enhances prominently following contrast agent infusion (Figure 26-8). The test

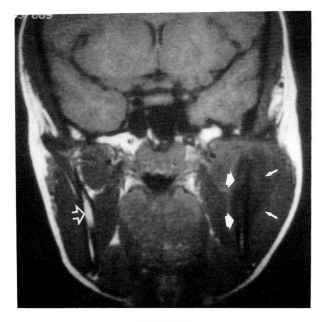

SE 600/25

*Figure 26-6.* Actinomycosis. This coronal T1-weighted MR scan shows the normal high-intensity mandibular marrow (open arrow) on the right; the marrow in the left mandibular ramus has been replaced by low-intensity material (wide solid arrows). There is an associated low-intensity area (thin solid arrows), which represents an abscess within the left masseter muscle bordering the ramus of the mandible.

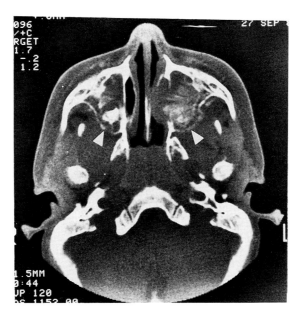

*Figure 26-7.* Metastatic neuroblastoma. Axial CT scan of the sinuses shows irregular bone destruction of the posterolateral walls of the maxillary sinuses (arrowheads). There is expansion of the left maxillary sinus both posterolaterally and medially. Within this expanded sinus lies an array of spiculated bone characteristic of metastatic neuroblastoma.

605

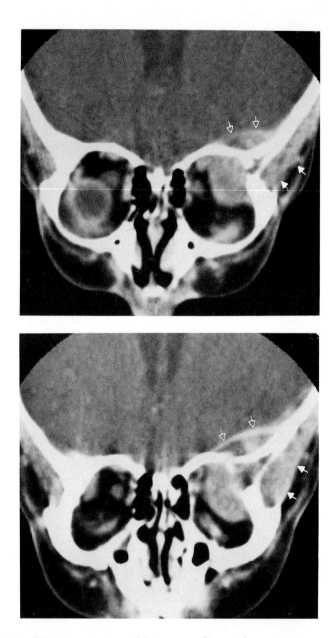

*Figure 26-8.* Metastatic neuroblastoma. Coronal postcontrast CT scans of the orbits in a young boy with left proptosis and bulging sclera show an enhancing soft tissue mass that involves the lateral portion of the upper left orbit. The tumor expands the sutures and extends through the endocranial osseous surface into the epidural space of the left anterior cranial fossa (open arrows) and beyond the exocranial surface into the left temporalis muscle (closed arrows).

images do not show evidence of such a soft tissue mass, and there is no evidence of irregular bone destruction.

## Question 108

Concerning dentigerous cysts,

   (A) a tooth remnant is identified in the cyst wall
   (B) most are located in the maxilla
   (C) extracystic soft tissue masses are typical
   (D) they are often multilocular

A cyst is an epithelium-lined cavity that typically contains fluid, blood, or semisolid material. Cysts frequently occur in the mandible or the maxillary alveolar ridge below the maxillary sinus. They appear radiographically as unilocular or multilocular lucent areas of various sizes and definitions. The relationship of the cyst to a tooth is an important feature for the differential diagnosis. Developmental cysts are subdivided into nonodontogenic and odontogenic types.

Nonodontogenic cysts lie in the jaws but do not contain tooth derivatives. Fissural nonodontogenic cysts arise along lines of fusion of embryonic structures. These cysts, like odontogenic cysts, are lined by epithelium and contain liquid or semisolid materials. An example of a fissural cyst is the nasopalatine or incisive canal cyst, which arises in the incisive canal from epithelial remnants. These cysts are always located in the midline and are usually ovoid (Figure 26-9). A similar lesion is the globulomaxillary cyst that occurs off the midline and lies between the lateral incisor and canine teeth.

Odontogenic cysts derive from embedded remnants of odontogenic epithelium. The radicular or periodontal variety evolves after the eruption of the involved tooth. It is caused by continued inflammatory stimulation of the epithelial cells in the periodontal membrane. As these epithelial cells continue to generate, a cyst forms around the root of the tooth (hence the name "periodontal"). The growth rate of periodontal cysts is variable. In all cases, the involved tooth is carious. Rarely, secondary infection leads to destruction of adjacent bone with secondary osteomyelitis.

Radiographically, a radicular or periodontal cyst appears as a cystic projection around the root of the tooth. Mandibular radicular cysts commonly displace the inferior alveolar canal inferiorly. When this lesion

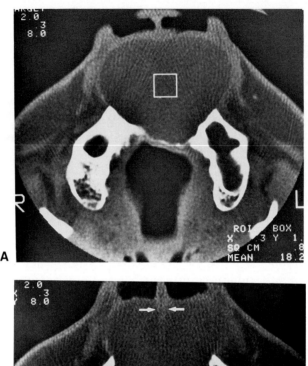

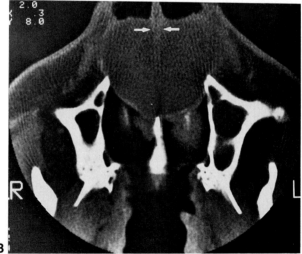

*Figure 26-9.* Fissural cyst. Axial CT scans of the maxilla show a large developmental fissural cyst of the premaxilla. The mass markedly expands the incisive canal and represents a nasopalatine duct cyst. There is no evidence of a tooth or tooth remnants within the cyst. (A) The attenuation value within the region of interest is 18 HU, indicating the presence of low-density material within the cyst. (B) The cyst is limited superiorly by the nasal septum (arrows), which causes its outline to be somewhat "heart"-shaped.

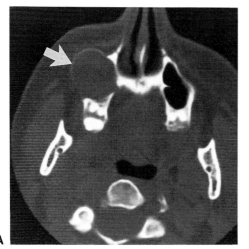
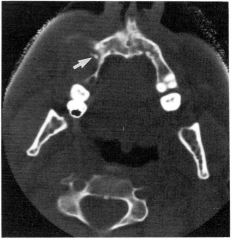

A                                                                          B

*Figure 26-10.* Residual radicular cyst. Axial CT scans of the maxilla show an odontogenic cyst in the right alveolar recess of the maxilla (arrow in panel A). Only a small remnant of a tooth root remains within the cyst (arrow in panel B). This was a carious tooth, and the findings are typical of a radicular cyst.

is large, it may appear in the maxilla as a cystic projection within the maxillary sinus above the root of a tooth, or the tooth may fill the maxillary sinus. The para-apical growth may continue even after a nonvital tooth has been extracted, in which case the cyst is usually referred to as a residual cyst (Figure 26-10).

After the radicular cyst, the dentigerous cyst is the most common type of odontogenic cyst, making up about 17% of all cysts found in the jaw. The dentigerous cyst arises from the enamel organ after the crown of the tooth has been partially or completely formed. This feature makes it possible to identify the unerupted tooth along with the surrounding cyst **(Option (A) is true)** (Figure 26-5). The cyst forms as a result of a fluid collection within the cell layers of the reduced enamel epithelium or between the crown and the enamel epithelium. The resulting cyst either completely surrounds the crown or, less commonly, attaches to one side of the crown. This cyst affects only the permanent teeth.

Dentigerous cysts are found primarily in adults during the third and fourth decades of life. They are initially asymptomatic and are often coincidentally discovered during a routine radiographic examination of the teeth. If they are left untreated, progressive enlargement of the jaw

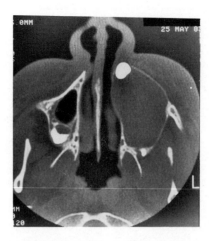

*Figure 26-11.* Dentigerous cyst. The osseous walls of the left maxillary sinus are expanded and thinned by a cystic lesion. A normally formed canine tooth is seen anteriorly near the midline.

may occur, with resultant facial asymmetry. These cysts are slightly more common in men than women. About 70% occur in the mandible, and 30% occur in the maxilla **(Option (B) is false).** Dentigerous cysts most often involve the mandibular third molars and second premolars (Figure 26-5) and the maxillary canine and third molar teeth (Figure 26-11).

Dentigerous cysts contain clear, straw-colored fluid in which cholesterol crystals may be present, or there may be purulent material if infection has occurred. The cyst wall is composed of fibrous connective tissue that may contain small islands or rests of odontogenic epithelium. The lining is stratified squamous epithelium that is only a few cells thick. The epithelium may include mucus-producing cells and even ciliated cells. On rare occasions, the lining is keratinized.

The radiographic appearance is that of a well-defined, unilocular cystic lucency associated with the crown of a normally formed unerupted tooth that is usually displaced from its expected position. A distinct cortex surrounds most or all of the cystic lesion, and there is no extension into the surrounding soft tissues **(Option (C) is false).** The roots of adjacent teeth may be slightly resorbed by the lesion (Figure 26-3).

With very large dentigerous mandibular cysts, multilocularity is occasionally apparent; however, this is uncommon **(Option (D) is false).** Rarely, the epithelial lining of a dentigerous cyst undergoes malignant transformation into an ameloblastoma. The treatment of choice for dentigerous cysts remains marsupialization or careful enucleation including the tooth of origin. Vital erupted adjacent teeth should be preserved whenever possible.

## Question 109

Concerning aneurysmal bone cysts,

(A) in the craniofacial region, they are typically found in the maxilla
(B) fluid-fluid levels are a common feature
(C) they commonly arise after trauma
(D) the most common presenting symptom is painless swelling

Aneurysmal bone cyst is the current name for a lesion previously referred to as an ossifying subperiosteal hematoma. The term "aneurysmal bone cyst" is more radiographically descriptive than pathologically accurate. The etiology of aneurysmal bone cyst is unclear, and three theories have been proposed. The first theory suggests a causal relationship with previous trauma, with the trauma leading to a subperiosteal hematoma and finally the aneurysmal bone cyst, which is the end result of the process. A clear trauma history, however, is rarely present **(Option (C) is false).** A second theory proposes a vascular anomaly within the bone, which progresses to an aneurysmal bone cyst. The third theory hypothesizes a primary bone lesion that at some point is destroyed by hemorrhage, resulting in an aneurysmal bone cyst.

The third is supported by the high frequency of associated osseous lesions that may occur with an aneurysmal bone cyst. Approximately one-third of aneurysmal bone cysts are termed "secondary" because of an associated lesion, which is most commonly a giant cell tumor, osteosarcoma, solitary bone cyst, or nonossifying fibroma or fibrous dysplasia.

Aneurysmal bone cysts occur most frequently (>50%) within the long bones, favoring a metaphyseal location within the femur. They are rare in the craniofacial bones, where they occur more often in the maxilla than the mandible **(Option (A) is true).** Approximately 20% of aneurysmal bone cysts occur within the vertebral column. They are most common in the first decades of life, with 90% of all aneurysmal bone cysts seen in patients younger than 20 years and 90% of mandibular aneurysmal bone cysts seen in patients younger than 30 years. There is a slight female predominance.

Pathologically, aneurysmal bone cysts are blood-filled cavernous spaces with fibrous septa. Septa containing bone and endothelial linings with a preponderance of multinucleated giant cells have also been reported. The surrounding bone, although frequently thinned, is usually intact, and soft tissue extension is rarely seen. The overall bone is expanded, frequently producing a clinical mass or focal swelling. This swelling is the most common presenting symptom of a mandibular aneurysmal bone cyst **(Option (D) is true).** Pain, which is the most common presenting complaint of a nonmandibular aneurysmal bone cyst, is present in the mandible in only about 25% of patients. Fewer than 10% of patients with mandibular aneurysmal bone cysts present with additional complaints such as trismus, malocclusion, or cranial nerve deficits.

Radiographically, aneurysmal bone cysts characteristically appear as expansile, bubbly, lytic lesions of bone. They are typically eccentric with trabeculations within the lucency. Periosteal new bone may be present along the margins of the lesion. This reactive bone is usually associated with a pathologic fracture and thus may complicate the imaging appearance. Mandibular aneurysmal bone cysts typically displace the adjacent teeth without causing resorption of their roots (Figure 26-1).

CT evaluation of aneurysmal bone cysts reveals an expansile mass of mixed soft tissue density surrounded by a thin shell of cortex or, in extreme cases, only a periosteal membrane. Periosteal new bone is more readily discernable by CT than by radiography. On sufficiently narrow CT window settings (+40 to +80 HU), fluid-fluid levels are seen within most cysts **(Option (B) is true).** These fluid-fluid levels are better seen on MRI. Patients must remain motionless for a short period (approximately 10 to 15 minutes) before scanning to allow for maximal separation of the fluid components. Fluid-fluid levels are not pathognomonic of aneurysmal bone cysts and may also be seen in patients with telangiectatic osteosarcomas. Bone scintigraphy of aneurysmal bone cysts shows increased activity. Angiography may reveal multiple abnormal small arteries that supply the lesion and show uneven tumor staining of the overlying cortex, cyst contents, or both.

MRI can conclusively demonstrate multiple well-defined cavities containing fluid-fluid levels (Figure 26-12). There is great variability in the signal intensities on both T1- and T2-weighted images owing to the different ages of the contained hemorrhagic and proteinaceous products. Additional MR features include both small diverticulum-like projections arising from the walls of the larger cysts and a dark line surrounding the lesion. These additional features permit differentiation of aneurysmal

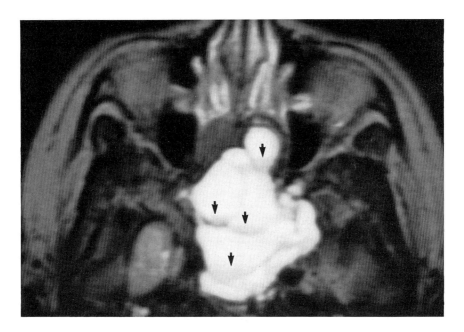

*Figure 26-12.* Aneurysmal bone cyst. Axial T2-weighted MR scan shows a mass in the sphenoid sinus and posterior nasal fossae. The lesion is composed of multiple cysts, which have fluid-fluid levels (arrows). (Reprinted with permission from Som et al. [3].)

bone cysts from telangiectatic osteosarcomas. Intravenous administration of gadolinium DTPA results in intense enhancement of the lesion.

Multiple treatment approaches are available for aneurysmal bone cysts. Radiation therapy was previously used as a noninvasive, cosmetically pleasing modality. However, irradiation is not currently used since most patients are young and radiation therapy may result in a significant rate of secondary malignant tumors. Cryotherapy can be used when a lesion is easily exposed and there are no surrounding nerves that can be damaged. When cryotherapy is used, there is a low recurrence rate (8%). Curettage has frequently been recommended, but recurrence rates are as high as 50%. Surgical excision provides the only complete treatment of the lesion, and when it is adequately performed, recurrence is extremely rare. With mandibular aneurysmal bone cysts, excellent functional and cosmetic results can be obtained from partial mandibulectomy and immediate reconstruction.

# Question 110

Common imaging features of mandibular actinomycosis include:

(A) periosteal reaction
(B) involvement of adjacent soft tissues
(C) low signal intensity of the medullary cavity on T1-weighted images
(D) expansile lesion
(E) cervical lymphadenopathy

Actinomycotic infection typically enters the soft tissues of the cervicofacial area from the mouth after dental extraction or minor oral trauma. It typically presents as a slowly enlarging, relatively symptomless, firm, woody mass beneath the skin, usually over the angle of the mandible. The skin overlying the lesion may become purplish red, and occasional areas of fluctuation may form. Actinomycosis spreads by direct invasion, and so there is rarely any adenopathy in the regional lymph nodes **(Option (E) is false).** Patients with actinomycosis often develop one or more sinus tracts that drain a thin, watery discharge containing characteristic "sulfur granules." These small yellow granules represent colonies of organisms composed of filamentous bacilli that appear similar to the hyphal form of many fungi.

The radiographic findings of mandibular actinomycosis are nonspecific, usually consisting of diffuse radiolucencies of various sizes with only occasional evidence of reparative bone. The CT findings are also nonspecific. There may be periostitis **(Option (A) is true)** with marked bone sclerosis and erosion of the mandible. Such a permeative destructive process is consistent with either osteomyelitis or a neoplasm (Figure 26-13). Soft tissue disease in addition to bone disease is the rule **(Option (B) is true).**

The MR findings of mandibular actinomycosis may be more diagnostic. Even though the medullary cavity is filled with pus or fluid, there is no evidence of expansion of the mandible **(Option (D) is false).** Early on, the normal marrow in the medullary cavity is replaced by fluid or pus. This changes the normally high T1-weighted signal intensity of the fatty marrow to low signal intensity caused by the watery fluid **(Option (C) is true)** (Figures 26-6 and 26-14A). After contrast agent infusion, any inflammatory change causes enhancement of the adjacent soft tissues. On T1-weighted scans, an abscess cavity has an enhancing rim surrounding a low-intensity central portion (Figure 26-14B).

Actinomycotic cellulitis is associated with significant surrounding fibrosis, which makes penetration of antibiotics difficult. Despite this,

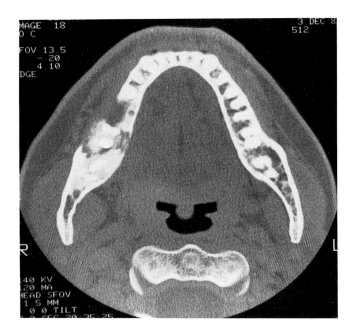

*Figure 26-13.* Actinomycosis. There is a combined sclerotic and lytic lesion in the body of the right hemimandible. The lesion causes destruction of the cortical margins and the adjacent tooth sockets.

medical therapy emphasizes intense, prolonged antibiotic therapy, with penicillin being the drug of choice. Surgical intervention may be necessary to remove abscesses, granulomatous tissue, or fistulous tracts whenever the infection does not respond to antibiotic therapy.

*Anton N. Hasso, M.D.*
*Monika L. Kief-Garcia, M.D.*
*Paul S. Kim, M.D.*

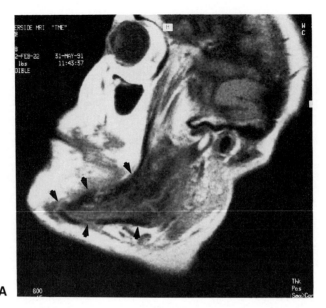

SE 700/15

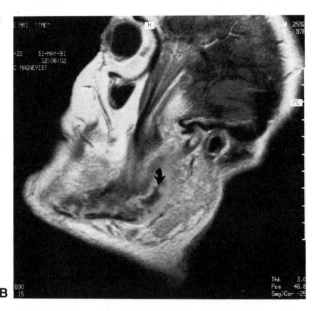

SE 700/15

*Figure 26-14.* Actinomycosis. Noncontrast and postcontrast oblique sagittal T1-weighted MR scans of the left hemimandible show an infiltrative process involving the bone. (A) The process replaces the normal high-intensity mandibular marrow with low-intensity fluid or pus (arrowheads). (B) Following contrast infusion, a small abscess cavity is visible near the angle of the mandible (arrow). Note the extensive enhancement of the adjacent soft tissues, consistent with cellulitis.

# SUGGESTED READINGS

## ANEURYSMAL BONE CYSTS

1. Hudson TM. Fluid levels in aneurysmal bone cysts: a CT feature. AJR 1984; 142:1001–1004
2. Hudson TM, Hamlin DJ, Fitzsimmons JR. Magnetic resonance imaging of fluid levels in an aneurysmal bone cyst and in anticoagulated human blood. Skeletal Radiol 1985; 13:267–270
3. Som PM, Schatz CJ, Flaum EG, Lanman TH. Aneurysmal bone cyst of the paranasal sinuses associated with fibrous dysplasia: CT and MR findings. J Comput Assist Tomogr 1991; 15:513
4. Zimmer WD, Berquist TH, Sim FH, et al. Magnetic resonance imaging of aneurysmal bone cyst. Mayo Clin Proc 1984; 59:633–636

## AMELOBLASTOMA

5. Hasso AN, Vignaud J. Pathology of the paranasal sinuses, nasal cavity and facial bones. In: Newton TH, Hasso AN, Dillon WP (eds), Computed tomography of the head and neck, vol III. New York: Raven Press; 1988:7.1–7.32
6. Miles DA, Kaugars GE, Van Dis M, et al. Oral and maxillofacial radiology: radiologic/pathologic correlations. Philadelphia: WB Saunders; 1991
7. Schultz SM, Twickler DM, Wheeler DE, Hogan TD. Ameloblastoma associated with basal cell nevus (Gorlin) syndrome: CT findings. J Comput Assist Tomogr 1987; 11:901–904
8. Waite DE. Textbook of practical oral and maxillofacial surgery, 3rd ed. Philadelphia: Lea & Febiger; 1987:209–211

## DENTIGEROUS CYSTS

9. Bhaskar SN. Synopsis of oral pathology, 7th ed. St. Louis: CV Mosby; 1986
10. Craig RM, Wescott WB, Correll RW. A well-defined coronal radiolucent area involving an impacted third molar. J Am Dent Assoc 1984; 109:612–613
11. Moore JR. Surgery of the mouth and jaws. Oxford: Blackwell; 1985
12. Waite DE. Textbook of practical oral and maxillofacial surgery, 3rd ed. Philadelphia: Lea & Febiger; 1987
13. Weber AL. The mandible. In: Som PM, Bergeron RT (eds), Head and neck imaging. St. Louis: CV Mosby; 1991:379–405

## MANDIBULAR ACTINOMYCOSIS

14. Feder HM Jr. Actinomycosis manifesting as an acute painless lump of the jaw. Pediatrics 1990; 85:858–864
15. Helm FR, Gongloff RK, Wescott WB. Bilateral mixed density lesions in the body of the mandible. J Am Dent Assoc 1987; 115:315–317
16. Podoshin L, Rosenman D, Fradis M, Wallish G. Cervicofacial actinomycosis. Ear Nose Throat J 1989; 68:559–561

17. Silverman PM, Farmer JC, Korobkin M, Wolfe J. CT diagnosis of actinomycosis of the neck. J Comput Assist Tomogr 1984; 8:793–794
18. Topazian RG, Goldberg MH. Oral and maxillofacial infections, 2nd ed. Farmington, CT: WB Saunders; 1987:403–407
19. Yenson A, deFries HO, Deeb ZE. Actinomycotic osteomyelitis of the facial bones and mandible. Otolaryngol Head Neck Surg 1983; 91:173–176

NEUROBLASTOMA

20. Angstman KB, Miser JS, Franz WB III. Neuroblastoma. Am Fam Physician 1990; 41:238–244
21. Bernstein ML, Leclerc JM, Bunin G, et al. A population-based study of neuroblastoma incidence, survival, and mortality in North America. J Clin Oncol 1992; 10:323–329
22. Long DM. Current therapy in neurological surgery. Toronto: BC Decker; 1989
23. Sutton D. Textbook of radiology and imaging, 4th ed. Edinburgh: Churchill Livingstone; 1987
24. Wende S, Aulich A, Nover A, Lamksch N, et al. Computed tomography of orbital lesions. A cooperative study of 210 cases. Neuroradiology 1977; 13:123–134
25. Zimmerman RA, Bilaniuk LT. CT of primary and secondary craniocerebral neuroblastoma. AJR 1980; 135:1239–1242

*Notes*

# Index

Where there are multiple page references, **boldface** indicates the main discussion of a topic.

Bruch's membrane, 103
Buccal spaces, 488
   masticator space abscesses and, 495, 496

## C

Calcifications
   esthesioneuroblastomas, 58, 66–67
   of the eye
      Coats's disease, 71, **98–100**
      coloboma of the optic disk, 71, 72–73,
         **104–6, 108**
      drusen of the optic nerve head, 71–72,
         73, **102–4**
      retinoblastomas, 71, **73–78, 80–81, 84–**
         **91**
      retinopathy of prematurity, 73, **110–13**
   optic nerve gliomas and, 567
   salivary gland tumors, 13, 378
Capillary hemangiomas, 492
Carcinoma. *See also* Squamous cell carcino-
         mas
   adenoid cystic, 546
   colon, 10
   esophageal, 447
   high-grade parotid gland, 181–82
   laryngeal, 17–26
   low-grade parotid gland, 181
   metastatic
      differential diagnosis
         branchial cleft cysts, 538–39
   mucoepidermoid, 545–46
   nasal cavity, **461–62**
   nasopharyngeal, **45, 47–48, 50**
      differential diagnosis
         adenoidal hypertrophy, 39
         cellulitis of the retropharyngeal
            space, 39
         necrotizing otitis externa, 35, 37, 39
         rhabdomyosarcoma of the nasophar-
            ynx, 39
   paranasal sinuses, **461–62**
   parotid gland, 11–12
   tongue, 433–47
Carcinoma ex pleomorphic adenoma, 12–13
Carotid aneurysms. *See also* Intrapetrous
         carotid artery aneurysms
   differential diagnosis
      parapharyngeal space schwannomas,
         368, 370
Carotid artery. *See* Aberrant carotid artery
Carotid body tumors, 512, **546–48**
   differential diagnosis
      branchial cleft cysts, 538
Carotid space, 42
Castelman's disease, 545

Cavernous hemangiomas, 492
Cavernous lymphangiomas, 494
Cavernous sinus thrombosis, 219, 391
Cellulitis
   orbital, 219
   retropharyngeal space
      differential diagnosis
         nasopharyngeal carcinoma, 39
      tonsillitis and, 43
Cerebellar abscesses, 389
Cerebritis, 400
Cerebrospinal fluid leaks, 390–91
Cervical lymphadenopathy, **542–45**
Cholesteatomas, **333–35, 339–40**
   differential diagnosis
      temporal bone hemangiomas, 327
   hearing loss and, 509
Cholesterol cysts. *See* Cholesterol granulo-
         mas
Cholesterol granulomas, **272–74**
   differential diagnosis
      aberrant carotid artery, 501
      petrous apex chondrosarcoma, 267–68
Chondrosarcomas, 130
   differential diagnosis
      obstructed laryngoceles, 285, 287
   laryngeal, **294**
   petrous apex chondrosarcomas, **275–76**
      differential diagnosis
         cholesterol granulomas, 267–68
         glomus jugulare tumors, 261, 266–67
         intraosseous epidermoid tumors, 268
         intrapetrous carotid artery aneu-
            rysms, 268
Chordomas
   petrous apex chondrosarcomas and, 276
Cigarette smoking, 45
Cleft palate
   Apert's syndrome, 195
   Crouzon's disease, 189
   hemifacial microsomia, 200
   Pierre Robin syndrome, 194
   Treacher Collins syndrome, 199–200
Cloverleaf skull configuration, 202
Coats's disease, 71, 78, **98–100**
Coloboma of the optic disk, 71, 73, 78, **104–**
         **6, 108**
Colobomatous cysts, **104–6, 108**
Computed tomography
   aberrant carotid artery, 513, 515
   aneurysmal bone cysts, 612
   branchial cleft cysts, 5, 7–8
   cholesteatomas, 335, 339
   cholesterol granulomas, 273
   chondrosarcomas, 261
   Coats's disease, 99–100

False cords, 17
Fat suppression, **462–71**
Fibrosarcoma, 130
Fibrous dysplasia, **128–30, 132**
  differential diagnosis
    Langerhans cell histiocytosis, 121, 123
    meningiomas, 126, 128
    mucocele of the sphenoid sinus, 119,
      121
    mucormycosis, 123–24
Fissure nonodontogenic cysts, 607
Fissures of Santorini, 35
Focal otogenic encephalitis, 399–400
Follicular cysts, 316
Fossa of Rosenmüller, 45
Fractures
  3-D CT and 2-D CT comparison, 207–8
Frontal sinusitis, 526
Fuch's coloboma, 104

# G

Gender factors
  aneurysmal bone cysts, 611
  Coats's disease, 98
  dentigerous cysts, 610
  dysthyroid orbitopathy, 241
  epidermoid cysts, 314
  extramedullary plasmacytomas, 67
  hemangiomas, 492
  hemifacial microsomia, 200
  juvenile angiofibromas, 455
  Langerhans cell histiocytosis, 136, 138
  lymphoepithelial parotid cysts, 165
  nasal cavity and paranasal sinus carcino-
    ma, 461
  optic nerve sarcoidosis, 590
  optic nerve sheath meningiomas, 563
  optic neuritis, 586
  pleomorphic adenomas, 178
  retinoblastomas, 75
  rheumatoid arthritis, 354
  synovial chondromatosis, 357
  Warthin's tumors, 168, 181
Genetic factors
  Apert's syndrome, 194
  Crouzon's disease, 188
  hemifacial microsomia, 200
  meningiomatosis, 414, 430
  neurofibromatosis, 421, 423
  Norrie's disease, 98
  paragangliomas, 548
  Pierre Robin syndrome, 194
  retinoblastomas, 75
  Treacher Collins syndrome, 197
  Warburg's syndrome, 95

Geographic factors
  aspergillosis, 528
  nasopharyngeal carcinomas, 45
Giant cholesterol cysts. *See* Cholesterol
    granulomas
Giant lymph node hyperplasia, 545
Glaucoma, 76–77
Globulomaxillary cysts, 607
Glomus faciale tumors
  differential diagnosis
    temporal bone hemangiomas, 326–27
Glomus jugulare tumors, 512, 546
  differential diagnosis
    petrous apex chondrosarcoma, 261,
      266–67
Glomus tympanicum tumors, 512, 546
  differential diagnosis
    aberrant carotid artery, 501, 504
Glomus vagale tumors, 513, 547
  differential diagnosis
    parapharyngeal space schwannomas,
      367
Glossopharyngeal nerve, 443–44
Gradenigo syndrome, 273, 389, 405
Granulomatous disease, 545
Graves' disease, 220, 240–41, 242–44
  differential diagnosis
    orbital myositis, 224–25
Guillain-Barré syndrome, 585

# H

*Haemophilus*, 216
Hand-Schüller-Christian disease, 136
Hardwood furniture makers
  adenocarcinoma of the paranasal sinuses
    and nasal fossae and, 10
Head shape
  Apert's syndrome, 194
  craniosynostosis of the skull, 202
  Crouzon's disease, 188
  hemifacial microsomia, 200
  Treacher Collins syndrome, 197–98
Hearing loss
  aberrant carotid artery and, 507
  acoustic neuromas and, 509
  atresia of the external auditory canal and,
    507, 509
  cholesteatomas and, 509
  conductive, 506, 507, 509, 510, 513, 515
  facial nerve sheath tumors and, 510
  glomus jugulare tumors and, 512–13
  nasopharyngeal carcinoma and, 45, 47
  neurofibromatosis 2 and, 427
  otosclerosis and, 507
  recurrent meningitis and, 390–91

Larynx *(cont'd)*
  supraglottic laryngectomy contraindica-
      tions, 21, 23, 25–26
  supraglottic region, 17
Lateral sinus thrombosis, 391, 394
LCH. *See* Langerhans cell histiocytosis
Leptomeningeal metastases, **428–29**
  differential diagnosis
      neurofibromatosis 2, 412
Leptomeningitis, 390, 586
Letterer-Siwe disease, 136
Leukemia, 534
Leukokoria, 76, 86–87
Lingual nerve, 443, 546
Lipomas
  differential diagnosis
      abscesses, 483, 485
      denervation atrophy, 478, 480
      lymphangiomas, 480, 483
      malignant schwannomas, 477
      simple ranulas, 310
      fat-saturation technique for diagnosis,
          471
Lyme disease, 352, 359, 585
Lymphangiomas, **493–95**
  differential diagnosis
      lipomas, 480, 483
Lymph nodes, 315
  giant lymph node hyperplasia, 545
  metastatic tumors, 542–45
  tuberculosis, 544
Lymphoepithelial parotid cysts, **172–74**
  differential diagnosis
      abscesses, 169
      non-Hodgkin's lymphoma, 168–69
      sarcoidosis, 165–66, 168
      Warthin's tumors, 168
Lymphomas
  differential diagnosis
      neurofibromatosis 2, 420
Lymphoplasmacytic tumors, 251, 254

# M

Magnetic resonance imaging
  adenocarcinoma of the head and neck, 10
  aneurysmal bone cysts, 612–13
  aspergillosis, 528
  branchial cleft cysts, 8, 537
  carotid body tumors, 548
  Chemsat, 463
  cholesteatomas, 339–40
  cholesterol granuloma, 273
  chondrosarcoma, 261
  Coats's disease, 99–100
  coloboma of the optic disk, 108

Magnetic resonance imaging *(cont'd)*
  epidermoid tumors, 278–79
  facial nerve schwannomas, 8
  fat suppression, **462–71**
  fibrous dysplasia, 119, 129
  glomus jugulare tumors, 266–67
  hemangiomas, 492–93
  high-grade parotid gland tumors, 181–82
  intrapetrous carotid artery aneurysm,
      275
  leptomeningeal metastases, 429
  lipomas, 477–78
  low-grade parotid gland tumors, 181
  lymphangiomas, 494–95
  lymphoepithelial parotid cysts, 165, 173
  mandibular actinomycosis, 614
  meniscus, 151–52
  mucoceles, 134–35
  nasal polyposis and mucocele, 53–55, 59
  nasopharyngeal carcinoma, 48
  necrotizing otitis externa, 37, 40–41
  neurofibromatosis, 411, 413
  normal parotid gland, 175–76
  obstructed laryngocele, 285
  optic nerve gliomas, 579
  optic nerve pseudotumors, 592–93
  optic nerve sarcoidosis, 591
  optic nerve sheath meningiomas, 553,
      572, 575
  optic neuritis, 587, 589
  orbital lymphomas, 247–48, 250–51
  parapharyngeal space schwannomas,
      365, 367
  parotid gland abscesses, 169
  parotid gland sarcoidosis, 166, 168
  persistent hyperplastic primary vitreous,
      94–95, 98
  petrous apex chondrosarcoma, 276
  pleomorphic adenomas, 3, 15, 178–79
  pseudotumors, 231, 233, 240
  retinoblastoma, 85–87, 89–91
  retinopathy of prematurity, 94, 112–13
  signal void, 519, 521, 524, 532
  sinonasal melanomas, 65
  sinonasal region tumors, 461–62
  sinonasal secretions, 531–32
  squamous cell carcinoma, 449
  STIR, 463
  temporomandibular joint, 343, 345
  toxocariasis, 89
  true vocal cords, 28–30
  Warthin's tumors, 168, 181
Malignant adenopathy. *See* Reactive or ma-
      lignant adenopathy
Malignant schwannomas, **488, 490–91**
  differential diagnosis

Malignant schwannomas *(cont'd)*
  lipomas, 477
Mandible involvement in tongue carcinoma, 439–40
Mandibular actinomycosis, 604, **614–15**
Mandibular radicular cysts, 607, 609
Mandibulofacial dysostosis. *See* Treacher Collins syndrome
Masticator nerve, 488, 491
Masticator space anatomy, 488
Mastoiditis
  acute, 383, 385, 386
    complications, 389–91, 394–400
  coalescent, 388, 389
Maxillary dental infections, 526
Maxillary sinusitis, 526
McCune-Albright syndrome, 128
Melanomas
  sinonasal, **64–65**
    differential diagnosis
      nasal polyposis and mucocele, 56–58
Meningeal artery, 515
Meningiomas
  differential diagnosis
    fibrous dysplasia, 126, 128
Meningiomatosis, **429–30**
  differential diagnosis
    neurofibromatosis 2, 414, 416
Meningitis
  leptomeningitis, 390
  optic neuritis and, 586
  otogenic, 390
Meniscus. *See* Temporomandibular joint
Mental retardation
  craniosynostosis of the skull, 202
Middle meningeal artery, 515
Middle turbinate aeration. *See* Concha bullosa
Midline mass in the floor of the mouth, **315–16**
Mondini-type anomaly, 391
Monostotic fibrous dysplasia, 128, 129–30
Morning glory disk anomaly, 108
MPD syndrome. *See* Myofacial pain dysfunction syndrome
Mucoceles, **132–35.** *See also* Ranulas
  nasal polyposis and mucocele
    differential diagnosis
      esthesioneuroblastomas, 58–59
      extramedullary plasmacytomas, 59
      melanomas, 56–58
      squamous cell carcinoma, 55–56
  sphenoid sinus
    differential diagnosis
      fibrous dysplasia, 119, 121

Mucoepidermoid carcinomas, 545–46
  calcification, 13
Mucormycosis, 528
  differential diagnosis
    fibrous dysplasia, 123–24
Multiple melanoma
  extramedullary plasmacytomas and, 59
Multiple myeloma
  extramedullary plasmacytomas and, 67
Multiple sclerosis, 585, 586–87
  optic neuritis and, 556
*Mycobacterium*, 216
Myofacial pain dysfunction syndrome, 351–52, 359
Myositic orbital pseudotumors
  differential diagnosis
    dysthyroid orbitopathy, 213–14
    orbital lymphoid tumors, 214
    orbital metastasis, 214
    orbital rhabdomyosarcoma, 215

# N

Nasal fossae
  adenocarcinoma of, 10
Nasal polyps, **63–64**
Nasopalatine cysts, 607
Nasopharynx
  carcinoma of, **45, 47–48, 50**
    differential diagnosis
      adenoidal hypertrophy, 39
      cellulitis of the retropharyngeal space, 39
      necrotizing otitis externa, 35, 37, 39
      rhabdomyosarcoma of the nasopharynx, 39
Necrotizing otitis externa, 35, 37, 39, **40–41,** 350–51
*Neisseriaceae*, 216
Neuroblastomas
  differential diagnosis
    aneurysmal bone cysts, 604, 607
Neurofibromatosis 1, **421–23**
  malignant schwannomas and, 490–91
  optic nerve gliomas and, 553, 578
  optic nerve sheath meningiomas and, 566
Neurofibromatosis 2, **423–25, 427–28**
  differential diagnosis
    leptomeningeal metastases, 412
    lymphomas, 420
    meningiomatosis, 414, 416
    ruptured dermoid cyst, 413–14
  optic nerve sheath meningiomas and, 566
NF-1. *See* Neurofibromatosis 1
NF-2. *See* Neurofibromatosis 2
Node of Rouvier, 47

NOE. *See* Necrotizing otitis externa

Non-Hodgkin's lymphoma
  differential diagnosis
    lymphoepithelial parotid cysts, 168–69
    nasopharyngeal carcinomas and, 45
    orbital lymphomas and, 247

Noninfectious orbital inflammations. *See* Orbital inflammations

Nonodontogenic cysts, 607

Norrie's disease, 95, 98

## O

Obstructed laryngoceles, **287–88, 290**
  differential diagnosis
    chondrosarcomas, 285, 287
    squamous cell carcinoma, 285
    thyroglossal duct cysts, 287
    tuberculosis, 287

Odontogenic abscesses, 495, 496–97

Odontogenic cysts, 316, 607

Olfactory neuroblastomas. *See* Esthesio-neuroblastomas

Ophthalmic vein thrombosis, 219

Optic hydrops, 580

Optic nerve gliomas, **578–81**
  differential diagnosis
    optic nerve sheath meningiomas, 553, 555

Optic nerve pseudotumors, **592–93**

Optic nerve sarcoidosis, 589–91
  differential diagnosis
    optic nerve sheath meningiomas, 556–57

Optic nerve sheath meningiomas, **562–63, 566–67,** 572, 575
  differential diagnosis
    optic nerve gliomas, 553, 555
    optic nerve sarcoidosis, 556–57
    optic neuritis, 556
    orbital pseudotumors, 557, 559

Optic neuritis, **585–87, 589–91**
  differential diagnosis
    optic nerve sheath meningiomas, 556

Optociliary shunts, 553, 566, 567

Oral cavity anatomy, 301

Orbital cellulitis, 219

Orbital infections, 216–17

Orbital inflammations. *See also* Abscesses
  acute and subacute idiopathic apical orbital inflammations, 227–29
  anterior orbital pseudotumors, 221–22
  diffuse orbital pseudotumors, 222–24
  lacrimal adenitis, 229, 231
  orbital infections, 216–17
  orbital myositis, 224–25, 227

Orbital inflammations *(cont'd)*
  orbital pseudotumors, 220–33
  perineuritis, 231, **592–93**
  subperiosteal phlegmon and abscess, 217, 219

Orbital leukemia, 254

Orbital lymphoid tumors
  differential diagnosis
    myositic orbital pseudotumors, 214

Orbital lymphomas, 220, **247–51, 254**

Orbital metastasis
  differential diagnosis
    myositic orbital pseudotumors, 214

Orbital myositis, 225, 227
  differential diagnosis
    Graves' disease, 224–25

Orbital pseudotumors, **220–21,** 591
  acute and subacute idiopathic apical orbital inflammations, 227–29
  anterior orbital pseudotumors, 221–22
  differential diagnosis
    optic nerve sheath meningiomas, 557, 559
  diffuse orbital pseudotumors, 222–24
  lacrimal adenitis, 229, 231
  myositic
    differential diagnosis
      dysthyroid orbitopathy, 213–14
      orbital lymphoid tumors, 214
      orbital metastasis, 214
      orbital rhabdomyosarcomas, 215
    orbital myositis, 224–25, 227
  perineuritis, 231, **592–93**

Ossifying subperiosteal hematomas. *See* Aneurysmal bone cysts

Osteoarthritis. *See* Degenerative arthritis

Osteogenic sarcoma, 130

Osteomyelitis, 485, 497

Otitic brain abscesses, 398–400

Otitis externa. *See* Necrotizing otitis externa

Otitis media, 43. *See also* Serous otitis media
  acute, 383–85, 389
  chronic, 136
  facial nerve paralysis and, 330

Otogenic meningitis, 390

Otosclerosis, and hearing loss, 507

Oxycephaly, 202

Oxygen, and retinopathy of prematurity, 110

## P

Paget's disease, 129

Papillary cystadenoma lymphomatosum. *See* Warthin's tumors
Papillitis, 585
Paragangliomas. *See* Carotid body tumors; Glomus faciale tumors; Glomus jugulare tumors; Glomus tympanicum tumors; Glomus vagale tumors
Paraglottic space, 17
Paranasal sinus adenocarcinoma, 10
Parapharyngeal space, **378–80,** 488
 schwannomas, **371–73**
  differential diagnosis
   carotid aneurysms, 368, 370
   deep-lobe parotid tumors, 368
   glomus vagale tumors, 367
   minor salivary gland tumors, 367–68
Paratracheal nodes
 lymphatic drainage, 26
Parotid gland
 adenocarcinomas
  differential diagnosis
   pleomorphic adenomas, 3
 carcinoma, 11–12
 description, 174–76
 lymphoepithelial parotid cysts
  differential diagnosis
   abscesses, 169
   non-Hodgkin's lymphoma, 168–69
   sarcoidosis, 165–66, 168
   Warthin's tumors, 168
 metastasis to
  differential diagnosis
   pleomorphic adenomas, 8
 tumors, **174–76, 178–79,** 181–82, **376–78,** 545
  differential diagnosis
   parapharyngeal space schwannomas, 368
Parotid space, 488
Perineural extension, 443, 444
Perineuritis, 231, **592–93**
Periodontal cysts, 316, 607, 609
Perisinus abscesses, 389
Persistence of the primitive stapedial artery, 515
Persistent hyperplastic primary vitreous, 78, **92–95, 98**
Petrosal sinus thrombosis, 391
Petrous apex chondrosarcomas
 differential diagnosis
  cholesterol granulomas, 267–68
  glomus jugulare tumors, 261, 266–67
  intraosseous epidermoid tumors, 268
  intrapetrous carotid artery aneurysms, 268

Petrous apicitis, 405
PHPV. *See* Persistent hyperplastic primary vitreous
Pierre Robin syndrome
 differential diagnosis
  hemifacial microsomia, 194
Plagiocephaly, 202
Plasma cell tumors. *See* Lymphoplasmacytic tumors
Pleomorphic adenomas, **12–15**
 differential diagnosis
  adenocarcinomas of the parotid gland, 3
  branchial cleft cysts, 5, 7–8
  facial nerve schwannomas, 8
  metastasis to the parotid gland, 8
 location, 176, 178
 salivary gland tumors and, 375
Pneumatized middle turbinate, 133
Polyostotic fibrous dysplasia, 128, 129, 130
Premature infants
 retinopathy of prematurity, 73, 78, **110–13,** 110–13
*Pseudomonas*, 216
*Pseudomonas aeruginosa*, 40, 350
Pseudotumors. *See* Optic nerve pseudotumors; Orbital pseudotumors
Pterygoid muscle, 546

# R

RA. *See* Rheumatoid arthritis
Radiation therapy
 aneurysmal bone cysts, 613
 edema of the retropharyngeal space and, 43, 45
 malignant schwannomas, 491
 nasopharyngeal carcinoma, 48, 50
 optic nerve gliomas, 581
 3-D CT and, 208
 tongue carcinoma, 446
Radicular cysts, 316, 607, 609
Ranulas, **309–12,** 315
 differential diagnosis
  submandibular space abscesses, 304
 plunging
  description, 309–10
  differential diagnosis
   cystic lymphangiomas, 311
   reactive or malignant adenopathy, 312
   second branchial cleft cysts, 311
   suprahyoid thyroglossal duct cysts, 312
 simple
  description, 309

Tonsillitis, 43
Toxocariasis, 78, 84, 585
   differential diagnosis
      retinoblastomas, 88–90
Toxoplasmosis, 585
Tram track sign, 567
Traumatic arthritis, 353
Treacher Collins syndrome, **197–200**
   differential diagnosis
      hemifacial microsomia, 190, 192, 194
Trilateral retinoblastomas, 76
True vocal cords, 17
   axial image through, 28–30
   lymphatic drainage, 26
Tuberculosis
   differential diagnosis
      obstructed laryngoceles, 287
   lymph node involvement, 544
Tumefactive pseudotumors. *See* Diffuse orbital pseudotumors
Turricephaly, 202

# U

Ultrasonography
   orbital lymphomas, 247
   retinoblastomas, 78
Uveoparotid fever, 13, 590

# V

Vagus nerve, 365, 371, 373
Ventricle of the vocal cord, 29
Venus sinus thrombophlebitis, 394
Visual loss
   optic nerve gliomas, 553, 578
   optic nerve sarcoidosis, 589
   optic nerve sheath meningiomas, 566
   optic neuritis, 559
   orbital pseudotumors, 559
Vitamin B$_2$, 586
Vocal cords. *See* False cords; True vocal cords
von Recklinghausen's disease. *See* Neurofibromatosis 1
von Willebrand's disease, 534

# W

Warburg's syndrome, 94, 95
Warthin's tumors
   description, 179, 181
   differential diagnosis
      lymphoepithelial parotid cysts, 168
   location, 178
Wegener's granulomatosis, 220, 221